# HOW TO STAY PRETTY & TRIM

Editorial Director     Arthur Hettich
Editor     Marie T. Walsh
Art Director     Joseph Taveroni
Beauty Consultant     Mary Milo
Associate Editor     Jean Maguire
Art Associate     Walter Schwartz
Editorial Assistant     Ceri E. Hadda
Production Manager     Norman Ellers

A New York Times Company Publication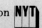

# contents

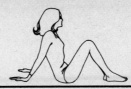

**5 - 13** Your Hair: from Good Looks to Great Looks
    **6** Have Healthier, Shinier Hair
    **8** Create a Super Evening Hairdo
    **10** Haircuts that Flatter Your Face
    **11** Choosing the Haircut that's Right for You
    **12** Highlight Your Hair
    **13** Guide to Home Hair Coloring
**14 - 31** Be Your Own Special Beauty
    **16** Have Glowing Skin
    **16** Save Your Face
    **22** Balance Your Face with Makeup
    **26** Makeup Tricks to Enhance Your Features
**32 - 47** Shape Up! Special 16-Page Exercise Section
    **48** 70 Most-Asked Summer Beauty Questions
    **52** How to Get the Perfect Tan
    **53** How to Have a Lovelier-Sounding Voice
    **54** Face and Body Hair — What to Do about It
    **56** Have a Professional-Looking Manicure and Pedicure
    **56** New for Spring
    **58** Herbs for Beauty and Health

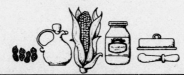

    **60** Diet Entrées You'll Love
**63 & 72** Dinner Menus
    **74** Mouth-Watering Salads
**77 & 84** Luncheon Menus
    **86** Desserts Your Waistline Won't Show
**89 & 94** Breakfast Menus
    **97** Appetizer Recipes
    **98** Breakfast Recipes
    **100** Super Slim Soups
    **114** Good Nutrition for Good Health —
        Family Circle's Guide
        to the Nutritive Value of Food
    **116** What Does RDA Really Mean to You?
    **117** Your Calorie Counter
    **120** Mary Ann Crenshaw's Eating for Beauty
    **122** Exploding Some of the Vitamin Myths
        by Jane Heenan
    **123** Dr. Jean Mayer's Guide to Better Nutrition
    **127** Cook's Guide
    **127** Buyer's Guide
    **127** Credits
    **128** Recipe Index

4

Soft and natural is the greatest look for hair. Hair shouldn't be just *there*, but should be a part of you—moving, changing, looking alive. A pretty hairdo, a becoming hair color, a decorative ornament can do a lot to perk up your looks and your mood, but the important thing is whether or not it all fits in with the total you—your overall appearance, personality, life-style—and makes the statement *you* want to make. Right now, ask yourself some questions about your hair. Do you like the way it looks? The way it feels? Is the color right for you? Do you always seem to be fussing with it because it never falls right? Can it go from a day to an evening look with just a few touches of your comb? Are you more concerned with the latest style or do you just want to work on making your hair more lustrous and vibrant-looking? No matter what your answers, you'll find lots of ideas here—covering everything from ways to have shinier, healthier hair to reshaping your face with the right haircut. Also included: complete guide to home hair coloring and tips for summer care. Now—make your hair all you want it to be.

## YOUR HAIR: FROM GOOD LOOKS TO GREAT LOOKS

*pretty & trim*

# HAVE HEALTHIER, SHINIER HAIR

If you happen to be on Madison Avenue and 48th Street in New York any day from Monday through Saturday, you're likely to encounter women with some of the loveliest hair in the world . . . hair so shiny and healthy-looking that every strand catches a gleam of sun as it floats in the wind, some so long it reaches down to the knees. If you follow one of these ladies to the second floor of the building near the corner of the block, which is where she's sure to be going, you'll find out why her hair looks as it does. For there is the salon of the famous hair-care expert responsible for these luxurious manes, George Michael of Madison Avenue, to whom women come from all over the world to have their hair treated, pampered and conditioned back to life.

As soon as you enter the salon, you can tell that hair is a serious business here. There's none of the sophisticated equipment, piped-in disco music and colored lights found in many modern salons; instead, women are brushing their own hair in modestly decorated surroundings, while others are having special conditioning treatments or being shown how to comb their hair so that not one strand is broken. Each client has her problems personally evaluated and is issued a list of instructions for home care which advise her, among other things, to use only wide-tooth combs, natural bristle brushes, creamy shampoos and different conditioners in summer and winter. But perhaps the most unusual thing about the salon is that absolutely *no* one is being given—or asking for—the latest haircut. Only blunt cuts are offered.

What does all this have to do with shiny, beautiful hair? A lot, according to George Michael, who presides over his salon in kingly fashion and who loves nothing better than to talk about what it takes to transform dull, lifeless locks into a vibrant crowning glory. And whether or not you agree with all of what he says, you listen, for it's impossible to argue with this man who is at once opinionated, stubborn, charming and witty. You also give him your undivided attention because he's been achieving amazing results with hair for over 20 years now—especially long hair, has a medical degree, and perhaps most important, because you can't help wanting your *own* hair to look as gorgeous as that of the living testimonials you see in his salon! (His clients include, among other famous personages, Faye Dunaway, Liv Ullman, Valerie Harper and model Samantha Jones).

When you come to George Michael for advice about your hair, he greets you warmly, looks you straight in the eye and says something completely disarming like "How come you're so beautiful?" While you try to think of an answer, you notice that he's a tall, impressive-looking man with strong features and that his own hair is quite plentiful, with only a hint of gray, although he's 57.

But he also lets you know that he means business. The next thing he does is scrutinize your hair under a special, powerful light, while firing questions at you about your general health. If (heaven forbid) you happen to be wearing your hair pulled back with a rubber band or some other device of which the master doesn't approve, he's liable to snip the offending piece off instantly, and with a mischievious glint in his eye, give you a stern lecture on what you're doing wrong with your hair: "You must *never* wear rubber bands. And furthermore, you must stop mistreating your hair. You get up in the morning to wash your hair and you only have 20 minutes, so you throw on some shampoo, scrub it like a pair of dungarees, you rake a comb through the tangles, put the blow dryer on the hottest setting and then curl it in five minutes with boiling hot curlers that have teeth in them. Then your hair falls out or breaks off and you wonder why. Well, those are some of the reasons why."

Now that you've been told what you're doing wrong, the next lesson involves learning what to do right. Michael feels that any woman can have great-looking hair—and without spending hours in beauty salons. It's simply a matter, he insists, of understanding how physical and emotional factors affect your hair, simplifying your routines so you don't abuse it with constant processing or improper handling—*and* forgetting all the misconceptions you may have heard about hair before. Some of his theories have caused quite a stir in the beauty field—in fact, he's in disagreement with many stylists on what constitutes proper hair care—but this doesn't bother him a bit. "Do you see my customers complaining?" he challenges. You don't.

Before Michael will even begin to discuss maintenance and daily care, he insists that you first know something about the relationship between the condition of your hair and your general health. He explains that although the *amount* of hair you have —its thickness or thinness—is determined largely by heredity, there are other factors affecting hair, many of which you can control. "People always ask me what to do, but you have to know the *why*," he announces, pounding his fist on his desk for emphasis. "The only part of your hair that is alive is the root. Once hair grows out of the follicle, it's dead matter. You have to treat it carefully, because it's fragile, but the source of healthy roots comes from within the body. You can give your hair all the treatments in the world, but it won't be beautiful if you're unhealthy in general."

A well balanced diet plays an important part in contributing to the hair's growth and lustre, Michael points out. He prescribes lots of protein-rich foods and fresh vegetables and fruits—good sources of vitamin B, which is a hair booster. To retain vitamins, he recommends that vegetables be undercooked. An occasional supplement of brewer's yeast (high in vitamin B) also does good things to the hair.

Michael has also found that sudden changes in life-style, emotional upsets and dramatic climatical changes tend to be reflected in the condition of your hair, and enjoys telling the following story to illustrate his point: "I had a gorgeous woman come into my salon —a former Miss Sweden—and she'd always had beautiful hair. When she came to me for the first time, it started falling out, almost as if I had jinxed her. She asked me what I did to her, and everyone laughed. But *I* found out what was wrong. She was here without friends or family, upset about being jobless and couldn't get used to the water and pace of life. The climate and altitude are also quite different in Stockholm. This combination caused a sudden change in her metabolism, which affected her hair."

Generally, if you're not abusing your hair in any obvious way and it's still dull and lifeless, Michael says, there may be a problem physically that won't always be evident in the way you feel. If you suspect anything is wrong, he advises, "see a doctor for tests. You can't tell by yourself because some imbalances, especially a slight thyroid deficiency, will affect your hair but not necessarily your general health."

Tension, the next topic of discussion, is perhaps the worst enemy of healthy hair. When you tense up, your scalp tightens also, making it difficult for the blood to circulate properly. Setting aside a few minutes a day when you can just sit back and relax is always a good idea, but if you can't seem to slow down, Michael offers this suggestion: "When things get too crazy, stop for a minute and do this exercise: Sit down, put your head in your lap and massage your scalp in slow motions—10, 15 or 30 times in one minute. This will loosen up your scalp and relax you, as well. Those who follow this advice rarely even have headaches."

His method for massage is this: Slide your fingers under your hair, press firmly and move your scalp back and forth, *not* in circular motions, which can tangle the hair. Also, don't slide your fingers over the scalp—keep them in place. Pay special attention to the area near the front hairline, where the hair is weakest.

Pregnancy is another condition that affects the hair, but it is after the child is born, not *during* pregnancy, that these changes take place—usually in the form of hair loss. This has a lot to do with a repatterning of life-style, Michael feels. "Before you conceive, you may be washing your hair every day, smiling all the time, having a lot of good times, and your metabolism is functioning at a very high level," he likes to say (and who can argue with that reasoning?). When you become pregnant, you usually slow down because you tire more easily.

You may quit your job, sleep more and start gaining weight—and all of this slows down your metabolism. But the hair won't be affected yet, because a woman's body has a remarkable way of revitalizing itself during pregnancy because of the unborn child. In fact, her hair is usually better at this time.

"After your baby is born, you're suddenly very active once more—taking care of the child and resuming your normal activities—and your metabolism again undergoes a change. This constant fluctuation finally takes its toll, and you may experience more hair loss than usual." Michael feels you can counteract this however, by taking it as easy as you can—get plenty of rest, proper nourishment and ease back gradually into your normal routines. This is *not* a good time, he says to bleach your hair, give it a permanent or expose it to other chemicals, since your hair should first have a chance to adjust to the changes your body has been undergoing.

Many women who come to Michael are also concerned about the effects of birth control pills on their hair. Michael claims that if you're healthy to start, the Pill can cause some loss of hair because it upsets the hormonal balance in your body. But, if your hair improves, it's possible that you had a slight imbalance before you started taking it. If hair loss is extreme, he recommends that you talk to the doctor about switching to another brand of Pill, or changing your method of contraception entirely.

Aside from specific health conditions that have an effect on hair, Michael explains that there are also certain periods of life when hair goes through a change and when some shedding can be expected: during puberty, when the hormones are changing; around age 22, the time of transition from adolescence to adulthood; about the ages of 26 and 34—which he refers to as "peaks in the pre-menopausal stage"—and at menopause. But there's usually nothing to worry about, since these losses generally don't last very long. "During these periods there's a hormonal imbalance in the body, and it's perfectly normal to lose some hair. As the body adjusts to its changes, the losses will decrease."

If you're particularly concerned about hair loss, the following test may

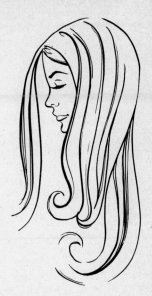

help you determine whether losses are actually increasing: Each day for 10 consecutive days, collect any hair that's fallen out—from your comb, brush, sink, clothes—and place in an envelope marked for that day. Also enter on the envelope briefly what you've done that day—including any upsets, anxieties, pressures—and any medication you've taken. Put the envelopes aside and skip the following month. The month after that, repeat the test with 10 more envelopes, and then compare the two months. If there's obviously more hair in the second set of envelopes, bring this to your doctor's attention. The notes you've recorded may also help him in diagnosing your problem.

Now that you know something about how hair functions, Michael says, you're ready for a daily program of hair care. He prefaces his advice with this caution, though: "Never go to extremes. One person neglects her hair completely, while another overdoes everything—shampooing, conditioning, cutting, bleaching to excess. You have to find a medium and then stop worrying."

CUTTING. Haircutting, or rather, *not* cutting, reflects a pet theory of Michael's that has created quite a bit of controversy. While most stylists are more than happy to apply the scissors, Michael doesn't believe in much cutting at all. He recommends that ends be trimmed every two months, but—here's another bombshell—he *refuses* to cut the hair in layers. Bangs are also out. If you come to the salon with a hairdo like this, he'll insist that you grow it to one length. He'll cut the

*(Continued on page 31)*

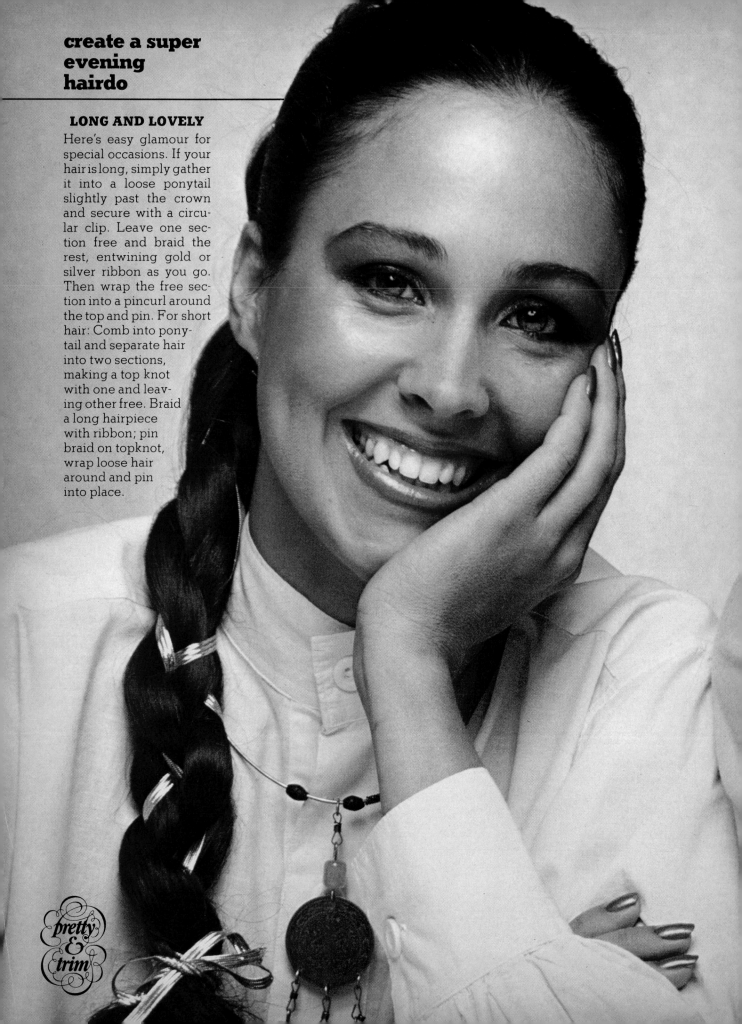

# create a super evening hairdo

## LONG AND LOVELY

Here's easy glamour for special occasions. If your hair is long, simply gather it into a loose ponytail slightly past the crown and secure with a circular clip. Leave one section free and braid the rest, entwining gold or silver ribbon as you go. Then wrap the free section into a pincurl around the top and pin. For short hair: Comb into ponytail and separate hair into two sections, making a top knot with one and leaving other free. Braid a long hairpiece with ribbon; pin braid on topknot, wrap loose hair around and pin into place.

pretty & trim

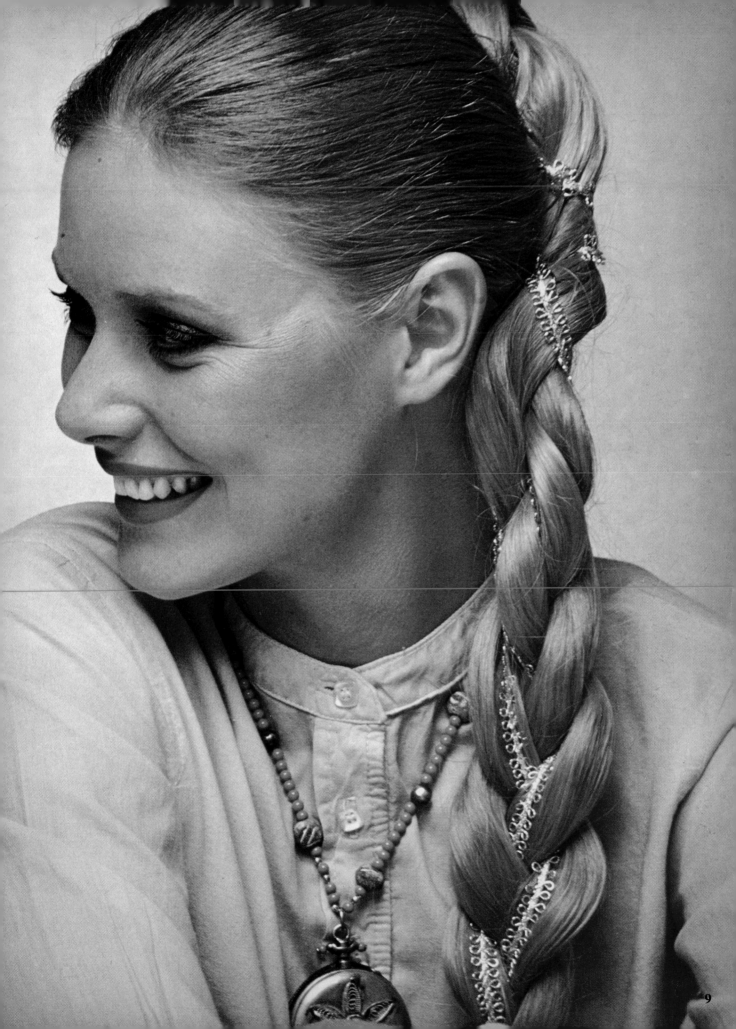

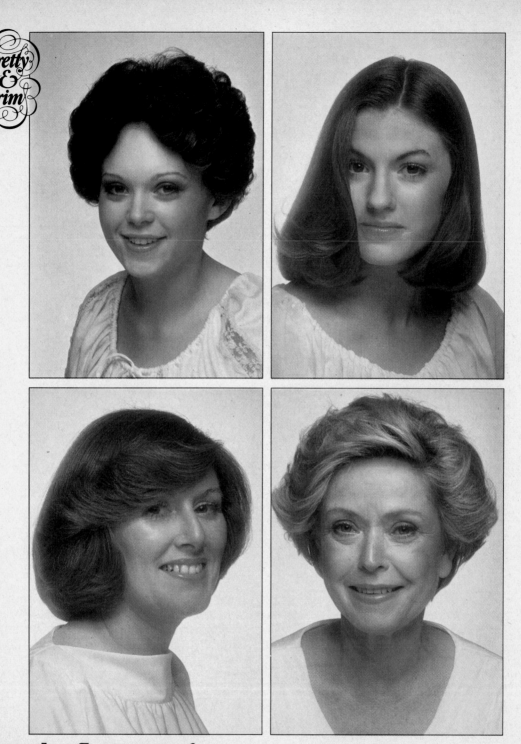

# haircuts that flatter your face

**TAPERED** and full, this cut (top, left) slims a round face. Our model has naturally curly hair which she'd been pulling down too close to her face for a thinner look. Hairstylist Jak Cronin cut it short—no more than 2 inches all around—to enhance her rosy good looks. Care is easy with a blow dryer or curling wand; if hair is straight, a permanent can give added fullness. **EASY-FLOWING** hairdo (top, right) softens a strong jaw. Style gives a young, carefree look, but can be curled for a more sophisticated effect. **SWEEPING BANGS** across the forehead give the illusion of a shorter face (bottom, left). This model's hair was cut to chin length, tapered at sides for softness and blunt cut at back for underturn to flatter her longish face. **BREEZY**, side-swept hairdo (bottom, right) is created with long layers around the face and short ones at the crown, giving texture to fine hair. Fullness at the sides delicately frames a heart-shaped face. (For help in choosing the style that's right for your face, see page 11.)

# CHOOSING THE HAIRCUT THAT'S RIGHT FOR YOU

Hair that looks natural and pretty can do much to improve your face shape. But any hairdo you choose should enhance the distinctive features that individualize *you*. Some women look most beautiful when they emphasize a unique face shape or an irregular feature. Others of us feel happier if our hairdo (and makeup) somewhat corrects or modifies a particular feature or our overall face shape.

Shown here are some of the more common face shapes with guidelines for achieving the most flattering hairstyle. But realize that these are suggestions only—while most hair stylists take into account the shape of your face when cutting your hair, he or she will also consider the texture and condition of your hair and the effect of the hairdo on your overall figure. The amount of time you're willing to spend on your hair is important, too, for you'll want a hairdo that's compatible with the way you live.

To analyze *your* face shape, start with a makeup-free face. Pull your hair back out of sight, away from your face (put on a high turtleneck to hide your throat if need be) and, looking directly into a mirror, try to visualize the outline—hairline, jaw, chin—as a circle, an oval, a square, an oblong or a heart. If you have an oval-shape face, you're lucky—just about any hairdo looks well on this shape.

**ROUND FACE,** probably the most common of all face shapes, appears thinner and longer with a full hairdo that gives volume at the crown and at the sides and cuts down on forehead width.

• For a *full round face*, the hair should *not* be worn close to the head, but should be built out to lift the crown, and tapered so the face is surrounded by a halo of hair that lengthens the face.

• For a *small round face*, hair should always be away from the face, off the forehead but still building up to the crown; hair should be off the sides of the face as well, with neckline tapered.

**SQUARE FACE** needs softening and looks best with a cut that has movement and hangs straight to a point just below the chinline.

**OBLONG FACE** is enhanced by a hairdo that falls around the jawline.

• For a *thin long face*, the hair should be full and rounded at the jaw, built up at the sides and shaped to be almost square with no greater length at the back of the head. The long face needs fullness at the sides—and bangs. If thick, the hair can be straight at the sides.

• For a *narrow face with a long chin,* the hair should fall to the chinline and be no longer than the chin when curled—and in this case, the hair *should* be curly.

**HEART-SHAPE FACE** tends to be wide at the cheekbones, thus looks well with side-swept waves that clear the forehead and add fullness at the sides. This makes the face appear narrower.

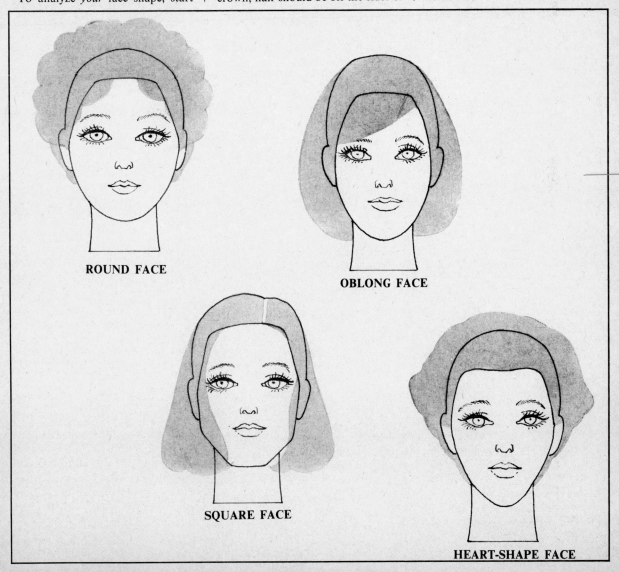

ROUND FACE

OBLONG FACE

SQUARE FACE

HEART-SHAPE FACE

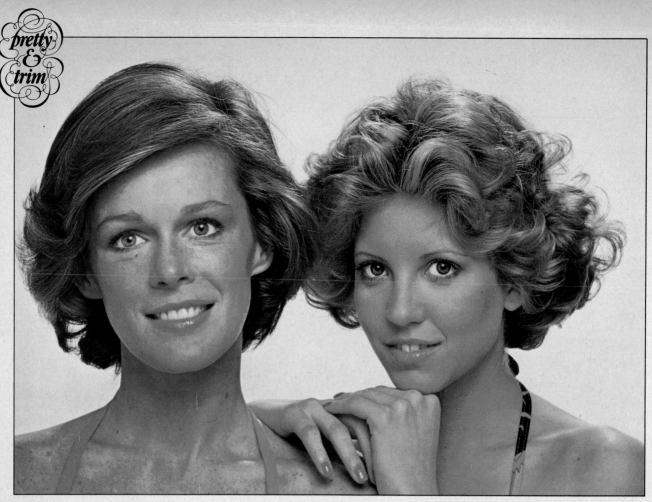

"**Changing your hair color** can be one of the most dramatic differences you make in your looks—even if the change itself is not daring," says New York colorist Leslie Blanchard. Highlighting alone can do wonderful things for your hair—and flatter your face shape, too. Lighter hair around the face is becoming to nearly everyone. • For long hair play the highlighting throughout the hair to give movement and color • For short hair, highlight around the edges to give design to the cut (*above, left*). Or choose strands already lightened by the sun and lighten them more (*above, right*) • In red hair, natural or colored, highlights flatter skin tones • If hair is mousy, you can lift the color of the whole head with a one-process tint, holding out the lighter strands by wrapping them in foil; lighten these strands further for gradations in color • Highlight gray in very dark hair by rinsing the gray strands to a sparkling white with temporary color • Enriching your natural color with a semipermanent coloring (lasts through four to six shampoos), in a shade lighter than your own color, will also highlight any gray • Very dark hair that is healthy and shiny creates its own highlighted look but it can be given red or gold variations by lightening selected strands.

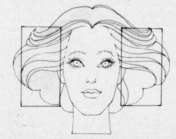

For a high forehead, start highlights a little behind the natural hairline at the temples and lighten more at one side than at the other for width in the eye area.

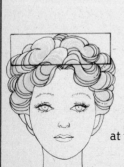

For a narrow face, place highlights at the sides for width at the cheekbones.

If your face is full, highlight at the top of the head to make the face appear slimmer, longer.

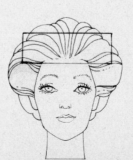

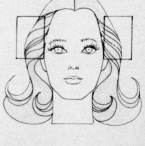

When forehead is low, put highlights at the front hairline for added height.

# GUIDE TO HOME HAIR COLORING

| WHAT IT IS | WHAT IT DOES | IF HAIR IS NATURAL COLOR | IF HAIR IS PREVIOUSLY COLORED |
|---|---|---|---|
| **HIGHLIGHTING—DOES NOT CHANGE OVERALL HAIR COLOR** | | | |
| **Hair painting:** Lightener applied by painting selected strands of hair. 30-min. process; redo in 3–4 months. | Lightens selected strands of hair with subtle color for a sunlit look and can define lines of hairstyle. | Most effective on hair that is medium brown or lighter. | Do not use on lightened and toned or frosted hair. |
| **Fingerpainting:** Lightener applied with fingertips to desired strands. 30-min. process; repeat in 2 months or less. | Lightens selected strands of hair for reddish-brown or golden highlights, depending on natural hair color. | For medium-brown hair or darker. | Do not use on color treated hair. |
| **Frosting:** Thin strands of hair are drawn through perforated cap and first lightened, then, when necessary, toned. Processing time—1 to 2 hours. Repeat in 6 months. Patch test. | Lightens selected strands for dramatic blond contrasts throughout the hair or wherever streaks are wanted. | For dark brown to dark blond hair. | Do not use on hair that has been color treated. |
| **TEMPORARY HAIR COLORING (LASTS TILL NEXT SHAMPOO)** | | | |
| **Lotion rinse** or **spray-on color:** Applied after each shampoo. | Enriches color, gives body, blends in gray. Hides yellowing in gray or white hair. | Use golden shades for glow; reddish shades for warmth. | Use as color refresher, to tone down brassiness, to blend in new growth. |
| **SEMIPERMANENT COLOR (LASTS UP TO SIX SHAMPOOS)** | | | |
| **Foam-in** or **shampoo-in:** Processing time—20-30 minutes. Repeat after 4 to 6 shampoos. Patch test. | Enriches color, covers gray, gives body. Does not lighten. Shades range from black to blond, including grays and white. | Use in a shade near your natural hair color to enrich color or cover gray. Choose in a slightly lighter shade to achieve a highlighted effect. | Do not use on tinted or lightened hair. |
| **HENNA (LASTS FOUR TO SIX WEEKS)** | | | |
| **Henna Pack:** Plant product in form of white powder is boiled in water and applied as a warm pack. 45-min.–1-hr. process. Repeat in 4–6 weeks. | Gives reddish color to brunette hair or picks up color in reddish hair. Adds body. Useful to those who are allergic to other products. | Best on natural auburn or brunette hair. Do not use on natural blond hair or hair that has been permanented or straightened. | Do not use on lightened or previously colored hair. |
| **ONE-PROCESS PERMANENT HAIR COLOR (COLOR LASTS TILL HAIR GROWS OUT)** | | | |
| **Shampoo-in tint:** Applied to entire head each time. Processing time—20 minutes. Retouch every 4 to 6 weeks. Patch test. | Lightens or deepens color, covers gray. Adds body, shine. Most include conditioners for added body; color ranges from black to blond. | If you want to go a few shades lighter, use the palest shade. For brightness and a color lift, choose a shade a little lighter than your own. To enrich color, choose a darker or warmer (reddish) shade. For body only pick a shade near your own color. | If you have been using a semipermanent color, you can safely change to a shampoo-in tint. Just wait till after six shampoos to remove the semipermanent color. If you want to change from two-process to one-process color, consult your hairdresser. |
| **Lotion tint:** Applied by applicator or brush to entire head the first time; after that, only new growth is retouched. Processing time—30 minutes. Retouch in 4 to 5 weeks. Strand test. Patch test. | Lightens several shades and deepens color to any shade you want. Maximum gray coverage. Color range from black to blond. | If you want to lighten several shades or cover resistant gray hair, the tint is preferred to shampoo-in permanent color. You can go from light brown to golden blond with the lightest shade of lotion tint. | You can change from shampoo-in tint to a lotion tint if you want more lightening or better coverage of gray. You can also go from semipermanent coloring to one-process lotion tint if you wait till after six shampoos. Get a hairdresser's advice on other changes. |
| **TWO-PROCESS PERMANENT HAIR COLOR (LIGHTENING AND TONING)** | | | |
| Hair is first **lightened** (process one) and then **toned** (process two) to give the desired blond or light-red shade. Processing time—1 to 2 hours (longer for resistant hair). Retouch 3–4 weeks. Strand test. Patch test. | Lets those with darker hair get any light blond or light red shade. Hair must be lightened to the correct degree of yellow or pale yellow to take the toner (color). May make hair more manageable, give body. | Choose two-process blonding only if you have the time and willingness to keep the new growth treated, if your skin tones are compatible with pale-hair colors, and if your hair is in good condition. | You can change from semipermanent or permanent hair coloring to two-process hair coloring, but we suggest you consult a hairdresser. |

# BE YOUR OWN SPECIAL BEAUTY

## your face is showing!

And *what* does it show? It *should* show that you care about it a lot—enough to treat it kindly by doing the right things with your skin and your makeup so that it always looks the best it possibly can. For the face that you show the world says much about who you are and what you think of yourself and, of course, you want to keep that statement positive. While not everyone can have perfect features and a naturally flawless complexion, it's a shame that more women don't realize their own special beauty potential and make the most of what they have. And it's always there—just waiting to be tapped. For instance, did you know that you can dramatically enhance your facial contours, eyes and mouth

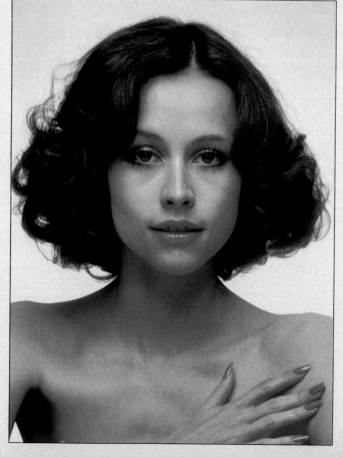

—with just a few dots of color added in strategic places? Or play up a feature you're not totally happy with, instead of hiding it, for a more appealing look? And that's not all you can do—there's a lot more. But first, you need to have the healthiest, smoothest skin you can get because all the makeup in the world won't camouflage a complexion that's less than what it should be. Pay attention to what your skin is telling you. If it's looking good, you're doing the correct things, so be sure to stay with it. If your skin is giving you problems, it's a sign that something is going wrong. Once you find out what it is, and what to do about it, stick faithfully to the program of care your skin requires to look its most beautiful.

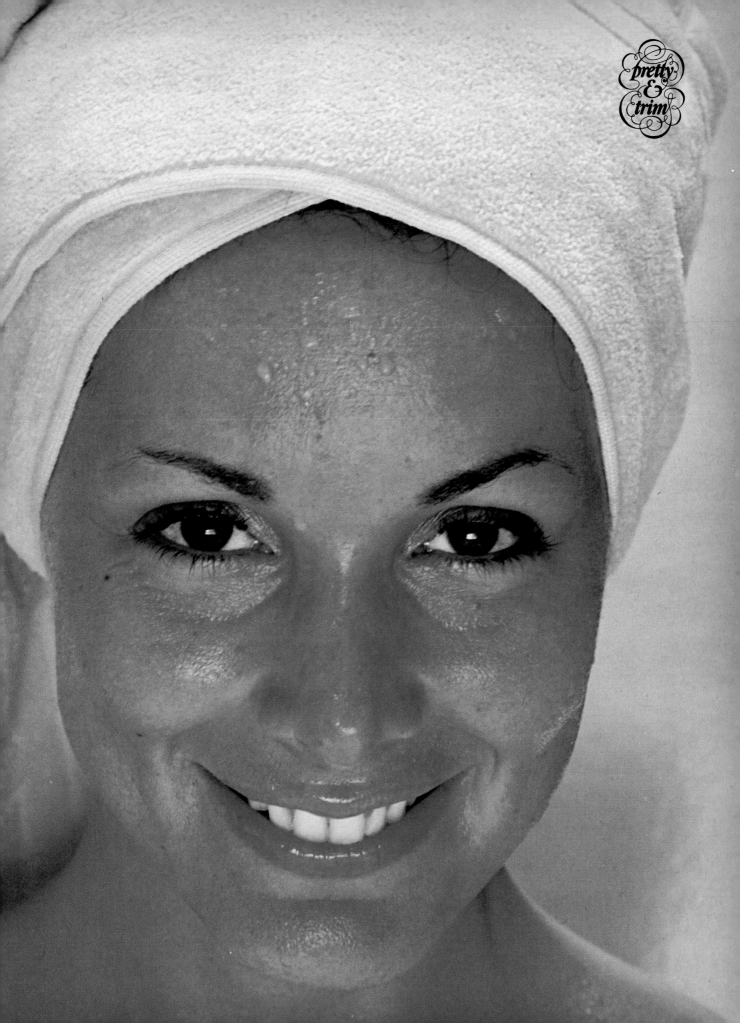

Clear, clean skin is healthy skin. And healthy skin is beau-

# HAVE GLOWING SKIN

tiful skin. Achieving a smooth, vibrant-looking complexion is not difficult, but it does require that you take a close, careful look at your own skin and its needs—and give it the best possible care.

Healthy skin has its own built-in beauty treatment: Natural moisture keeps the skin smooth; skin oils soften the skin and prevent moisture from evaporating while protecting the skin from infection. The best thing you can do for your skin is to keep the natural moisture system working well.

**DIAGNOSE YOUR SKIN.** The first step toward caring for your skin properly is finding out a bit more about it. Oily skin tends to be softer and less wrinkle-prone than dry skin. But some areas can be too oily—and this type of skin is apt to collect grime. Or your skin may be too dry and have a tight, itchy feeling. It's also possible that your skin has dry, oily and normal areas—all at the same time.

A cosmetic mask that can also be used as a face firmer can help you determine what kind of skin you actually do have. Paint the mask on, let it set, peel off and examine it, according to label directions, for areas that show flakiness (dry skin), smoothness (normal skin) or darkness (oily skin).

You can also diagnose your skin by dabbing various areas with cosmetic blotting papers (or eyeglass cleansing tissues). Go to bed with a freshly washed, uncreamed face. In the morning before washing your face, do the blot test. Really dry areas will produce no shine on the tissues. Excess oil comes off on tissue and makes it almost transparent, while normal skin shows a slight trace of shine. The middle of the face—forehead, nose and chin—usually tends to be oiler than the rest of the face. Dry and normal skins need more protection than oily skin, but in cleansing, there is not that much difference.

**CLEANSING.** A thorough cleansing, morning and night, is essential to healthy skin. Always remove all traces of makeup at bedtime—never be tempted to sleep with your makeup on. The following steps should be a part of your daily routine:

• Wash with soap and water but use a superfatted (moisturizing soap) for dry and possibly for normal skin. Wet the face with warm water, rub the soap against the face to create a film and work it into a lather.

*(Continued on page 55 )*

These facial exercises take less time than putting on makeup. If you do them for only two minutes a day, you'll be helping condition your face, eyelids and neck. They won't totally prevent sag, but they may help you look younger.

Let's face it—we all worry about wrinkles, sagging chins, frown lines and crow's feet. But now, maybe, we can stave them off—with exercise. These are the exercises suggested for his own patients by Dr. William H. Friedman, a specialist in facial surgery at Mount Sinai Hospital, N.Y. A combination of isotonic and isometric techniques, the exercises are designed to give your face a more healthy appearance.

Following the directions and illustrations here, start at the collarbone and continue in a rhythmic, wavelike motion up to the forehead. Then reverse, beginning with the forehead and working down. This way you'll be exercising both the skin-related neck muscles and the main areas of the face.

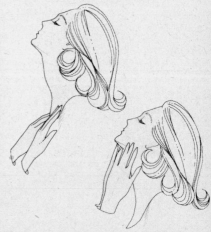

To help prevent horizontal lines on throat and neck: Place hands at collarbone; push down and stretch chin up. Then move hands to jawline and push upward.

Muscles of expression are used less as we go from youth to adult-

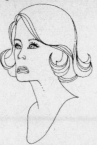

hood. To help preserve jawline: With mouth slightly open, move the corners of the lips downward. Relax. Then holding the lips together with the fingers, try to repeat the movement.

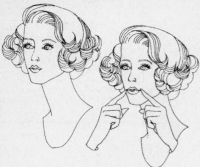

For lines surrounding the mouth: Purse the lips as if you were about to whistle. Relax. Then, pressing the index fingers to the lip margins, try to do the same thing again. Keep touch firm but gentle.

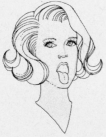

To help tone the musculature under the chin: Open the mouth and extend the tongue as far as possible. Then draw in the tongue and close mouth.

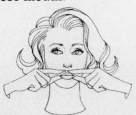

To help tone the lip area and prevent fine wrinkling: Press fingers against the face above and below the mouth so lips are held against the teeth. Attempt to open the mouth. Close and repeat.

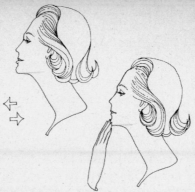

To help tone the middle third of the face: Flex the jaw muscles by clenching teeth; then release slightly and move jaw back and forth, following arrows. Relax. Press fingers to chin and try again.

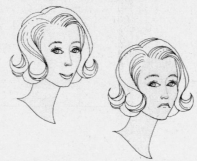

To tone cheek/nose area: Close the mouth and move the upper lip down over the lower lip. Relax. Press fingers to the lip edges and repeat. Reverse procedure, with lower lip over upper lip.

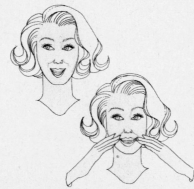

To further tone the middle third of face: With mouth slightly open, move lips and cheeks diagonally upward toward temples. Relax. Now press fingers to lip edges and try to repeat the motion.

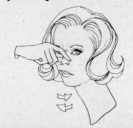

To help prevent wrinkles on the nose: With the thumb on one side and the index finger on the other side of the nose, gently press. Then wrinkle the upper part of the nose and at the same time move the tip from side to side.

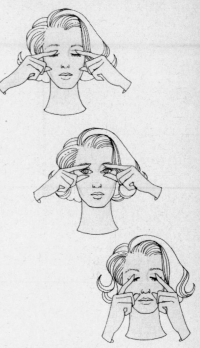

To help eyelid skin: With eyes open, place tips of your index fingers on lids and gently close the eyelids with fingertips. Relax. Now holding eyelids open with fingertips above and below, try to close the eyes. Finish by holding fingertips on your eyelids while attempting to open the eyes.

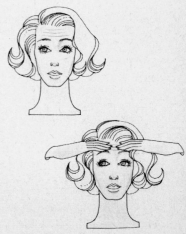

To help prevent frown lines in the forehead area: Move the eyebrows upward to wrinkle the forehead. Relax. Then press brow lines down with fingers of both hands, and against this resistance, try again to wrinkle the forehead.

Makeup: George Newell                                    Photographs: Ron Schwerin

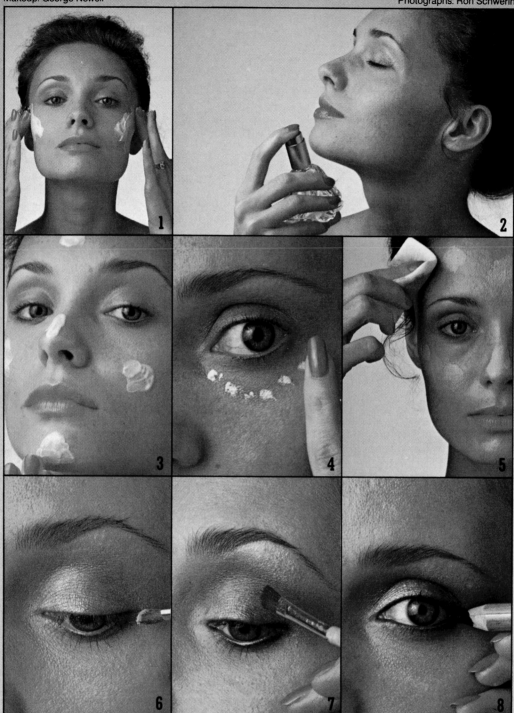

Part of the knack of keeping makeup on is to use the right products. For instance, oily skins need an astringent, dry skins a light toner. Also, if you have oily skin, you normally need a moisturizer only on under-eye area and cheeks, and you should always use a waterbased foundation, followed by an oil-blotting lotion. For blusher, a combination of cream plus powder is the longest lasting for all skin types, as is powder eye shadow. The best tip for everyone: the "ice cube set" (photo opposite). Once your makeup is on, including powder, pat an ice cube gently over your face. The cold will help set makeup and remove excess powder, and give skin a fresh, dewy glow.

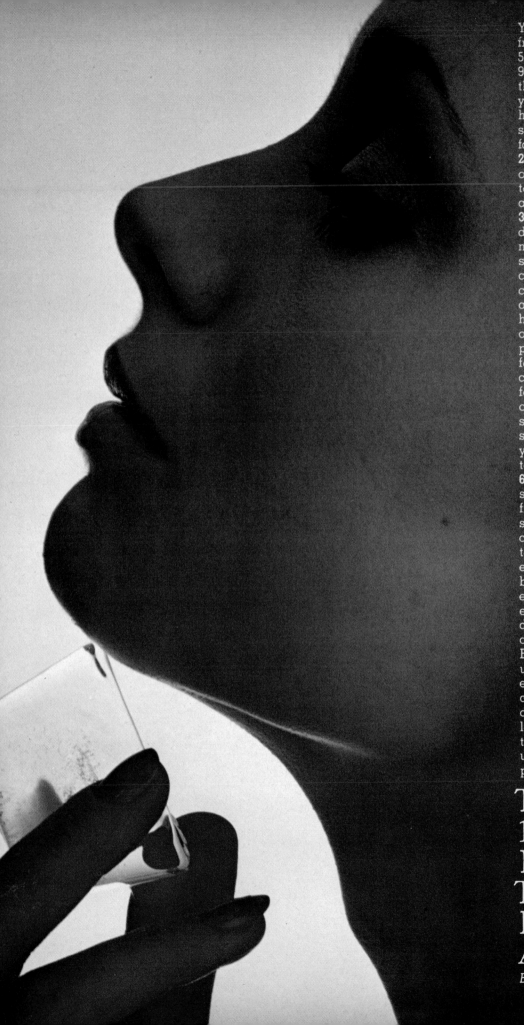

Yes, you can look as fresh and polished at 5:00 P.M. as you did at 9:00 A.M. The trick is the way you apply your makeup. Here's how: **1.** Before you start, cleanse your face thoroughly. **2.** Then, lightly spray on a refrigerated toner with an atomizer bottle. **3.** While skin is still damp, dab on moisturizer and smooth. **4.** Dot a cream concealer carefully under eyes and blend until you have an invisible film of coverage. **5.** Next, place large dots of foundation on nose, cheeks, chin and forehead. Smooth all over face with a slightly dampened sponge, making sure you blend all the way to ears and jawline. **6.** To make-up eyes, start with a slightly frosted shadow in a shade of brown that's close to your skin tone. Apply over entire upper lid and blend up into eyebrow. **7.** Cover entire upper lid with a deeper brown, or colored, shadow. Brush color out and up toward corner of eyebrow; stroke more color in crease for definition. **8.** Line lower lashes as close to lid as possible, using a deep brown eye pencil. Smudge with cotton

# THE 10-MINUTE MAKEUP THAT LASTS ALL DAY

*By Barbara Winkler*

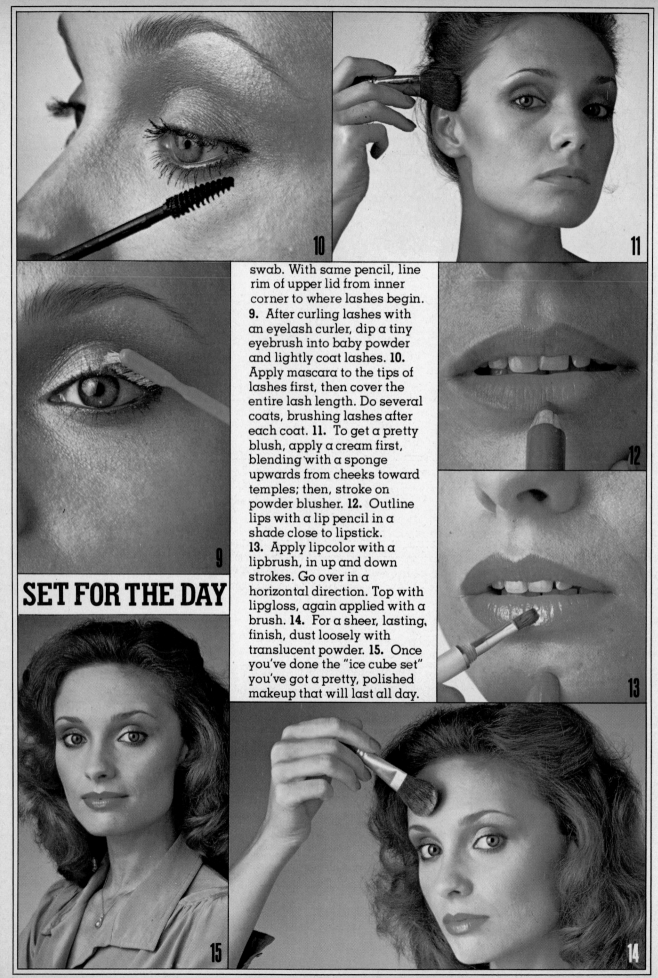

swab. With same pencil, line rim of upper lid from inner corner to where lashes begin. **9.** After curling lashes with an eyelash curler, dip a tiny eyebrush into baby powder and lightly coat lashes. **10.** Apply mascara to the tips of lashes first, then cover the entire lash length. Do several coats, brushing lashes after each coat. **11.** To get a pretty blush, apply a cream first, blending with a sponge upwards from cheeks toward temples; then, stroke on powder blusher. **12.** Outline lips with a lip pencil in a shade close to lipstick. **13.** Apply lipcolor with a lipbrush, in up and down strokes. Go over in a horizontal direction. Top with lipgloss, again applied with a brush. **14.** For a sheer, lasting, finish, dust loosely with translucent powder. **15.** Once you've done the "ice cube set" you've got a pretty, polished makeup that will last all day.

## SET FOR THE DAY

*Barbara Winkler is co-author of* The Working Woman's Body Book.

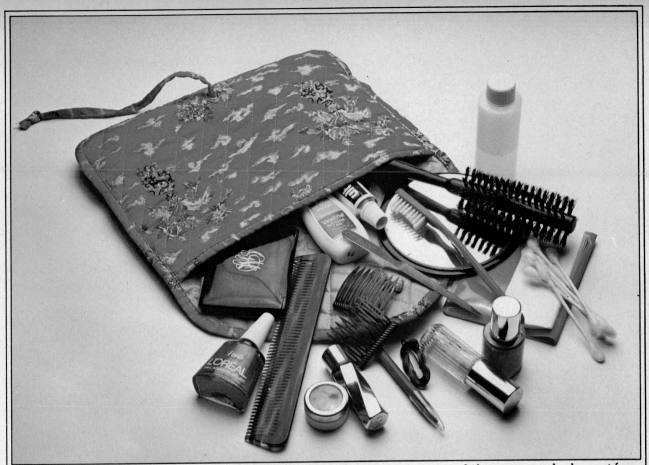

# DESK DRAWER MAKEUP KIT

This is an essential if you want to look great from 9 to 5. Buy either a makeup case or a clear plastic box, and use it to stow the following items: Comb and brush, mirror, toothbrush and toothpaste, hand lotion, cologne, nail polish, remover, cotton swabs, oil blotters or tissues, toner or astringent, barrettes or decorative combs, tweezers, breath freshener; plus, extra makeup such as foundation, blushers and lipstick.

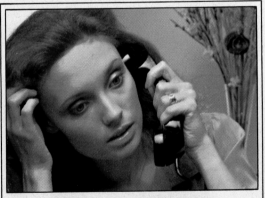

## DO'S & DON'TS FOR OFFICE LIGHTS

DO stick to subtle eye shadow colors. Anything too bright will look garish. DON'T wear opaque base or heavy powder. It will give you a masklike look. DO use a foundation that matches your skin shade as closely as possible. DO blend eye shadow up and out toward brows so you avoid a "circle" of color on lids which is very obvious when you look down. DON'T use a white highlighter or concealing cream. Use a beige or peach toned one.

## LUNCHTIME PICK UPS

- If you have oily skin, pat face with oil blotters, then lightly apply a bit more foundation over forehead, nose and chin.
- If you have dry skin, blend a dot of moisturizer with foundation and apply lightly over face.
- Check eyes and re-line with pencil, if needed.
- Since lips are always the first to go, redo carefully.

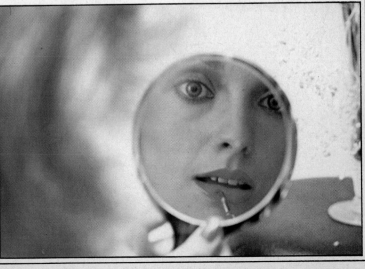

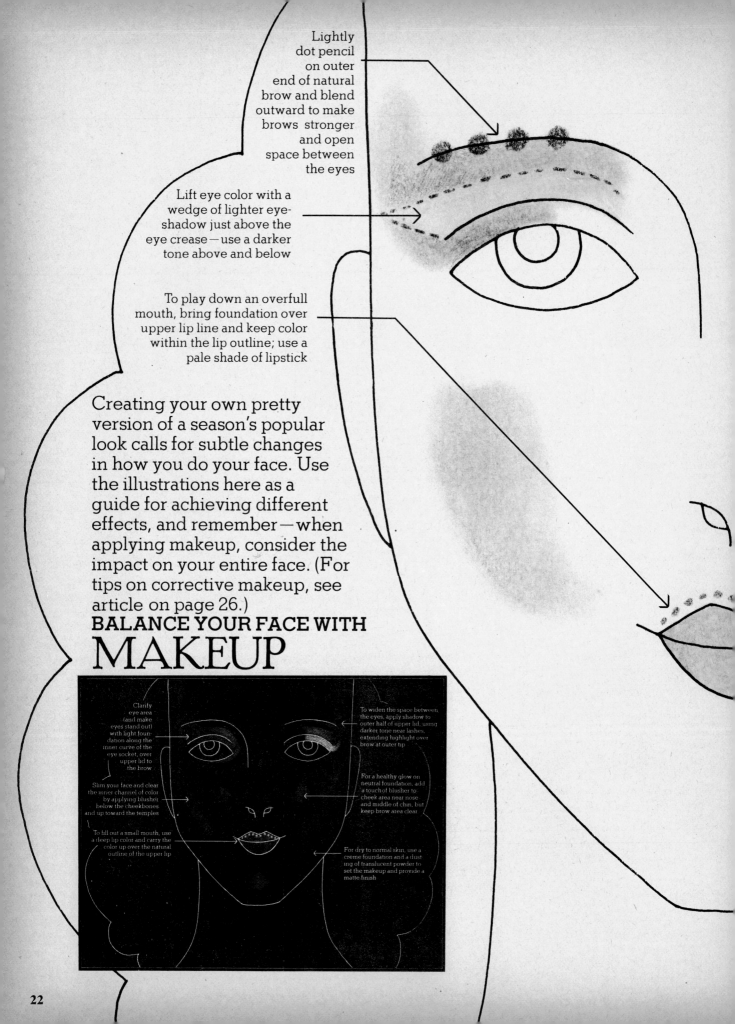

Lightly dot pencil on outer end of natural brow and blend outward to make brows stronger and open space between the eyes

Lift eye color with a wedge of lighter eye-shadow just above the eye crease — use a darker tone above and below

To play down an overfull mouth, bring foundation over upper lip line and keep color within the lip outline; use a pale shade of lipstick

Creating your own pretty version of a season's popular look calls for subtle changes in how you do your face. Use the illustrations here as a guide for achieving different effects, and remember — when applying makeup, consider the impact on your entire face. (For tips on corrective makeup, see article on page 26.)

## BALANCE YOUR FACE WITH
# MAKEUP

Clarity eye area (and make eyes stand out) with light foundation along the inner curve of the eye socket, over upper lid to the brow

To widen the space between the eyes, apply shadow to outer half of upper lid, using darker tone near lashes, extending highlight over brow at outer tip

Slim your face and clear the inner channel of color by applying blusher below the cheekbones and up toward the temples

For a healthy glow on neutral foundation, add a touch of blusher to cheek area near nose and middle of chin, but keep brow area clear

To fill out a small mouth, use a deep lip color and carry the color up over the natural outline of the upper lip

For dry to normal skin, use a creme foundation and a dusting of translucent powder to set the makeup and provide a matte finish

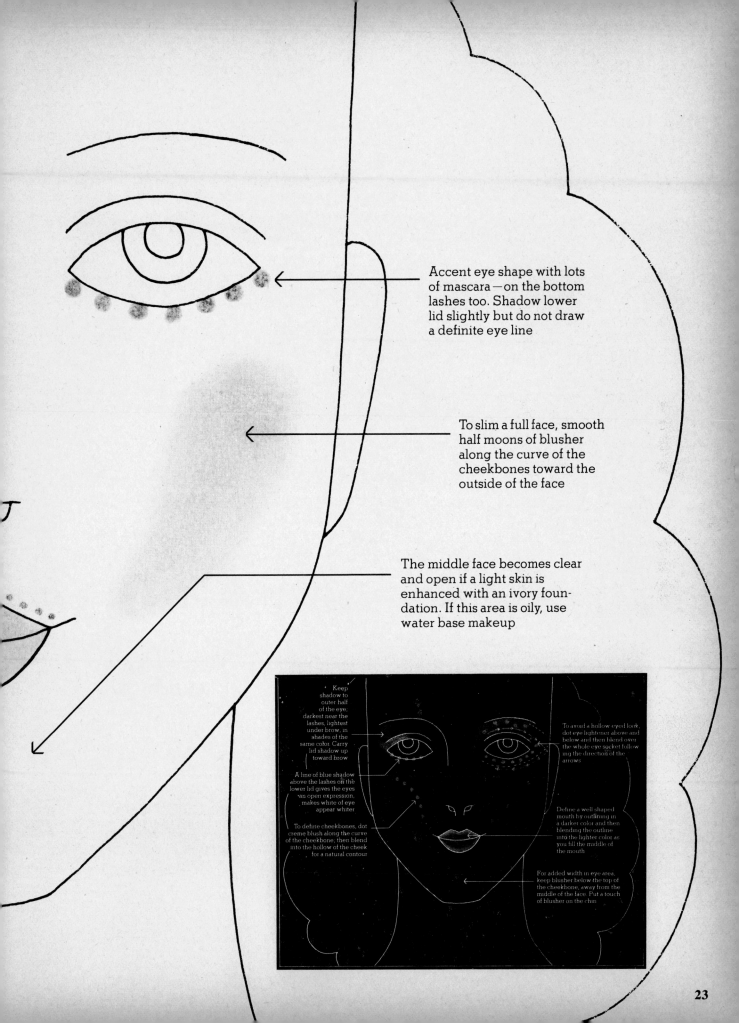

Accent eye shape with lots of mascara—on the bottom lashes too. Shadow lower lid slightly but do not draw a definite eye line

To slim a full face, smooth half moons of blusher along the curve of the cheekbones toward the outside of the face

The middle face becomes clear and open if a light skin is enhanced with an ivory foundation. If this area is oily, use water base makeup

Keep shadow to outer half of the eye, darkest near the lashes, lightest under brow, in shades of the same color. Carry lid shadow up toward brow

A line of blue shadow above the lashes on the lower lid gives the eyes an open expression, makes white of eye appear whiter

To define cheekbones, dot creme blush along the curve of the cheekbone, then blend into the hollow of the cheek for a natural contour

To avoid a hollow eyed look, dot eye lightener above and below and then blend over the whole eye socket following the direction of the arrows

Define a well shaped mouth by outlining in a darker color and then blending the outline into the lighter color as you fill the middle of the mouth

For added width in eye area, keep blusher below the top of the cheekbone, away from the middle of the face. Put a touch of blusher on the chin

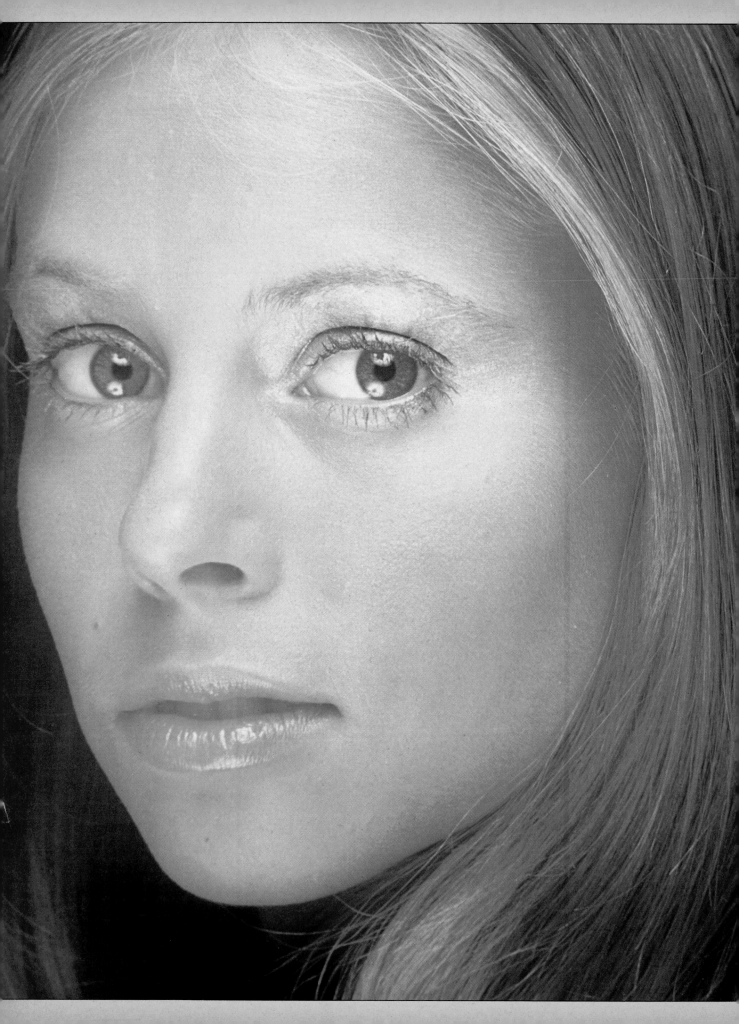

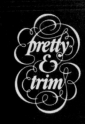

At some point you get tired of being just another pretty face and want your look to make a real statement. Makeup color is the key. Pick up the light in your hair with light in your face. For evening (*left*), achieve the look of flawless skin with a luminous makeup in a see-through tint, with golden notes to echo hair highlights and eyes that shimmer in color. In daytime makeup, go with your own

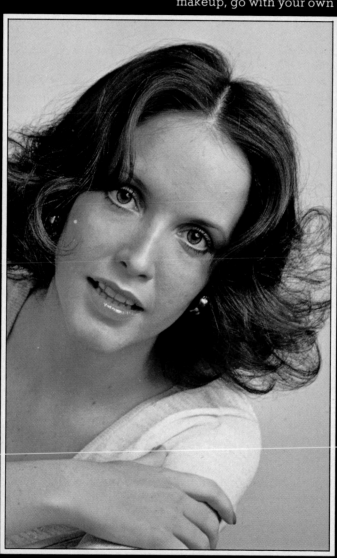

color but enhance it. Tone down ruddy notes with beige-tone foundation so the complexion appears translucent (*see above*), with lip and eye color picking up deep red highlights in the hair. Sallow skin needs added color, so tinted foundation is a must; lips should be vibrant and the eyes need to be emphasized with lots of mascara.

# MAKEUP TRICKS TO ENHANCE YOUR FEATURES

A bit of color well placed—a line here, a smudge there—can go a long way in transforming your looks. Here makeup artist Stan Place shows you how to make the most of your face, brows, eyes and mouth with a few easy touches.

For today's look, says Stan, color is put on the outside of the face, leaving the middle free except for a bright accent on the mouth. This creates an illusion of wider space between the eyes. Color accents are not well defined, but become soft, blurred images. Shades are neutral and beiged, as if a little brown had been added. There are smoky tones in eye makeup and lips are creamy and gentler in color, with less shine and no frost.

With this natural look, you should aim for a flawless complexion.

## LIGHTS AND SHADES

Be careful about using light and shade on the face—too much can look garish. But if you need some redefinition, and do this correctly, highlights and contouring can be effective.

Contour makeup *shading* should be only a shade darker than your foundation, light in texture, gently applied and well blended, so it is not apparent. Contour only the lower part of the face, the nose and the eyes as a start. Then stand away from the mirror and look at your face. Does it look older? Better sculpted? More interesting? Probably all three. It won't look *older* once color is added.

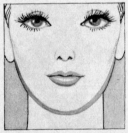

**Firming the jawline:** Use shading under the chin from behind the earlobe around and underneath the natural chinbone and down onto the neck, to the first ring in the throat.

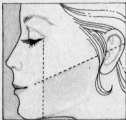

**Hollowing the cheeks:** Shading belongs on the outside plane of the face and should come no closer to the middle of the face than the outside corner of the eye. It should go as far as the back teeth. If you were to draw an invisible line from the middle of the ear to the outside corner of the mouth, you'd work under that line.

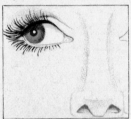

**Shaping the nose:** An "invisible" shadow, stripped down the top edge on each side of the nose can give the illusion of a straighter, narrower, better chiseled nose. Keep it off the widest part of the nostril and away from the bridge of the nose. It should run from the top of the brow down the top sides of the nose, leaving a clean stripe in the middle. The narrower the stripe, the narrower the nose will appear. The broader the stripe, the wider the nose will appear.

**To shorten the nose:** A shadow just under the lower tip of the nose can create the illusion of a shorter nose. Make it very delicate.

Highlight should be only a shade lighter than your foundation. Apply it, if necessary, only on the under-eye circles, top of cheekbones, forehead or jawline. Pearl, gold or frost highlights can be placed on the height of the cheekbone or under the eyebrow—they should not be white. A pearlized version of your basic makeup color—eye makeup or blusher—usually gives enough light.

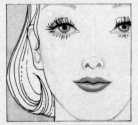

**To make the cheekbones prominent:** Highlight the top of the cheekbones; add a highlight under the browbone and a thin line down the very middle of the nose.

**Jawbone:** Highlight along the jawbone makes it seem more prominent.

**Lines at side of mouth:** So-called smile lines from the side of the nose to the outside corners of the mouth can be lightened by placing a small dot of highlighter cream at the crease of the nose. Do not blend the cream in the length of the crease.

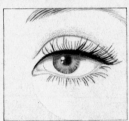

**Circles under eyes:** Do not wrap a lightener all around the eyes, because it can make the eye look small. Some kind of circle is normal—part of the bone structure. If the hollow is very dark, a little highlight cream patted on in three light dots under the lower lash line and blended only halfway out and around can help.

**Nose creases:** A bit of cream at the outside edge of the nose fold, carefully blended so that it doesn't collect in the crease, highlights this area.

## ROUGE AND BLUSHERS

Although rouge adds color to the face, it can also either highlight or contour, often working even better than lights and shades in redefining the face.

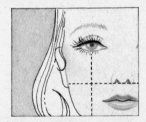

Rouge basically goes on the cheekbones, but should be kept toward the outside of the face, never coming closer to the middle of the face than just below the middle of the eye.

There is one exception: If you have a cute, pert face, you can add a touch of blusher to the tip of the nose to shorten it a little. On the cheeks, the rouge should usually not be dropped below the base of the nose.

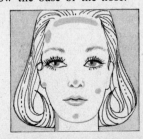

If you do not have too broad a *forehead,* you can add rouge to the temple, to make the forehead more prominent and to warm the eyes.

A little rouge around the *hairline* adds a warm halo to the face and helps make the forehead seem lower.

Rouge on the *chin* helps shorten the face a bit.

If you are wearing an absolutely beige makeup that has little color, you can use rouge in the *hollow of the cheeks* as if it were a contour. But it should be in a dusky or tawny tone.

Rouge on the *earlobes* or on the side of the neck or throat helps create a warm glow.

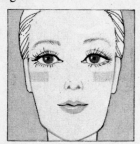

**Long face:** Place rouge in a horizontal bar, directly across the cheekbones.

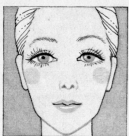

**Diamond-shape face:** Place rouge in a circle on height of cheekbones to the outside of face.

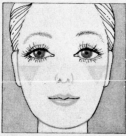

**Round face:** Triangles of rouge should be placed to the outside of the face, as shown.

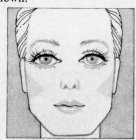

**Square face:** Triangles of rouge can be lower than suggested above and carried all the way to outside of face, as shown.

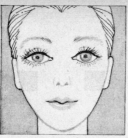

**Heart-shape face:** Place squares of rouge in the middle of the high cheekbones, toward the outside of the face, not too close to eyes.

## SHAPELY BROWS

Your eyebrows do more than anything else to set the expression of your face. Nature gives us brows of different shapes, thicknesses and colors. The shape depends on the natural browbone, and we have to work within the natural contour. But improvements can be made.

In color, brows should usually be a full shade lighter than your hair color (and should not exactly match it) unless you happen to be light-blond or silver-white or gray-haired. Then the brows should be no more than a shade darker than the hair. Usually a half shade darker is enough.

Brows can be lightened with liquid brow makeup or bleached with a special eyebrow bleach. *Never* use hair dyes on the brows.

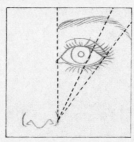

**Shaping the brows:** Brows should be the proper length, fullness and shape to best frame your eyes and fit within the contour of your whole face. Whatever you do with them, remember you are locked in by the form of your bone structure, so measure them in relation to your other features.
• Place a pencil vertically at the side of your nose at the widest point of the base, so it extends over the inside corner of the eye and across the inner tip of the brow. Mark this point with a brow pencil. This is where your brow should begin.
• Move the pencil so that it goes from the base of the nose across the outer corner of the eye to cross the brow. Mark this point with a brow pencil. This is the *minimum* length of the brow. It can be longer.
• From the base of the nose, move the pencil till it crosses the outer rim of the iris (the colored part of the eye)

as you look straight ahead—and intersects the brow. Mark this point with a brow pencil. This is ideally the highest point of the arch.
• Repeat with other brow.

Brows should be about the same thickness or thinness along the entire length, diminishing only slightly along the outer tip.

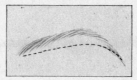

Tweeze the hairs between the inner tips of the brows, and under the brow, to get a clean shape. Pluck only stray hairs above the arch.

When the space between the brows is clean and the space below the arch shaped, start tweezing at the outer tip to find the length that is most becoming to you, but be careful not to tweeze beyond the mark for minimum brow length.

## BEAUTIFUL EYES

Eye makeup colors should always be considered an accessory to whatever outfit you are wearing. For today's look, choose monochromatic values —lighter to deeper shades of a single color—to highlight, shadow and even to smudge at the lash line for an accent that is not really a line, but does emphasize the eye shape.

It is mascara, not liner, that does the most to shape your eyes. Apply to lower lashes first and give them a chance to dry. Then do the upper lashes, moving from one eye to the other, building up about three coats so they look thick and full. For a more curled look, push upward on your lashes with your mascara case between coats, and hold for a second.

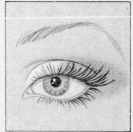

**Contouring:** The new trend in eye makeup calls for highlighting the inner corner of the lid to create the illusion of width between the eyes. For contouring and to further accent this illusion of width, place shadow on the outer half of the upper lid, starting at mid-point and tapering off beyond the outer corner. The eyes look more wide open with soft colors blended around the eye, without hard edges to reveal where the color begins and leaves off.

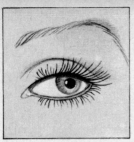

Sometimes a bit of rouge placed near the arch of the brow to the outer tip *above* the eyebrow will create a warmer, bright-eyed look. So will a little touch of blue as an inner liner placed at the base of the lashes. This lightens the eye, makes it seem brighter and more sparkling.

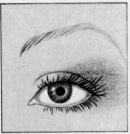

**Making small eyes seem larger:** Always use eye makeup in a shade darker than the color of the eyes—and never use pale, frosted colors. Use little definition around the eye so that it seems to float in a pool of color. Keep the brows thin and highly arched and spaced as far above the lashes as possible. Shadow should not go all the way to the brow line; only about half way. Then elongate and round it out at the outer corner.

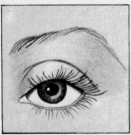

**Making deep-set eyes fuller:** This eye needs a light color all at one level, from the lash line all the way to the brow, but don't extend shadow too far beyond the outer corners.

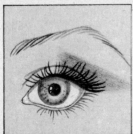

**Round eyes:** Here the shadow can be extended well beyond the outer tip so the eyes don't look so protuberant. From the middle of the upper lid at the lash line, extend the shadow up over the crease to about a quarter inch from the brow and outward, tapering to a point at the level of the eye tip and extending almost to the socket bone. Brows for this eye should be long and thin.

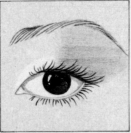

**Flat eyes (no fold in lid):** Use a highlighter on the upper lid in the inner half of the eye, with darker shadow on the outer half of the upper lid and a lighter level of the same shade below the brow. Extend the shadow in a bar at the outer tip.

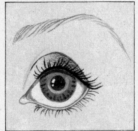

**Bulging eyes:** Play down by using dark, smoky-brown shadows, starting about a quarter of the way across from the inner tip of the upper lid and covering the lid to the crease. Use a little liner to make the lash area appear darker.

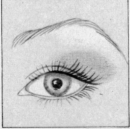

**Long, narrow eyes:** Carry the shadow up in a rounded shape over the eyelid, nearly to the crease line, starting at the middle of the upper lid. Use a flat shadow in the socket of the eye or a smoky highlighter under the eyebone.

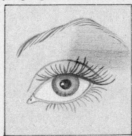

**Slanted eyes:** Keep eye makeup to a minimum. If you use any, it should be soft cream on the eyebone over a very small area. If you add color on the lid itself, keep it very close to the lashes, and above it use a neutral matte color.

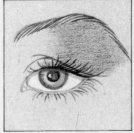

**Overhung eyes:** These look best with dark-brown shadow all the way up to the brow, starting about a quarter of the way in from the inner corner.

## LOVELY MOUTH

Your lips are the color accent on your face. Pale lip colors make the mouth seem less important, while a bright color calls attention to the mouth. For today's look, avoid high gloss and shine. Use a creamier lipstick for a softer appearance.

Outlining the lips in a dark color defines the mouth, but the natural light that falls on the lip outline is a white or paler light. Therefore, if you want to line your lips to create the most flattering light, use a paler, softer color than the regular lip color for lining.

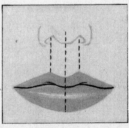

If your upper lip has a *cupid's bow,* be sure the highest point of each curve is directly under the opening of the corresponding nostril. The lowest point of the lower lip should be directly under the tip of the nose. This helps the mouth fit the shape of the face and makes the nose look straighter.

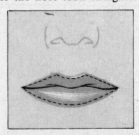

**For thin lips:** You can slightly extend the shape of the mouth by using a lip brush or lip pencil and going just barely over the outer rim of the lips. Too much will look artificial, but a slight filling out can make the mouth *(Continued on page 54)*

# 16 Steps to Take for a Good Night's Sleep– Without Pills

**1.** Get more exercise during the day. But don't exercise before bed.
**2.** Live by your natural rhythms. Don't go to bed until you're sleepy.
**3.** Eliminate noise with carpeting, drapes and so on.
**4.** Make sure the bedroom isn't too hot or too cold.
**5.** Have a snack that's not sweet. Milk is good.
**6.** Don't drink too much alcohol during the day.
**7.** Take inositol, a vitamin B. A 2000-mg. tablet at bedtime acts as a natural sleeping pill.
**8.** Establish a go-to-bed ritual such as brushing your hair.
**9.** If music helps you go to sleep, have an automatic timer connected to your radio. Don't play it all night. Music keeps you from sleeping deeply.
**10.** Don't let problems get to you. Pick just one and think it through.
**11.** Think of something pleasant that happened that day.
**12.** Sleep less. Maybe you don't have insomnia, you simply need less sleep than others.

## FOUR EXERCISES TO GO TO SLEEP BY

**1.** Create a picture in your mind. A soft, silent snow scene; a pastoral painting of horses grazing along a meadow.
**2.** Think of downward movement. Picture yourself floating, like a feather, from a cloud.
**3.** Close your eyes and relax your body as completely as you can, starting from your toes and relaxing every muscle right up to your scalp. Then count slowly from 10 to zero. Tell yourself that when you reach zero you will be asleep.
**4.** Talk yourself to sleep. Tell yourself your eyelids are growing heavy, heavier, heavier; that you are relaxing more and more, deeper... and deeper... your eyelids are heavy; that you are getting sleepier and sleepier.

# High-Vitality Drinks from High-Energy People

*By Mary Ann Crenshaw*

Do you wonder why some of the busiest, most "on-stage" people in the world—those who ought to be dog-tired a lot of the time—seem to have boundless energy? Did you ever think they must have a bit of magic potion at their elbows? You're right! When asked what kept them hale, hearty, healthy and bubbling through their 10-to-16 hour days, these energetic folk told us about the "magic" drinks they use to keep their vitality never-flagging. Here are their secret recipes.

Linda Clark, author of many books on nutrition and beauty, says her "everything drink" is so satisfying it gives you a lift you can feel within 10 minutes. And if you drink it before meals, you feel less hungry, and that helps to bring about weight loss—an added bonus.

## LINDA CLARK'S EVERYTHING DRINK

1 teaspoon brewer's yeast flakes*
(work up to several tablespoonfuls)
1 glass fruit juice or water

Stir together.
*Available in health-food stores.*

Dr. Robert C. Atkins, who wrote *Dr. Atkins' Diet Revolution*—and practically started one—has a current best-seller, *Dr. Atkins' Super Energy Diet*. He considers his energy drink a meal in itself—it's so filling often his patients feel no need to eat after drinking it.

## DR. ATKINS' EXTRA-ENERGY DRINK

1 tablespoon powdered milk protein*
1 tablespoon cold-pressed safflower oil
2 tablespoons lecithin granules
½ teaspoon brewer's yeast
   Vanilla extract to taste
   Artificial sweetener to taste
   Club soda or Perrier water to add froth.

Blend and pour into a tumbler. For variety you can put in an ounce of heavy cream and ¼ cup (no more) of blueberries or strawberries and still adhere to Dr. Atkins' low-carbohydrate, energy-giving, weight-losing regime.
*This must be without carbohydrate.*

*Mary Ann Crenshaw is the author of Shape Up For Super Sex.*

Charlotte Ford Forstmann, fashion designer, is onto the health bandwagon. For breakfast she has the traditional bacon and eggs. For lunch she takes this drink. It's nourishing and non-fattening.

## CHARLOTTE FORD'S HIGH-SPEED LUNCH

2 cups skim milk
2 tablespoons wheat germ
1 teaspoon honey
1 banana

Mix all ingredients in a blender.

Way Bandy, makeup wizard, tells us that this potion overcomes morning acidity and prepares his stomach for digesting whatever he eats during his on-the-move day.

## WAY BANDY'S WAKEUP DROPS

1 teaspoon apple-cider vinegar diluted in 1 glass of water

Drink first thing in the morning.

Kate Jackson, one of Charlie's Angels, soars on this drink's high protein. Use it as an energy-extender when skipping lunch.

## KATE JACKSON'S ANGEL JUICE

1 tablespoon carob powder
1 cup natural yogurt
1 tablespoon wheat germ
1 mashed banana
½ cup whole milk

Blend and chill.

Gayelord Hauser, the grand old man of healthy food, reminds us that herbal teas are an age-old recipe for relaxation as well as for a late day lift. He suggests you simply use two-thirds of your favorite tea leaves and one-third dried peppermint leaves for a delicious between-meal pick-up.

## GAYELORD HAUSER'S TRANQUILITEA

1 ounce dried peppermint leaves
1 tablespoon rosemary leaves
1 tablespoon sage leaves

Mix and store in tightly closed jar. Use one tablespoon of the mixture to a cup of boiling water. Let steep one minute, strain, sweeten with honey.

You've found the perfect hairdo, a pretty new makeup. What else do you need to be a glowing year-round beauty? Exercises for a great-looking figure and special tips for under-the-sun care. Turn page and find out how to jump, stretch and condition your body into shape, and then on to page 48 for most-often asked summer beauty questions answered, including how to protect your face, hair and hands when out in the sun, how to get the perfect overall tan—and more.

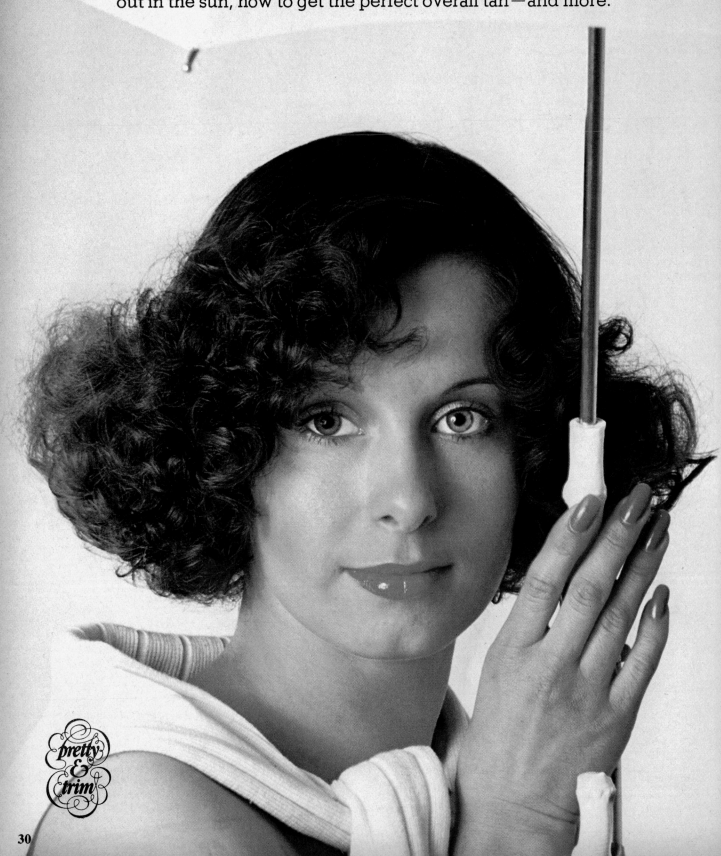

pretty & trim

30

*(Continued from page 7)*

hair short when someone requests this —albeit reluctantly—but only in a blunt cut that's fairly even all around. And chin length is the shortest he'll go. "When your hair is one length, you have a gorgeous sheen and gloss to it," he says convincingly. When you cut it in layers, it's like taking a hammer and knocking a mirror to pieces. The mirror will stop shining, and you'll just have broken lines.

He announces further that cutting the hair in layers actually causes more hair loss than you'd have normally: "The body always works to maintain a balance, and if you cut the hair into bangs or into a shag, the long part will begin to shed to balance out with the shorter part. So you always lose more hair when it is not one length."

Style-conscious women may not be too happy with this advice, but Michael explains that he's tested this theory on thousands of women and found it to be valid. He also points out that artfully arranged, hair cut in one length can be styled in many different ways. If you now have bangs or a layered cut, don't panic, however. Michael assures that you won't go *bald*—but he recommends that you start growing it out immediately!

**BRUSHING.** Daily brushing is a must, according to Michael. Although some stylists now believe that brushing isn't necessary, he dismisses these notions. "Brushing stimulates the scalp, distributes oils and gets rid of excess dirt and dust, so how can it be bad for you?"

The key is *how* you brush, he says. Never brush your hair in a hurry— this can cause breakage—or when it's wet, when it's at its weakest and easily stretched. Always use a natural-bristle brush—Michael recommends Kent's LHS #5—preferably one with a wooden handle and base, but never one with a rubber base, which creates static. Large, oval-shaped brushes with tufts that gradually get longer toward the center are best for long hair, while circular or curved brushes are fine for hair six inches or shorter, because these brushes require a twist-of-the-wrist motion that works best with short hair.

Since one of the most important reasons for brushing is to stimulate the scalp, Michael says the best time to do it is immediately after you get up in the morning—you've been in a horizontal position all night, and at this time there's more of a concentration of blood in the scalp than when you've been standing or sitting a few hours. Here's the way to do it: Plant both feet firmly on the floor, about a foot and a half apart, bend over until your head reaches the level of your waist, and brush your hair *slowly* from

the nape of your neck to the ends, smoothing your hair with your hand after every stroke. Also brush underneath, from the forehead out.

Brushing should be a gradual process, so start off with 20 a day and increase by 10 until you reach 100. Then drop off by about 20 strokes a day until you reach the amount you feel works best for your hair. If for some reason you skip a day, decrease the amount of strokes by 20 the following day, and build up again. Otherwise, you'll put too much stress on your roots

**ACCESSORIES.** In addition to a natural bristle brush, use only a wide-tooth comb; Speert #15 is the one used in the Michael salon. This kind is easier on the hair than one with narrow teeth, which tends to tear the hair and besides, doesn't last long.

Michael is firmly against rubber bands—even the coated variety—because they put too much tension on the hair and scalp. Ribbons are fine, but circular comb clips (usually found in tortoise shell) are probably the best, since they hold the hair in place without pulling.

**SHAMPOOING.** For both salon and home use, Michael favors Windsor Shampoo Concentrate by Helene Curtis (can be bought cheaply in beauty supply stores; mix one ounce shampoo to seven ounces water). He follows this with an application of Breck Creme Rinse (pink only) to make combing easier. Creamy shampoos, he feels, are better for the hair than the clear kind—especially for long hair—since they slide better and prevent friction and tangling.

You can shampoo as often as you like, provided you stick with gentle products. If you have long hair, however, realize that your ends tend to be dry even though your scalp may be oily. If you want to wash frequently, Michael suggests that you drench the ends with creme rinse before shampooing. Then shampoo the scalp and upper portion of the hair, without working the ends. The shampoo will slide over the creme rinse without penetrating the hair. After shampooing, apply creme rinse to the rest of your hair as usual, and rinse.

*How* you shampoo is as important as what you shampoo with, for as Michael quips, "You can't wash lingerie like you wash a pair of dungarees. The lingerie is delicate; it has to be washed gently, and it's the same with hair. If you scrub roughly, you'll tear it to pieces and cause a lot of split and broken ends."

The first shampoo should be a *gentle* sudsing to wash off surface dirt. The second time you lather, mas-
*(Continued on page 57)*

## DIET DO'S

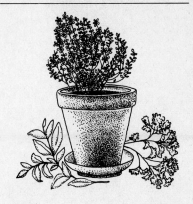

Guides for cooking with herbs:
• Keep herbs and spices in alphabetical order on the spice shelf and you will always be able to find them quickly.
• Use a new herb by itself the first few times you cook with it. Then you will learn how pungent it is, and how it blends with other foods.
• Give herbs time to season foods. If the cooking time is short, let the herb soak in part of the cooking liquid while preparing other ingredients.
• To determine the strength of an herb, crush a bit of it in the palm of your hand and sniff its aroma.
• Choose lean birds (chicken, turkey, game hen) instead of the fattier ones (duckling, goose).
• Pick young birds (broiler-fryers, for example) over the older; they have less fat and fewer calories.
• Choose light meat instead of dark (chicken breasts are particularly slimming).

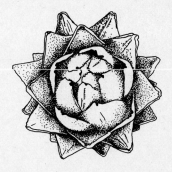

Dieters can enjoy artichokes with a free conscience. To cook them, trim all leaves with kitchen shears; scoop out the choke with a sharp spoon (a grapefruit spoon is perfect). Place in a kettle with a bit of lemon juice and a few whole allspice; add a 1-inch depth of water. Cover and bring to boiling; lower heat and simmer 30 minutes, or until tender. Cool in cooking liquid. Serve with thin slices of poached chicken breast and a little low-calorie salad dressing.

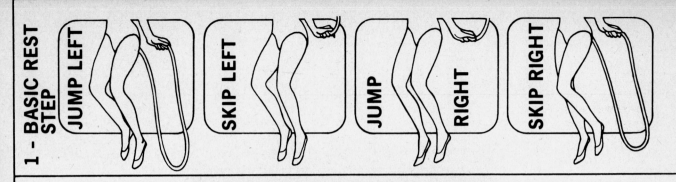

**1 - BASIC REST STEP** JUMP LEFT · SKIP LEFT · JUMP RIGHT · SKIP RIGHT

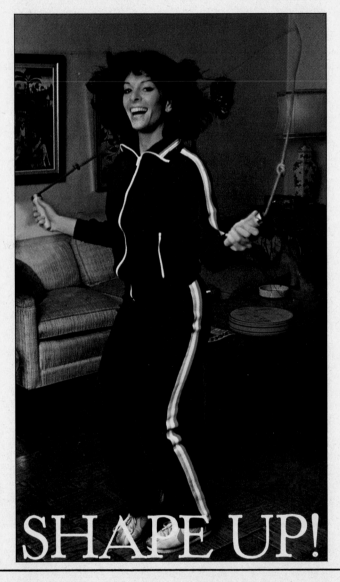

# SHAPE UP!

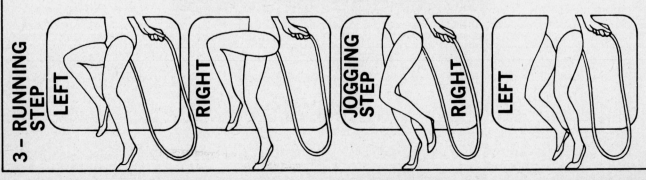

**3 - RUNNING STEP** LEFT · RIGHT · JOGGING STEP · RIGHT · LEFT

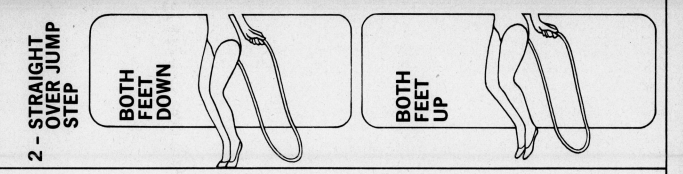

**2 – STRAIGHT OVER JUMP STEP**

BOTH FEET DOWN

BOTH FEET UP

The right exercises, done daily, will help you look — and feel — your best. In this special 16-page section you'll find exercises to fit your every need — from relaxing stretches to do when you're tired and tense to overall conditioners that help firm and tone your muscles. The more you exercise the better, but even a few minutes a day with any of these will help increase circulation, provide you with more energy and — give your body a more graceful, trim look.

### JUMP INTO SHAPE IN 4 EASY STEPS

Rope-jumping is a fun way to lose inches quickly. Bounce on the balls of your feet, with knees slightly bent, arms close to sides and wrists loose. Jump only high enough to clear the rope.

1. *Basic Rest Step:* Start with this for warming up. Jump over rope, landing on the ball of left foot. As the rope turns over your head, bounce again on left foot with a little hop, kicking the right foot out a bit. Then jump over the rope, landing on the ball of your right foot with a hop (or skip) while the left foot kicks out. Alternate feet, building to a steady rhythm.
2. *Straight-over Jump Step:* Jump straight over the rope, toes together, coming down lightly on balls of feet, knees slightly bent. Don't come down hard.
3. *Running Step:* Jump, alternating feet as the rope passes underneath, lifting knee as high as you can. (Another version of this is the "jogging step.") Run in place, landing lightly on the balls of the feet.
4. *Toe Tap:* Jump on the balls of both feet, with feet side by side, tapping the left toe onto the floor in front of the right foot. Jump, tapping the right foot out in front of the left foot. Keep alternating. Can also be done as a heel tap.

*(From Ms. Sidney Filson, who teaches jump rope in New York City. See photo opposite.)*

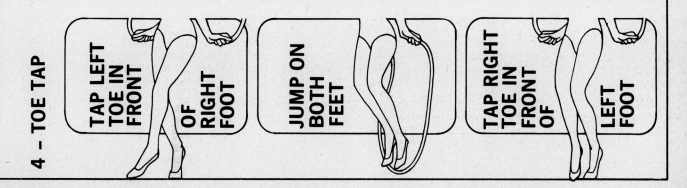

**4 – TOE TAP**

TAP LEFT TOE IN FRONT

OF RIGHT FOOT

JUMP ON BOTH FEET

TAP RIGHT TOE IN FRONT OF

LEFT FOOT

"The more you tune up your body with exercise, the more aware of it you'll become. And only when you're aware of how you're moving—where you're stiff and where your tensions are—can you change things for the better," says doctor of chiropractic and exercise expert Alan Levy. Dr. Levy and his partners Dick Shea and Laura Hoefler own and run the Levy Shea studio in N.Y., where everyday people exercise side by side with the famous in a program based on yoga and dance techniques. The exercises here are part of the program and consist of a lot of stretching to get your body working at its optimum efficiency. They're grouped into wake-up exercises to get you going in the morning, relaxation exercises to do anytime you feel tense and overall toning exercises to give you a greater degree of suppleness. Pay special attention to the breathing instructions; they're important to getting the most from the exercises. (The Levy Shea studio also offers a step-by-step exercise tape; see Buyer's Guide.) *Note:* It's wise to get your doctor's approval before beginning this or any other exercise program.

**Wake-up.** (1) Stretch and yawn, bringing arms over head in back of you. Then extend arms at sides and bring right knee into chest. Now bring right knee across body to your left so that ankle and knee touch bed. Try to keep right shoulder on bed. Hold; feel a stretch on right side; breathe deeply, imagining breath going into right side. Repeat with left leg. *4 times.* (2) Keeping arms at

# RELAX, STRETCH & TONE YOUR BODY

sides, bring both knees into chest. Swing knees over to left side, turning your face to right; hold; feel stretch on right side. Then bring knees tight into chest again and to right side, with face to left. *4 times.* (3) Sit up in bed; place soles of feet together, hands on knees; point elbows up toward

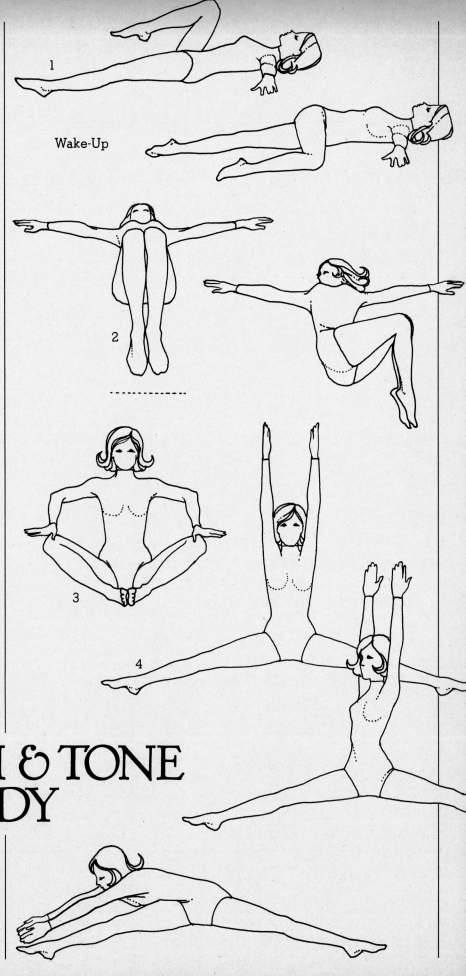

Wake-Up

1

2

3

4

ceiling. Keeping back straight, press down on knees with hands; as you press down, try to raise knees up. (Firms inner thighs.) *5 times.* (4) Get out of bed, sit on floor and open legs as wide as you can. Stretch arms straight over head, keeping back straight. Hold for a count of 5. Then twist, from waist up, to right side and bend over right knee, keeping back straight. (Bend over starting with low back rather than rounding middle and upper back.) Return to first position, twist to left side and bend over left knee. *4–5 times.* (5) Stand up with feet together; inhale deeply and allow arms to float above head. As arms come up, sense a stretch along sides of ribs, through armpits, upper arms, elbows, wrists, and fingers; place palms toward each other. Hold for a count of 5. (6) Bring legs apart, reach up to ceiling with left arm and allow right heel to come up off floor. Repeat with right arm and left heel to establish a rocking motion. Feel a sense of pull on each side as you reach up. *6 times.* (7) Bring legs about 2 feet apart, bend elbows slightly, with palms facing, and bend over as far as you can to the right. Breathe deeply, feel a stretch on left side and imagine breath going there. Hold for count of 10. Repeat on left side. Now come over to right side again and bounce several times from waist area; repeat on left side.

**Relaxation.** (1) Do this exercise in a quiet room. Stand very still with eyes closed, feet and hands together as shown. Imagine a line dropping from just behind the ear, through the middle of body, through center of hip joint to the arch of your foot, a little in front of your ankle bone. Sense the weight of your body being distributed equally over heels and balls of feet. Breathe deeply, inhaling and exhaling through nose, keeping head erect and neck relaxed. Don't allow your body to come too far forward or back. Imagine breath flowing through body to all your vital organs. Hold about 2 minutes. (2) To relax neck area, stand up, bend knees slightly and tuck your pelvis under; keep head erect. Bring right ear down toward right shoulder (don't move shoulders),

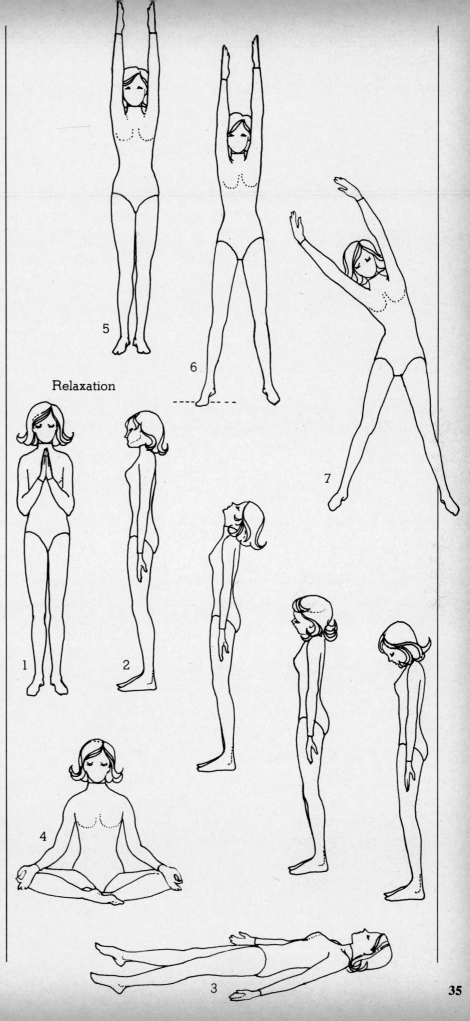

Relaxation

then bring head back, then to left shoulder, then forward, dropping chin on chest. Do complete head roll *5 times.* (3) Put on some soothing music and lie down on back with arms loosely at sides, palms facing upward, fingers relaxed and legs slightly apart. Breathe slowly and deeply through nose; feel yourself breathing to the rhythm of the music. Sense your body sinking into the floor with each exhalation; try not to concentrate on any one thought. Stay this way for about 5 minutes, breathing quietly with the music. (4) This is a meditative pose, frequently used in yoga, and should be done in quiet surroundings. Sit with eyes closed, back straight, legs crossed, backs of hands resting on knees. Place thumbs and index fingers together. Imagine a line dropping from behind ear, through center of body, and feel your thoughts and energies drawing inward. Feel "sit bones" making contact with floor. Hold for about 5–10 minutes.

**Overall toning.** (1) To work complete spine: Stand with feet together, arms stretched over head, palms facing forward. Starting with small of back, roll down spine until palms touch floor. (Until you become more limber, it's okay to bend knees as you come forward.) Hold for a count of 5, sensing feet making contact with floor. Now inhale and roll up your spine, keeping buttocks tucked under, and stretch back as far as you can. Feel a pull through abdomen, chest, arms and front of thighs. Then roll forward, exhaling, to first position. *3 times.* (2) For balance, back and backs of thighs: Stand up straight and pick a point in front of you that's eye level. Sensing both feet making contact with floor, and keeping eyes focused on point, bring right knee up to chest and grab lower leg with both hands. Pull thigh as tight into chest as you can, keeping back straight. Hold for count of 10. Repeat with left leg. (3) To correct round shoulders and relieve tension in neck and back: Stand with back straight and clasp hands behind back. Now bring shoulders back and arms away from you. Hold for a count of 5 and release slightly. *2 times.* (4) To stretch calf muscles: Stand about 2½ feet from wall, with legs straight, about 6 inches apart,

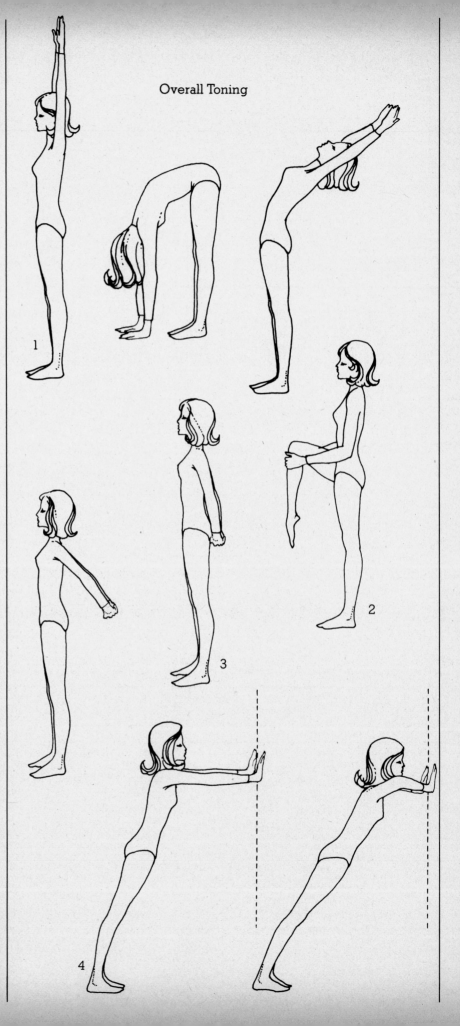

Overall Toning

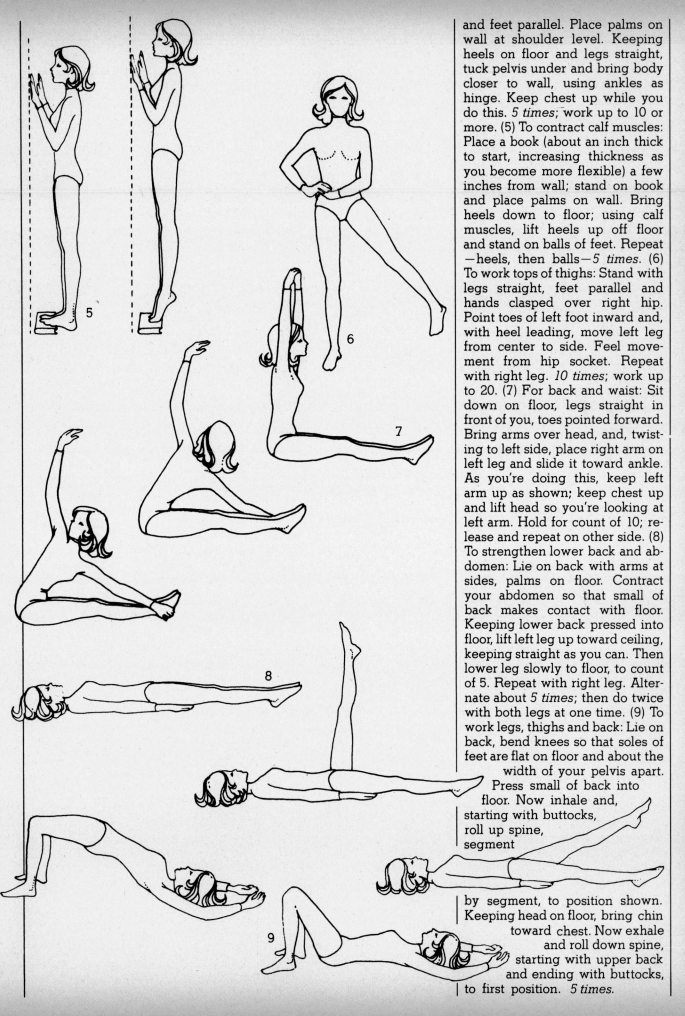

and feet parallel. Place palms on wall at shoulder level. Keeping heels on floor and legs straight, tuck pelvis under and bring body closer to wall, using ankles as hinge. Keep chest up while you do this. *5 times;* work up to 10 or more. (5) To contract calf muscles: Place a book (about an inch thick to start, increasing thickness as you become more flexible) a few inches from wall; stand on book and place palms on wall. Bring heels down to floor; using calf muscles, lift heels up off floor and stand on balls of feet. Repeat —heels, then balls—*5 times*. (6) To work tops of thighs: Stand with legs straight, feet parallel and hands clasped over right hip. Point toes of left foot inward and, with heel leading, move left leg from center to side. Feel movement from hip socket. Repeat with right leg. *10 times;* work up to 20. (7) For back and waist: Sit down on floor, legs straight in front of you, toes pointed forward. Bring arms over head, and, twisting to left side, place right arm on left leg and slide it toward ankle. As you're doing this, keep left arm up as shown; keep chest up and lift head so you're looking at left arm. Hold for count of 10; release and repeat on other side. (8) To strengthen lower back and abdomen: Lie on back with arms at sides, palms on floor. Contract your abdomen so that small of back makes contact with floor. Keeping lower back pressed into floor, lift left leg up toward ceiling, keeping straight as you can. Then lower leg slowly to floor, to count of 5. Repeat with right leg. Alternate about *5 times*; then do twice with both legs at one time. (9) To work legs, thighs and back: Lie on back, bend knees so that soles of feet are flat on floor and about the width of your pelvis apart. Press small of back into floor. Now inhale and, starting with buttocks, roll up spine, segment by segment, to position shown. Keeping head on floor, bring chin toward chest. Now exhale and roll down spine, starting with upper back and ending with buttocks, to first position. *5 times.*

These twists, shrugs and walks were worked out by exercise specialist Bonnie Prudden. They're designed to give your body greater flexibility and help you carry yourself more gracefully.

# AIDS FOR EASY MOVEMENT

**Waist twist.** Stand with feet apart and arms at shoulder level. Twist upper body left and right as far as possible (1), letting arms droop slightly, but always ending at shoulder level. Do 25 times. This slims waist and upper torso and releases tension in shoulders and upper back. Keep standing position (2) and, with knees straight, bend forward from hips. Pretend a small dwarf is standing in front of you and, keeping elbows bent, box his ears, first one side, then the other, 25 times as shown. This prevents unsightly lumps and stiffness.

**Shoulder twist for heavy or flabby upper arms.** Rest most of your weight on right foot, twist right arm under as far as possible (1) and watch thumb as it comes around. Feel pull in arm and shoulder. Then open and twist arm out and back (2), keeping eyes on thumb. Each time you open, take a breath in. Start with four of each on one side, then the other; next, alternate from side to side 8 times.

**Thigh twist for hip and leg tension, balance and gait.** Stand on right foot and twist left foot, leg, and hip inward (1). Twist foot, leg and hip outward (2). Start with a slow beat, doing eight with each leg. As you improve, step up the time.

**Shrugs to relieve tension in shoulder and neck.** Shrug up (1), pulling shoulders up to almost touch ears. Shrug down (2), pressing shoulders down to make a long neck. Shrug forward (3), rounding shoulders forward to stretch back. Shrug back (4), pressing arms back to stretch chest.

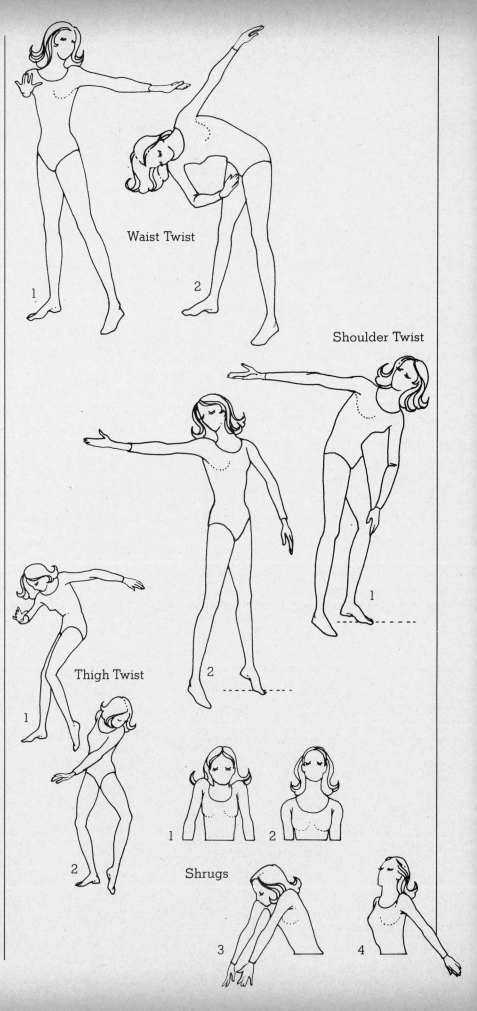

Waist Twist

Shoulder Twist

Thigh Twist

Shrugs

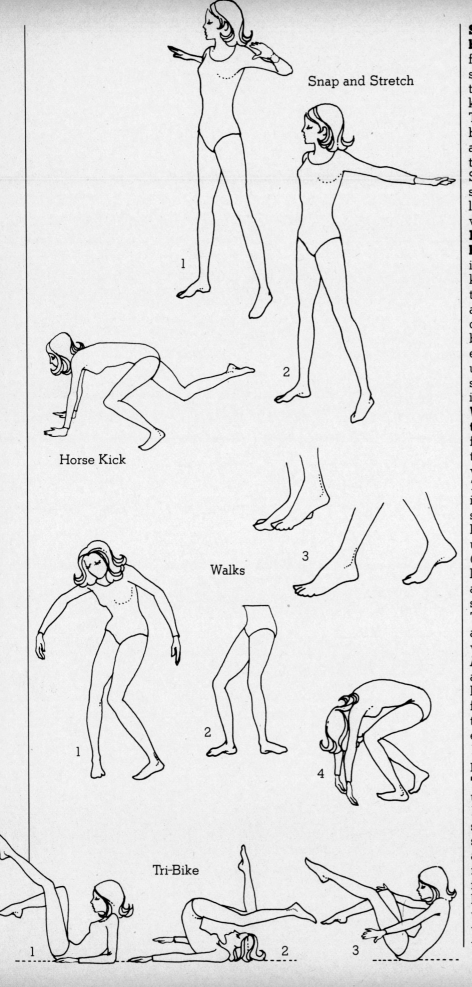

Snap and Stretch

Horse Kick

Walks

Tri-Bike

**Snap and stretch for round back or shoulders.** Stand with feet apart and raise bent elbows to shoulder level with fingertips touching. Snap elbows back (1), keeping hands at shoulder level. Then bring hands forward again, but don't stop at fingertip touch; allow hands to overlap (the farther, the better). This stretches back. Swing arms wide (2) to full back stretch. Be careful not to drop below shoulder. Do 8 to a set; start with 4.

**Horse kick for shoulders, arms, back, seat and legs.** Start out in the four-foot position, trying to keep arms straight. At first just try to run in place with little steps and to a beat. (If you haven't exercised in a while, you may feel breathless or hear ringing in your ears. This is normal.) As you get used to the exercise, take slower steps and kick legs higher, working to 16 times.

**Walks for feet, legs, hips and thighs.** *Turned-in walk* (1) is good for lower legs and flat feet. Turn toes in as far as possible as you walk. Take 16 steps.

*Turned-out walk* (2) is good for inner-thigh flab, abdominals, and seat. Walk with feet well apart, knees turned out, and seat tucked under for 16 steps.

*On-your-toes walk* (3) is a foot and leg strengthener; good for balance. Get up high on toes with a straight body. Keep head erect. Tighten muscles of thighs, seat, and abdomen. Take a small bounce with each step for 16.

*Dropover walk* (4) strengthens legs and back. Drop over well bent knees and walk with small steps, feet facing straight forward—not turned out. Try to get down far enough to drag fingertips. Take 16 steps. When you have completed walk series, start over.

**Tri-bike.** Lie back on elbows and use legs in a bicycle motion (1) for 16 circles. Then roll back onto shoulders and, supporting yourself at waist, do 16 more. When you are strong enough, push your legs farther over head (2), stretch arms flat, and bike in this position. Now balance yourself on seat (3) and, using no hand support, start biking with four circles and gradually work up to 16 circles. Relax.

With these exercises you can tone up and slim down while watching TV, sitting in your office or waiting for the laundry to dry. They were worked out by Marjorie Craig of the Elizabeth Arden salon in N.Y., who adapted some of her more rigorous exercises to ones you can do sitting down. (*Note:* The number of times at the end of each exercise is the suggested maximum; if you're really out of shape, start with fewer than the suggested limit.)

# EXERCISE SITTING DOWN

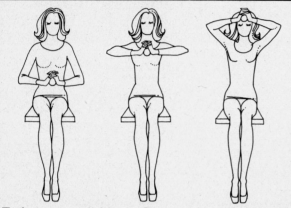

To firm arms and bust: Sit straight with stomach tucked in, feet together flat on floor. Hold a small sponge-rubber ball between palms, with fingers interlocked. With arms and elbows at waist level, press heels of hands against ball for a count of 5; relax. Move arms to shoulder height, press again for count of 5; relax. Finally, raise hands to forehead level and repeat. *10 times.*

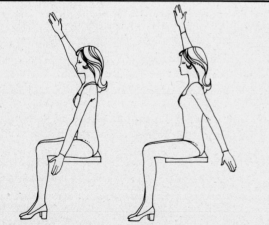

To straighten upper back and firm bust: Sit with feet and knees together, back straight, one arm up and slightly forward, other arm down as shown. Keeping this position, push both arms back in a chopping fashion, 5 times. Reverse arm positions; repeat. *6 times* for each arm change.

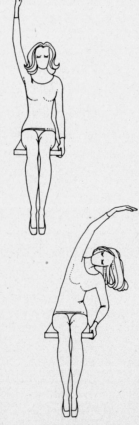

For waist, upper hips and upper back: Sit up straight, with stomach tucked in. Rest one arm on chair side, raise other over head as shown. Bounce to one side 3 times, curving raised arm over head; relax. Repeat using other arm. *6 times.*

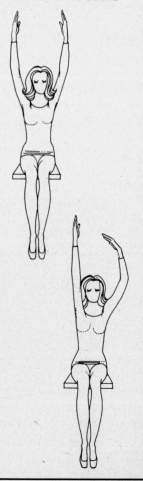

To stretch and relax waist, upper hips, abdomen and back: Sit straight, stomach tucked in, legs and feet together. Raise arms over head, as shown. Now stretch right arm as far up as possible; relax. Repeat, other arm. *10 times.*

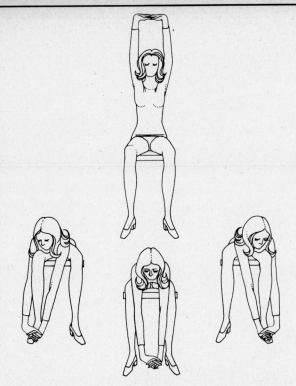

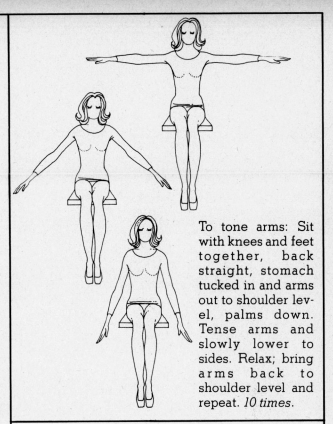

For waist, hips, thighs, back and chest: Sit with feet apart, stomach tucked in, arms raised above head, hands clasped and palms facing ceiling. Bend down and touch hands to toes of right foot; come up. Bend again, this time touching hands between feet. Come up, then bend and touch hands to left toes. Finish by coming up with hands over head; relax. *3 or 4 times.*

To tone arms: Sit with knees and feet together, back straight, stomach tucked in and arms out to shoulder level, palms down. Tense arms and slowly lower to sides. Relax; bring arms back to shoulder level and repeat. *10 times.*

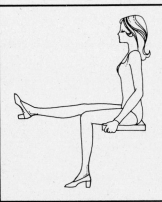

For leg tone: Sit straight with stomach tucked in and hands on chair. Place one leg on floor, bring other leg out in front of you, parallel to floor. Rotate raised leg in a circle (keeping leg slightly bent). Slowly circle in one direction, then the other. *15 times* for each leg.

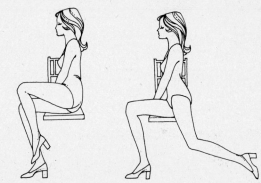

For buttocks and thighs: Facing sideways, sit on edge of chair with weight on right hip. Bring left knee up as far as you can, then straighten leg out behind you as shown. Rest hands on chair slightly in front of body for support. Turn and repeat with other leg. *10 times* for each leg.

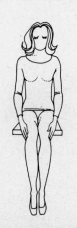 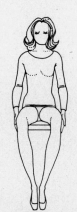 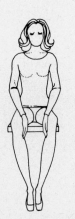 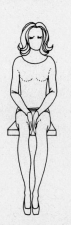

For legs and thighs: Sit straight, stomach tucked in, knees and feet together. Push hands firmly against outside of knees as you slowly spread knees. Relax. With knees apart, place hands inside knees and push as you bring knees together. *4 times* each way.

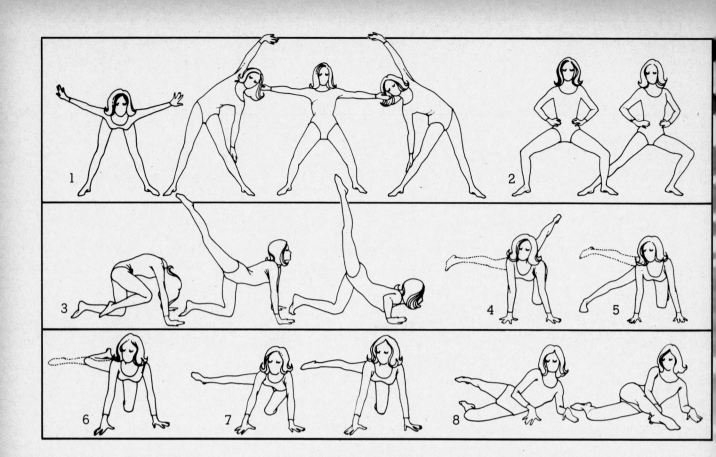

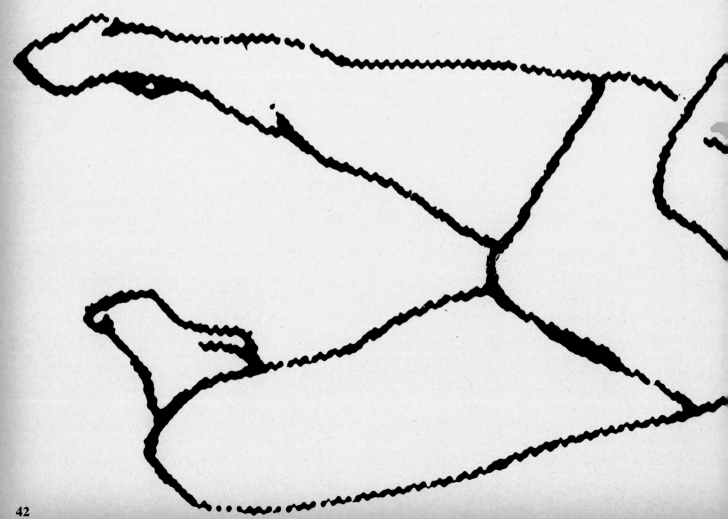

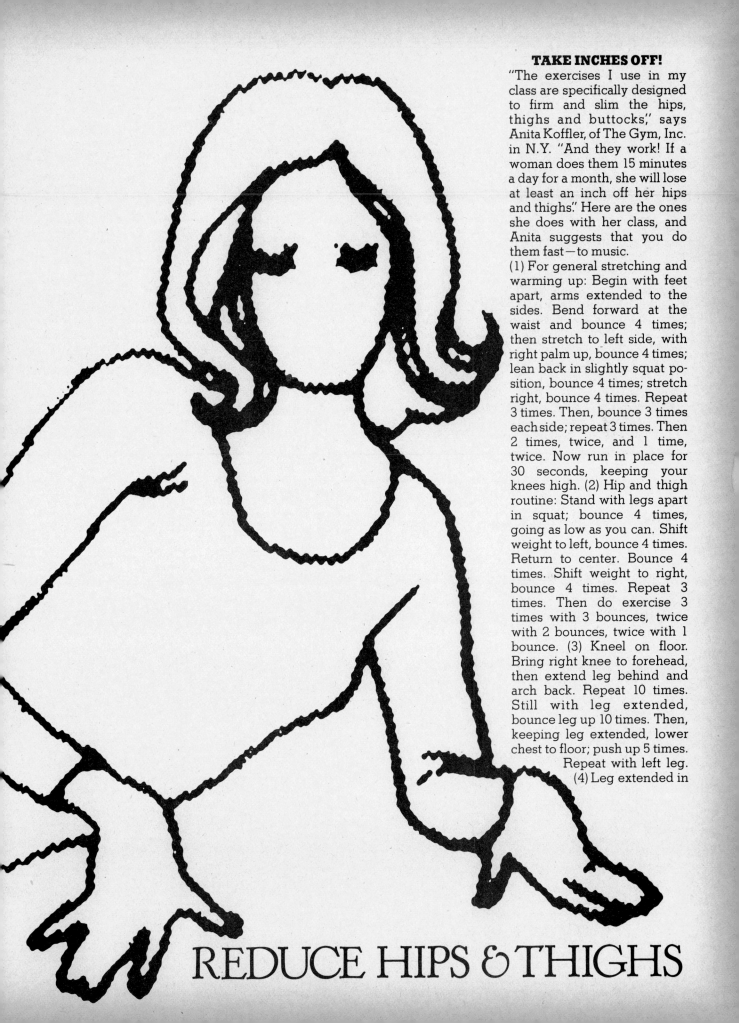

## TAKE INCHES OFF!

"The exercises I use in my class are specifically designed to firm and slim the hips, thighs and buttocks," says Anita Koffler, of The Gym, Inc. in N.Y. "And they work! If a woman does them 15 minutes a day for a month, she will lose at least an inch off her hips and thighs." Here are the ones she does with her class, and Anita suggests that you do them fast—to music.

(1) For general stretching and warming up: Begin with feet apart, arms extended to the sides. Bend forward at the waist and bounce 4 times; then stretch to left side, with right palm up, bounce 4 times; lean back in slightly squat position, bounce 4 times; stretch right, bounce 4 times. Repeat 3 times. Then, bounce 3 times each side; repeat 3 times. Then 2 times, twice, and 1 time, twice. Now run in place for 30 seconds, keeping your knees high. (2) Hip and thigh routine: Stand with legs apart in squat; bounce 4 times, going as low as you can. Shift weight to left, bounce 4 times. Return to center. Bounce 4 times. Shift weight to right, bounce 4 times. Repeat 3 times. Then do exercise 3 times with 3 bounces, twice with 2 bounces, twice with 1 bounce. (3) Kneel on floor. Bring right knee to forehead, then extend leg behind and arch back. Repeat 10 times. Still with leg extended, bounce leg up 10 times. Then, keeping leg extended, lower chest to floor; push up 5 times. Repeat with left leg. (4) Leg extended in

# REDUCE HIPS & THIGHS

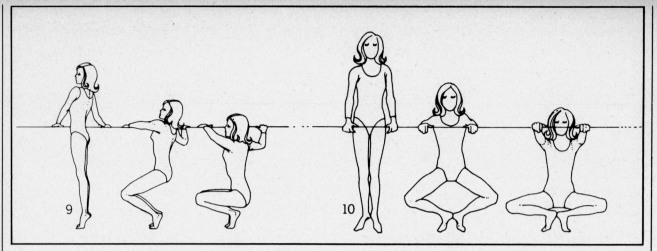

back, foot flexed, swing leg to the side and back, 10 times. Then, with leg extended to side, bounce up 4 times, and forward 4. Repeat, other leg. (5) Leg extended to side, foot flexed facing forward, lower leg to floor and raise, 10 times. With leg still extended, circle back and around 4 times. Repeat, other leg. (6) Leg raised, in bent-knee position at hip level, ankle slightly lower than hip, foot flexed, extend leg out to the side and back, 10 times. Repeat, other leg. (7) Leg extended to side, sit back on heel, then come back up to kneeling position, 5 times. Repeat, other leg. (8) Lie on side, resting on forearm. Lower leg is slightly bent. Swing upper leg backward and forward 10 times, toe pointed. Then bounce leg back 10 times. Repeat, other side. (9) This exercise should be done holding on to the back of a heavy chair or dresser, waist-high. Start on toes, hips at right angle to chair. Sink down halfway, keeping knees and ankles together, back straight. Hold for count of 10. Come back up, then down halfway again for another count of 10. Now drop all the way down to your heels, bounce up and down 10 times. (10) Similar to #9, but this time facing chair. This is specifically for inner thighs. Start on toes, keeping heels together at all times, back straight; sink to halfway position; hold for count of 10. Drop down to heels, then come halfway up again for another count of 10. Drop down to heels and bounce 10 times. This is the final hip and thigh exercise. Now run in place, jump and shake yourself out for a minute or so.

# 20 MINUTES OF SPOT EXERCISES FOR SPRING

Go gracefully from spring to summer with these amazingly effective spot-reducing exercises developed by Larry Lorence, owner of the Gala Fitness salon in New York. Larry, who has spent 30 years studying and teaching gymnastics all over the world, has worked out this 20-30 minute daily routine to keep the body well toned and in proportion. He suggests that you exercise on a mat or carpet in an open room.

**WARM-UP**

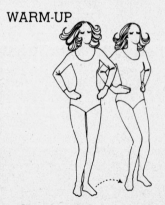

1. Stand with hands on hips, feet together and jump from side to side. (10 times)

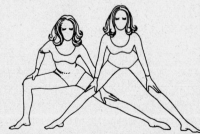

2. For legs, place feet apart and hands on knees. Bend right knee and then straighten. Alternate with left. (6 times each)

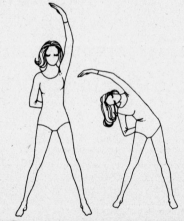

3. To tighten waistline, place feet apart in a normal stance with arms at sides. Lift left arm up, put right hand behind back and bend 4 times to the right. Now lift right arm and bend to left.

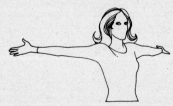

4. To straighten upper torso, stand with feet apart, arms stretched

sideways. With palms up, swing arms back and forth, keeping them at shoulder level. (10 times)

## WAIST AND STOMACH

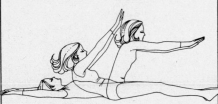

5. Lie down on back with arms above head. Swing into a sit-up, keeping legs straight. Lie down and repeat. Do these slowly, without jerky motions, to avoid injuring the back—emphasis is on stretching, *not* pulling. (6 times)

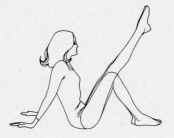

6. In a sitting position bend knees and support yourself with arms on the floor behind you. Extend your legs up and lower them slowly. If you find this difficult, move your hands further back to accommodate movement. (6 times)

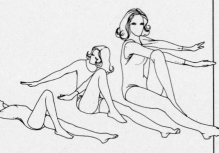

7. Lie down on back with one knee bent and sit up, moving arms to the right. Reach right knee with left elbow or shoulder 3 times. Now do 3 times on the left.

## BACK AND HIPS

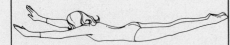

8. Lie down on abdomen with arms and legs straight. Raise arms and legs up and down off floor. Stretch muscles—don't arch. Do this 6 times to work shoulders, buttocks and backs of legs.

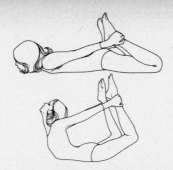

9. Lie on stomach, bend knees and catch ankles. Now, in one movement, stretch head, shoulders and legs upwards, pulling shoulder blades together. (4 times)

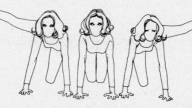

10. For hips, get on hands and knees and extend right leg sideways. Raise and lower leg 8 times. Repeat with left leg.

## ARMS

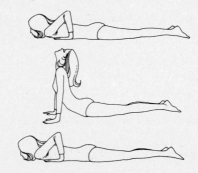

11. For back of arms, lie on stomach and push up with arms, keeping hips on floor. (6 times)

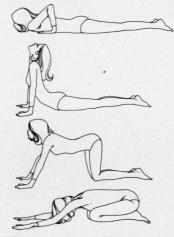

12. For a "fake" push-up, lie on your stomach with arms bent, hands resting beside shoulders

with elbows up, and hips and knees on the floor. Now straighten arms and lift hips in one movement. Then return to knees and reach heels with hips. (4 times)

## STAND TALL—WALK TALL

Good alignment can add an inch to your height and take 5 to 10 pounds off your appearance.

To align your body correctly, start with your feet and build each section properly on the one below till your body is balanced, with your head floating on top of your spine:

• Stand on balls of feet (not back on heels).
• Relax knees.
• Tuck buttocks under.
• Lift from diaphragm.
• Keep ribcage relaxed and free.
• Keep shoulders down and relaxed.
• Feel that head is aligned and floating on top of spine.

Practice this alignment in front of a mirror and try to keep it throughout the day when you walk, sit, stand, work, read, and so on.

"Once you're in tune with posture and carriage, you find it covers other body defects," says Lisa Doubloug, Woman's Spa Director at Palm-Aire, Pompano Beach, Florida. "And posture correction is a first step toward body awareness.

"In whatever you're doing, be aware of how your body works for you. When you walk, stride. When you sit and get up and go up and down stairs, use your legs. Also feel the movement of your hips and waist—when you brush your teeth, drive your car, watch TV, wash your hair. Tune into yourself.

"Striding is one thing you can do right away that does marvels for your figure and your face. Simply start from good posture position and walk easily, rolling along over the length of the whole foot. Increase slightly the length of your step and maybe lift your feet higher. Let your arms swing, your hips and waist move. Keep your chest and chin up and your head free. Gaze out straight ahead. This makes you feel and look important. It's a mood-lifter too, so your face becomes smoother, more serene."

To help you get the most slimming and firming in the least possible time we asked Jack La Lanne for a program that takes only 20 minutes, firms the soft spots and makes you feel good all over. Jack came up with his 9 best Trimnastics. Each exercise is multipurpose, but each also hits at a specific target area. Double up on those that firm the areas that concern you most.

# JACK LA LANNE'S 9 BEST EXERCISES

## DO THEM IN 20 MINUTES

Once you get into them, these exercises can be done in a total of about 20 minutes. In the beginning, work slowly, in front of a mirror if you can. Be very precise. You'll get the best results from each exercise if you think hard about the area you are working.

Stretch till you feel the pull in the target area:
*Point your toes…*
*Point your fingers…*
*Stretch that waist…*
*Think tall…*
*Think a flat tummy…*
*Think a high bust…*
*Think a firm bottom…*

Begin with only one or two run-throughs of each exercise—or as many as you can do perfectly and precisely in 20 minutes.

Stay at two or three repeats per exercise for a few days before increasing. Develop a regular, smooth rhythm. Each movement should flow into the next without a break.

When you've got one exercise right, increase the number till you can do the whole 9 in 20 minutes. It may take several weeks to work this program into an easy routine. But once you get there, you'll find these multi-purpose exercises easy, but never boring. And the results will be great—all over!

It's easier to get into a routine if you set aside a certain time each day for exercising. Or your program might include a variety of exercises to do at different times of the day. For instance, you might try working on these in mid-morning, since they're fairly vigorous, and then in late afternoon or early evening do some stretches for relaxation. Whatever you choose, it's important to stick with it.

Keep in mind that exercise firms and shapes the figure, but you need to diet to take weight off. Exercising while you diet helps keep your appetite down and your body firm and fit.

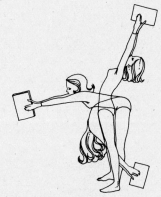

### 1. Dynamo swing
*Target area:* This will warm you up and work the entire body—thighs, hips, waist, abdomen, arms, shoulders, lower back, hands. And it does great things for heart and lungs.
*Start:* Stand straight, legs 12 to 18 inches apart, holding a two- to three-pound book with both hands.
• Bend all the way forward, head down, and swing the book between your legs as far back as you can. Keep arms straight.
• Swing the book back up over your head till you are bent in a back arch.
• Without a pause, swing again to forward position and repeat.
*Goal:* 40 swings in groups of 10.

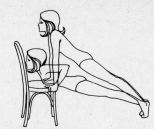

### 2. Chair push-up
*Target area:* Chest line and bust. Also works backs of arms and shoulders and the skeletal muscles of the lower back; firms the chinline; slims the legs.
*Start:* Place a straight-back armless chair against the wall. Crouch in front of it, grasping the sides of the seat with your hands and lean your chest on the chair seat. Now stretch your legs out behind you till you're braced against your toes.
• Push your torso straight up from the chair seat, elbows locked, till your arms are straight and your body forms a straight line. Keep chin high.
• Lower chest to touch chair seat.
• Immediately return to starting position and repeat.
*Goal:* 10 chair push-ups.

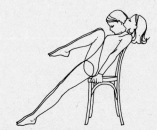

### 3. Knee lifts
*Target area:* Upper stomach, between bottom of rib cage and waist. Also works the arms, shoulders and top of thighs.
*Start:* Sit straight on the front edge of an armless chair, back stiff, knees together, feet on floor and grasp sides of chair. To get the full benefit of the exercise, do it *slowly.*
• Keeping knees together, toes pointed, bring your knees up to touch your chest. You may have to adjust your position to improve balance.
• Without a pause, return to starting position and repeat.
*Goal:* 10 knee lifts.

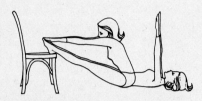

## 4. Slant sit-up

*Target area:* Abdominal muscles from waist to groin. Also works arms, shoulders, thigh tops and back.
*Start:* Stretch out flat on back on floor and rest heels on a kitchen chair (or the lowest rung), legs straight. Stretch arms up over head, resting on the floor, fingers pointed.
• Slowly sit up, arms still raised, knees locked, and bend forward till your fingertips touch your toes.
• Return to starting position, lowering shoulders to floor slowly; repeat.
*Goal:* 10 sit-ups.

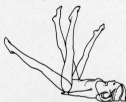

## 5. Leg scissors

*Target area:* Inner thighs. Also works back of buttocks, neckline, arms, shoulders, outer thighs and hips.
*Start:* Lie on the floor on your back, palms flat on the floor under your buttocks.
• Raise your legs straight up from the hips till they're at right angles to your body.
• Spread your legs to make the widest split you can.
• Bring your legs back toward each other and cross them scissors-fashion.
• Without a pause, spread legs wide again. Repeat.
*Goal:* 10 leg scissors.

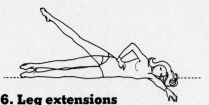

## 6. Leg extensions

*Target area:* Outer thighs. Also works fat pads at hip tops, sides of waist, arms and shoulders.
*Start:* Lie on the floor on left side, legs straight, one on top of the other, left arm extended straight out, right hand on hip, thumb forward.
• Lift your right leg 10 to 15 inches.
• Move the right leg back as far as it will go till it crowds the hip muscle. In this exercise, higher isn't better; the point is to crowd the hip muscle.
• Bring leg back to raised position and repeat. Don't rest between movements—and work precisely.
• Turn over and do the exercise on your right side.
*Goal:* 10 extensions each side.

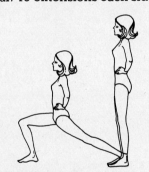

## 7. Fencer's lunge

*Target area:* Top of thighs. Also works inner thighs, hips, lower back and is great for posture.
*Start:* Stand with your back very straight, hands on hips. Step forward on your left foot and bend your knee way down, extending your right leg straight out behind as near to parallel with the floor as you can get without raising foot off floor.
Adjusting your balance is tricky with this one, but it's the best exercise for thigh tops.
• Jump into a reverse lunge, right leg forward, knee bent, left leg extended straight out. Keep your back straight.
• Repeat as rapidly as you can.
*Goal:* 10 lunges for each leg.

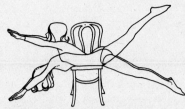

## 8. Arch-ups

*Target area:* Hips and those fat pads at the top of the hips. Also works lower back, top of thighs, legs, arms, shoulders and back of neck.
*Start:* Lie on your stomach across an armless chair, legs and arms straight out, toes and fingers touching the floor.
• Keeping arms and legs straight, raise them as high as you can, chin up, to make a reverse arch.
• Keeping arms and legs straight, return to start position and repeat slowly.
*Goal:* 10 arch-ups.

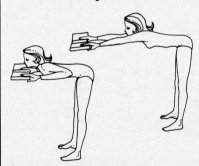

## 9. Arm extensions

*Target area:* Shoulders and upper back. Also works back of neck, firms lower neckline and chin, lower back, top of thighs, front of arms—and slenderizes your hands.
*Start:* Stand straight, legs apart 12 to 15 inches, with a 2- to 3-pound book in each hand.
• Head up and chin stretched forward, bend your torso forward at right angles to your waist till you can feel your stomach muscles pull; keep arms straight, elbows locked and tight to your sides.
• Energetically thrust both books forward as far as your arms reach.
• Bring elbows back to sides and repeat.
*Goal:* 10 arm extensions.

# 70 MOST-ASKED SUMMER BEAUTY QUESTIONS

**1. Does the sun dry the skin or make it oilier? I've heard both.** Sunlight does make the skin drier; those who are confused about this are probably mistaking increased perspiration for oiliness. However, in an oily skin—where the pores are plugged with oil deposits—the heat of the sun can loosen the deposits and make the oil flow more freely.

**2. Does sunshine help acne? How?** Sunlight reduces the bacteria content in pimples and helps the fat in plugged-up glands flow more freely, and this can help an acne condition. But, if a person with acne perspires heavily in the sun, this can irritate the skin.

**3. Humidity makes my hair flop. How do I overcome this?** A soft, loose body wave and a setting lotion with strong holding power will help.

**4. I'm a brunette and get a good tan. What would be a smashing summer makeup for me?** If you have a good tan, you should let your color come through. A deep peach foundation, with pink-bronze blusher gives glow to a tan. A dusky plum shadow on the upper lid (to the brows) with pale beige shadow in a wide band at the lash line above and below reverses the usual lid color pattern and makes the lashes show up more. Mouth can be a cheerful red with lip gloss in ginger brown.

**5. How can I stop my lips from getting dry if I'm out in the sun a lot?** Protect them. Evaporation of moisture from the lips causes dryness and can be prevented by wearing lip gloss, even creamy lipstick, and reapplying it often.

**6. I have little broken capillaries on my arms and legs. Can this be caused by sunbathing? What can be done about it?** Some people are genetically susceptible to this condition, and it can be aggravated by exposure to the sun, particularly if skin is very fair. If you have this condition or it runs in your family, avoid excessive exposure—and also avoid strong astringents and very hot or very cold water. Makeup can be used to hide the marks. In some cases, treatment with an electric needle can get rid of them, but

they may reappear.

**7. I've heard that if you take the Pill, you shouldn't sunbathe. Why?** Some women—not all—who take birth-control pills become particularly sensitive to the sun and may develop peculiar pigmentation when their skin is exposed to sunlight. This may also happen in pregnancy.

**8. Are photosensitivity and sun allergy the same thing? What is the cause?** Yes, they are the same thing. The ultraviolet rays of the sun aggravate certain people's skin more than others'. This can be a systemic allergic reaction or it can be produced by certain drugs, such as antibiotics.

**9. Do I need a mositurizer if I use a cream foundation?** Foundation actually goes on the skin better and is less likely to separate and streak if you use moisturizer.

**10. Do you put lip gloss under or over lipstick? I've heard both.** Always over. If you use gloss under lipstick, you can't control the intensity of the lip color, which is partly what glosses do. Put the creamy texture lipstick underneath and the gloss on top, but only in the center of the mouth so it won't smear the lip line.

**11. How do you cover up the white circles you get from wearing sunglasses?** Under-eye makeups—either powder or cake—in a beige tone work best.

**12. My eye makeup creases. Any way to prevent this in hot weather?** Cream shadows keep the eye skin moist-looking and are pretty because they come in strong colors, but they do tend to crease. Using a powder eye shadow in the same shade *over* your cream shadow corrects this.

**13. I try for a moist look and just come out greasy. What can I do?** You may have an oily skin and, if so, you do better to use a drying makeup base and then, after your makeup is complete, splash cold water over your face for a moist look. Finish with a frosted powder that reflects and diffuses light.

**14. Can I get swimproof false lashes?** Yes—they are accompanied with waterproof glue and can be used when you swim. But we think it is better *not* to wear

them when you swim. Instead, try waterproof mascara.

**15. I have body hair that shows when I wear a bikini. Should I shave it—or what? I've heard about wax depilatories. Can I do this myself?** Waxing, which delays the formation of stubble, is the preferred method for removing body hair (unless, of course, you want to go to the time and expense of permanent removal—electrolysis). Otherwise, shaving (you may have to do it daily if hair is dark) with a "feminine-hair" razor does the trick.

**16. My forehead perspires heavily. Is it safe to use an antiperspirant on your face? Or what do you do about it?** It is not good to apply an antiperspirant to the forehead—or any part of the face —because it could get into the eyes or irritate the skin. Absorbent powder on the forehead helps.

**17. I'm in the sun a lot in summer but not really lying on the beach. I get a pale section under my chin. How can I equalize the color?** The best way to even a tan is to use a sun block on the tanned areas and expose only the pale parts to the sun. We believe the best solution (if you don't sunbathe regularly) is to use a darker foundation or synthetic tanner to blend in the under-chin color.

**18. I get freckles on my shoulders that don't go away even in winter. How can I get rid of them?** Try a bleach cream and then protect your shoulders with extra-heavy use of a sun block. Often such freckles result from continual exposure of unprotected skin or a sudden severe burn. In boating, water-skiing or gardening, bare shoulders get more direct sunlight than the rest of the body and should be protected.

**19. Will tanning a fresh scar make it appear less noticeable?** No! Wait about six months; then the sun's rays may help. A fresh scar contains sensitive tissue that tends to become overpigmented with sunning and permanently tan. The surrounding skin will become bleached after a time, but not the overpigmented scar area.

**20. I'm fair-skinned and don't want a lot of tan. What is a good**

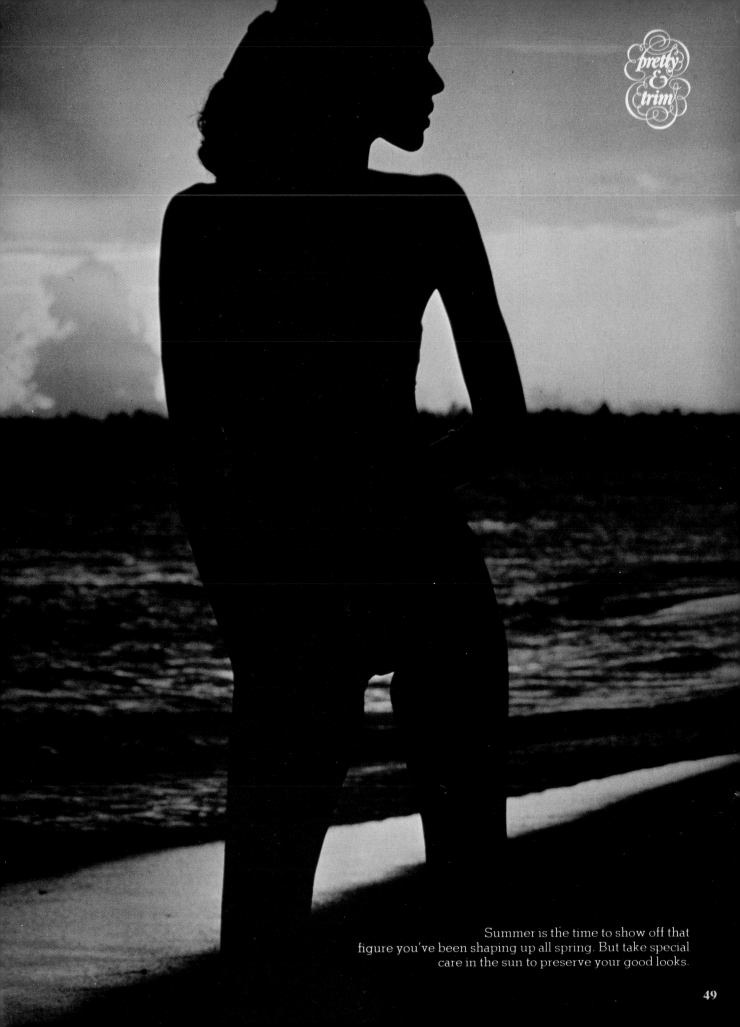

Summer is the time to show off that
figure you've been shaping up all spring. But take special
care in the sun to preserve your good looks.

outdoor look for me that won't appear artificial? Use a covering makeup as light as your skin tone (it can be your regular makeup) with translucent powder to help block the sun. Before powdering, apply cream blusher (pink) to a damp sponge and pat the sponge lightly on the cheeks for glow. For an outdoor look, use powder blusher (after powdering) on the cheeks and also under the brows, down the nose and on the throat down into the hollow. Brush the powder on lightly, just enough to give some color. Strong eye makeup in violet and a red lipstick help overcome any paleness. To give your face a real outdoor glow, use brown or tan powder over your makeup; press it on and brush off any excess.

**21. Can I wear my precurled fiber wig in the water?** No problem so far as getting it wet is concerned. Chlorine in a pool, however, may bleach and discolor a blond wig. However, we don't recommend that you swim in your wig.

**22. My face, arms and back tan right away, but my legs stay pale. What can I do to get an even tan?** You have to work at getting an even tan. Cover up the rest of the body and expose the legs (applying a sunscreen) till the color comes up to match. Meanwhile, you can even up with a leg makeup.

**23. I like pale pearly lipstick and frosted white nails with my tan. Is it really all that old-fashioned? I think it's a great look.** It is a great look and if you like it, wear it. But current fashion goes in for creamier, more muted colors; you might like these, too, if you experiment.

**24. I know I'm overweight around the hips—but I don't mind that so much as the fact that I have sort of dimpled indentations on my thighs. They embarrass me in a swimsuit. What are they? How can I get rid of them?** These "dimples" usually appear when underlying muscles are soft. Exercise, with weight loss, is the answer.

**25. Is it true that exercise in the water —like kicks and pull-ups—are more effective? I want to reduce my hips fast.** Yes. The weight of the water creates a drag, and your muscles have to work harder to do kicks and leg circles. The buoyant (lifting) effect of water often makes it easier for those with bone or muscle problems to exercise in water, because they don't have to put body weight on a painful joint.

**26. Beach sand makes my skin itch. What's the cause?** Sometimes insects in the sand or the irritating particles from jellyfish can cause such an itch. Or the abrasive materials in the sand rub on the skin and cause itching. Lie on a towel or a beach blanket.

**27. Is there any sun-safe hair coloring?** Not really. Sunlight bleaches any hair color, even natural hair. Today's new brunette shades, however, wear well in the sun.

**28. Is it harmful to the eyes not to wear sunglasses? I like to have them but I don't like to wear them all the time.** It is good to protect the eyes when in very strong sunlight—chiefly because exposure to daytime glare can lead to poorer vision in the dark and because we tend to squint to protect ourselves from glare. Dark lenses should not be used all the time, however, or worn indoors, as this could produce eye strain.

**29. Does a hair conditioner protect the hair against sun damage? If so, what kind—protein or creme rinse or what?** No, a conditioner doesn't protect against sun damage. Having hair in good condition to begin with, though, does protect it. Protein conditioners give more body and smoothness to dry, split, already damaged hair.

**30. Does a cold shower really keep you cooler? I hate cold showers.** Cold baths or showers help keep body temperature down, which is why cold compresses are applied to someone who has a sunstroke. But they certainly aren't necessary in normal life. A cool or tepid shower and particularly a 20-minute tepid bath (slightly below body temperature) is also cooling.

**31. Can you come up with a great outdoor makeup for a black girl?** You should let your skin color come through and use a cream base in deep bronze only to even the skin tone. We also suggest a sun block under this to prevent uneven darkening of the skin if you expect to be in the sun a great deal. Pat on brown powder in the middle of the face, between the brows, on the nose and around the mouth, so the skin there does not appear gray. Pat on a very thin transparent cream rouge around the cheeks and eyes, above the brows and on the forehead to give a glow. It nicely balances a bright eye makeup—sea green. A gold-flecked beige makeup can be used under the brow and under eyes to reflect light. Do lips in transparent chestnut with pink gloss.

**32. I've heard heat and perspiration are hard on lightened hair. What do they do?** Sun lightens the hair but perspiration plus heat can change the hair color and even cause greenish notes. This is particularly true with two-process hair color—lightening and toning.

**33. My skin seems to itch more in summer. What's the best way to relieve this?** With a washcloth, apply hot water (120° to 130° F.) to area for a few moments, repeating several

times. This is usually effective, unless there's some complicated cause of itching.

**34. Can you give us some pretty after-swim hairdo ideas?** If hair is medium to long, braid colored ribbons into the hair and let braids hang down at both sides. Or bring hair up off the neck into a high chignon and place a barrette below it. The prettiest summer hair is simple and off face and neck. Little barrettes keep hair in place.

**35. My feet get rough and dry in summer. What can I do about it?** If your feet get particularly rough and dry, you might check with a doctor about the likelihood of a fungus infection. Otherwise, pamper them with lotion and cream them nightly. Try a little foot powder between the toes and in your shoes, as perspiration may partly be the cause of the flaking skin.

**36. I have tiny white dots on my skin that don't tan. What are they?** This may be a condition known as "vitiligo." It appears most often in dark-skinned people; at least it is more noticeable when skin is dark. Or it could be a fungus infection known as "tinea versicolor." See your doctor and find out for sure.

**37. What's the really best treatment for a sunburn?** Use a lotion especially made for that purpose—one that is rich in lubricating moisturizers to replenish oils and that has soothing ingredients (such as calamine) and a cooling anesthetic.

**38. Do vitamin creams—vitamins E and A and D—really help the skin?** The skin produces its own vitamin D in the presence of sunlight, and this vitamin helps keep skin moist and young-looking, as does vitamin A. Some physicians believe that E vitamins also hold back the aging process of skin and, applied as ointment, speed the healing of burns. Medically, however, vitamin-cream applications to the skin are still controversial.

**39. How do you know what kind of sunglasses to choose—lens color? shape? frames?** Lens color should be chosen with glare in mind. Extra dark for times when one is on or near water, because water reflects sunlight. Lighter for other situations, such as walking and driving. Pale green or light brown is considered most restful. It is wise to buy unbreakable glass or plastic lenses as a safety measure. Frames should flatter the face—but there are no rules at all about this. Most women like "dramatic" sunglasses because they are an accessory as well as eye protection. Frames should be well fitted so the glasses stay on during active sports and play.

**40. I've heard that walking in sand is good for the feet. How?** It makes my

**foot skin rough.** Sand is an abrasive, like a pumice stone, and wears off the surface or flaking skin on the feet. Walking in sand is also good exercise for the feet. If sand makes the feet dry and rough, use a cream on the feet every night.

**41. I get a tan every summer—but now it doesn't completely go away in the winter. Is something wrong?** As one gets older, the skin changes and its reaction to tanning changes, too, so that a tan may last longer. Be sure to cream your skin well, wear a sunscreen when you are exposed to sunlight, and don't try to get a *deep* tan every season.

**42. Is all perfume out when you sunbathe? Or just some brands? I like fragrance.** Some perfumes and toilet waters contain substances that can create peculiar pigmentation on the skin when it is exposed to sunlight. A condition known as "berlock dermatitis"—brown spotting like a stain—can come from exposure of the skin while you wear certain fragrance preparations. As perfume formulas are well guarded secrets, it's hard to find out what particular perfumes would cause the problem.

**43. I'm a redhead and I freckle a lot. What makeup would be right for me? I don't necessarily want a lot of cover-up.** A translucent shine-stopping base will give you a minimum of cover while providing some warmth and protection from the sun. For a tan look, blend a tiny bit of ginger-tone cream eye shadow over the entire face. A golden blusher tone over the outside of cheeks and up under the eye (pat on) gives a wholesome glow.

**44. My hair's always a mess on the beach. What can I do about it?** It's hard to keep a hairdo on the beach. Get a simple, no-set haircut—one that can be combed dry and that will keep its shape in the wind. For medium to long hair, pull the hair back and tie with a ribbon. Or braid the side hair and put barrettes at the ends.

**45. Is too much sunshine hazardous to the breasts?** If your breast skin hasn't been previously exposed to the sun, it can get a bad burn, just as will any pale skin. It is not known if radiation from the sun in normal exposure is a factor in breast disease. One of the functions of skin is to protect inner tissue from the sun's radiation.

**46. Is it bad for the feet to go barefoot a lot—I mean around the house and yard, not just when swimming?** Many different skin infections can be picked up if you go barefoot, and you also run the hazard of cuts, splinters and bruises, as well as hardening of the skin on the soles of the feet.

**47. Is a lemon or vinegar rinse for the hair too drying in summer?** These aren't necessarily "drying." Lemon or vinegar is used as a rinse to soften the rinse water and remove any soap curd or to mildly bleach (lemon), or to restore hair acid balance. A conditioner used after you shampoo is better for dry hair.

**48. Does the complexion need different care in summer than in winter? I mean besides a sunscreen?** Yes—in winter, skin may become chapped and dry because of the cold and dryness of the air, and extra lubricants may be needed. In summer, the skin perspires more and needs to be cleaned oftener and even more thoroughly than in the winter.

**49. My permanent tends to get frizzy on the beach. What can I do to prevent this?** Use a hair set with a moisture-barrier—such as an instant conditioner—to control the frizz.

**50. Does salt water or chlorine dry out the hair? What can you do about it?** Yes, they are drying. A 30-minute conditioner—the kind you apply after a shampoo and leave on for 30 minutes and then rinse out—will help. (See article starting on page 6 for further summer hair care.)

**51. Should you use more or less makeup in summer?** Usually, if you have a nice tan, you can use less makeup in summer. You don't need the added color of foundation to overcome pallor. An under-makeup moisturizer is important in summer and winter. Opaque cover-up makeup and powder with covering ingredients serve as a sunscreen—enough at least for walking-around sun protection. A deep tan may call for more dramatic and colorful eye makeup, however.

**52. When you're on the beach and you want to have makeup on, how can you keep your face from burning? Will the makeup protect it? Won't a tanning lotion tend to change the color of the makeup?** Opaque makeup and makeup that contains a sunscreen give some protection. With translucent makeup, which does not offer this protection, you need a tanning lotion under the makeup. Tanning preparation can mix with the ingredients in makeup and change either the color or consistency; but if the preparation is applied first and allowed to dry, this is not a great problem. Pat makeup over the sunscreen—don't smooth it on—to prevent streaking.

**53. How can you cover a bad sunburn so you won't look like a lobster without doing more damage to the skin?** A bad burn requires comforting treatment—such as a sunburn lotion. Moisturizing lotions also help the skin, and an opaque makeup over the moisturizer can successfully hide redness. A little green under-makeup toner (even a bit of green cream eye shadow) helps overcome that florid look.

**54. Can the sun change the color of bleached hair? If it does—help! What can you do in a hurry? And will it change slowly over a few days or quickly?** Yes, the sun lightens the hair. How rapidly the change takes place depends on how long or frequent the exposure is. A temporary color rinse in an ash or silver shade will correct brassiness in lightened hair, but be sure to cover it when out in the sun.

**55. Does it look right to put red nail polish on your toes during summer when you're wearing sandals?** Bare toes should have polish on their nails—on the beach or in open shoes, and red is certainly pretty.

**56. If you have varicose veins, is there anything that will cover them so you can wear a bathing suit? Something that won't come off in the water?** There are waterproof makeups that effectively cover varicose veins. The covering stays on even if you swim.

**57. Should you eat more or less in summer?** This depends on your metabolism and whether you are more active in summer than in winter. Medically, the only summer food recommendation relates to eating more salt—sprinkle a little extra on your food rather than taking salt tablets—because you perspire more at this time of year.

**58. Will straightened hair get curly or frizzy by the ocean?** Curly, perhaps, but not necessarily frizzy. Straightened hair is never completely straightened—a little bend is left in to give the hair body. Moisture will make the hair revert to this little bit of curl.

**59. Will an Afro tend to mat near the water? Or is it easier to care for if you're going to spend time on the beach?** Yes, it will mat. Take along an Afro pic to restore your Afro on the beach. Afterward, a de-tangler will be helpful. An oil-base treatment is also good if hair gets overly dry.

**60. Does air conditioning dry out the skin? What will help? A humidifier?** An air conditioner absorbs the moisture in the air around it. When the moisture content is low, and if the skin is naturally very dry, air conditioning can make it uncomfortable. Use a moisturizer on the skin for protection. A humidifier helps when the air is very dry—a good idea in winter, when air is even drier.

**61. Is air pollution harmful to the skin? How? What can we do?** This is an increasing problem in skin care. All kinds of substances—soot, gases, bacteria—can irritate the skin. If you are in a highly polluted area (an urban area), clean your skin thoroughly and protect it with a moisturizer and a covering makeup (especially foundation) to keep the irritants from penetrating deeply into the pores.

**62. Does hairspray protect the hair against sunlight? Or is this a bad combination?** No, on both points. It does little to protect the hair and this is not necessarily a bad combination.

**63. Does chlorine in house water affect hair color? How can I get rid of it?** There is not enough chlorine in house water to affect hair color, so don't worry. Hard water, though, may make it difficult to rinse hair thoroughly. Detergent shampoos help.

**64. Does antiperspirant wash off when you swim?** The chemicals in antiperspirants work by affecting the skin itself and, though the effect wears off in time, the antiperspirants do not wash off.

**65. When is the best time to apply an antiperspirant to make it most effective?** At bedtime, right after washing and drying your skin. Sleeping hours give the chemical time to act on your skin cells and slow the perspiration.

**66. What is the difference between a deodorant and antiperspirant?** The difference involves the way they work. A deodorant just stops or covers odor; it does not stop the skin from producing sweat, which is what causes the odor. Antiperspirants actually interfere with the action of the glands and keep them from producing sweat and, therefore, eliminate odor by stopping wetness.

**67. How can I keep my makeup from caking in hot weather?** Use a translucent liquid makeup to avoid caking. If you need a covering foundation, put it on smoothly and remove excess; then powder lightly with translucent powder and brush off excess.

**68. Do certain clothes attract gnats and mosquitoes? How can you avoid insect bites?** There is some evidence that certain clothes colors attract gnats and mosquitoes. Use an insect repellent on exposed skin, wear long sleeves and leg coverings and avoid insect-infested areas as much as possible. Perfumes may attract stinging insects—bees and hornets. Oils and foods attract flies.

**69. Does drinking lots of liquids in summer make you perspire more?** No. You perspire because you're hot and your body is trying to cool off. You drink lots of liquids in summer to restore the water lost in perspiration.

**70. My tan fades fast—even between weekends—and my skin starts to look yellowish. What can I do?** A pinkish foundation on your face can overcome that sallow look. You can use a body makeup on your arms and legs between exposures to make you look tanned even when you're not. ∎

# HOW TO GET THE PERFECT TAN

The best-looking tan is smooth, even and glowing. No matter how dark your skin color, you shouldn't look like burnt toast. *All* skin is susceptible to the effects of sunlight, and no matter how easily or how darkly you tan, it does *not* protect you from burning or parching. For a perfect tan that won't damage your skin too much, follow this plan:

• Wear an adequate sunscreen while your tan develops—and afterward. A sunscreen doesn't filter out all the sun's rays, but it does help keep the skin from burning and allow you to stay out in the sun longer at each exposure.

• Start your tan with moderation. At first, limit your stays in the sun to the hours before 11 a.m. and after 3 p.m. —and limit the time of exposure according to your skin type and the sunscreen you are using. Read the label carefully.

• Renew your tan weekly, but don't try for a very deep tan. Your skin is constantly shedding, and new skin is paler unless tanning is kept up. No matter how deep your tan, you can still burn, so keep using sunscreen.

• Don't let your skin dry out; use an after-sun moisturizer.

**USE THE RIGHT SUNSCREEN.** Choose a reliable manufacturer and study the claims made for each type product. A *sun block* prevents the sun's rays from reaching the skin and prevents a tan. A *sunscreen* prevents the burning rays from reaching the skin and enables you to expose your skin for longer periods so that you can get a good tan. Cocoa butters and suntan oils may—or may not—have a sunscreen even if they're called "tanning aids." Check the label. If the product does not have a sunscreen, it lubricates the skin but does not protect against burning.

According to Dallas dermatologist Dr. Bedford Shelmire Jr., the most effective sunscreens are based on three types of chemical ingredients: PABA, the PABA derivatives, and the benzophenomes. Other acceptable sunscreens include homosalate, cinoxate, menthyl anthranilate, digalloyl trioleate and triethanolamine salicylate. However, the concentration of the sunscreen in the product is of equal, if not greater importance, and this information is also stated on the label.

**PUT YOUR SUNSCREEN TO WORK.** All sunscreens should be applied liberally, regardless of the ingredients. Provided you use a sufficient amount, you can use almost any sunscreen you wish and still receive maximum protection.

Always try to match your sunscreen product to your activity. All of them will eventually wash off with swimming or heavy perspiration, but some tend to adhere better than others. PABA sunscreens adhere fairly well after the alcohol base evaporates (PABA screens should be applied an hour before exposure), and the oily or greasy bases tend to resist rinsing. You should take extra care when using a sunscreen with a lotion or cream base, and reapply it after swimming or perspiring heavily.

**TANNING PROBLEMS.** Certain conditions make the skin extra sensitive to sun. If any of these apply to your skin, be extra careful:

• Fair-skinned people with a tendency to freckle should take special precautions, because their skin is most susceptible to light. Darker skins are generally thicker and have more protective pigment, but even black skin isn't completely immune from sun damage. The same changes will also occur in dark skin with prolonged exposure.

• About 25 percent of women of childbearing age develop a bluish-brown darkening of the face known as "chloasma." Pregnancy and birth-control pills make this condition worse. And sunlight may change the chloasma from mild to severe after even short periods of exposure. The benzophenome sunscreens are particularly effective in preventing the darkening caused by chloasma. These are also suitable for young women not subject to chloasma, as they're very effective in protecting the skin against damage that causes wrinkles.

• Even some of those under 30 get little round brown spots that don't go away—and these can show up even when there's been no exposure to sun. They are part of the "aging" process of the skin and overexposure to the sun or too rapid exposure can accelerate the process. This discoloration differs from chloasma, and should be called to the physician's attention.

• If skin is dry, the sun may make it drier. There are a number of excellent chemical sunscreens in moisturizing bases that are helpful. Most sunscreens have some moisturizing ability, and this increases as you go from the lotions to the creams to the oils to the greases. The exceptions are screens in alcoholic solutions. Here a separate moisturizer must be applied over the sunscreen.

*(Continued on page 54)*

# HOW TO HAVE A LOVELIER-SOUNDING VOICE

An attractive speaking voice is one of the greatest assets a woman can have. We not only *enjoy* listening to those whose voices are pleasantly clear and distinct, we're almost *drawn* to them because they seem to have a greater sense of confidence about themselves. But did you know that the best speakers—radio and TV announcers, singers, actors—are not doing anything extraordinary, but merely using the voices they had to start with in a more effective way?

How about *your* voice? Are you satisfied with the way it is, or can it use improvement? If you're not sure how it sounds, try listening to yourself on a tape recorder. If you sound breathy, too weak, too thin, or your words are slurred together, you may want to work at achieving a richer, more lovely, sound. The exercises here, developed by voice teacher James McClure, will help.

McClure, who coaches singers and actors in New York and New Jersey, and who is himself an accomplished singer and speaker, has perhaps, one of the most sensible approaches to voice improvement around. He says that most unattractive-sounding voices result purely from "not using the vocal instrument the way it was intended to be used. In other words, it isn't necessary to try and change or *disguise* your natural sound, just use it to the fullest and make it work for you in the right way."

The following are two basic concepts that should be understood—and felt—before you get into your daily routine of voice developing exercises, continues McClure. (Do all exercises standing up, as this helps your breath to circulate properly—important in voice improvement. Practice taking deep breaths and feel your chest lifting and ribs expanding. Try to maintain this rib expansion and deepness of breathing as you do the exercises.)

• For the voice to work properly, sound must be channeled through the right passage inside your head. To get an idea of exactly *which* passage, try triggering a yawn. As you draw in the air, feel it going upward, beyond the throat, to a point behind your nose. Now yawn again and try to bring the air even higher. This passage behind the face that the air is going through is what McClure calls the "inner space." Physiologically, this is really the pharyngal space (consists of the entire pharynx) which extends from a point right above the vocal chords to beyond your nose. It is this area that must be open and elongated when you speak, for "a beautiful voice

originates in this space," McClure explains. "When someone speaks poorly, it's because he or she is neglecting this area and letting the vocal chords and the mouth do all the work.

"Compare your voice to a guitar. If sound doesn't have an open space to travel through, it's like a guitar without the wooden box. You can pluck the strings and have sound, but it's the wooden box that gives the sound its rich quality."

He suggests doing the yawning exercise several times so the concept of the "inner space" becomes familiar.

• There are certain conditions that help keep this space open when you speak. Say the word "sing" and dropping your jaw slightly, hold the "ng" sound for a few seconds, without putting too much emphasis on either the "n" or the "g," but blending the two sounds together. Feel the hum of it rising into your head. Now, keeping your jaw lowered and your mouth and tongue relaxed, say the "ng" by itself —very softly. Hold for as long as you can—but don't force the sound. Keep it light and pleasant-sounding.(The voice should never feel as though it's being forced from the throat. It should be thought of more as a *drawing in* of sound.)

As you're doing this, imagine someone pulling a string from the top of your head and the sound following the string upward into your head. Also note what the "ng" does to the back of your mouth. Your soft palate (the rear of the palate) and the upper rear part of your tongue—what McClure refers to as the "back door" of the mouth—are meeting, but not tightly. It is this position that should be present as much as possible when you speak, because it helps to shape and open that important inner space, taking pressure off the vocal chords. What it also does, provided your mouth is open and relaxed enough, is help the sound project from your mouth without having to force it.

"I call this the 'megaphone concept,' " McClure says. "The reason a megaphone amplifies sound is due to the way it's shaped—sound is going into a narrow channel and coming out one that's much wider. If it were reversed, and the sound were going through the opposite way, the power would be decreased. So think of the back door of your mouth, when it's in the "ng" position, as the narrow part of the megaphone and the front of your open mouth as the wider part of the megaphone."

Understanding and feeling all this may take a little practice, so McClure

suggests that you spend a few minutes every day for several days with these exercises before going on to the next set—which actually help maintain the "ng" position when you speak. When you do them, include this variation: Instead of staying on the same pitch as you say the "ng," vary it, starting with the highest note you can reach and proceed down to the lowest, then reverse—so it sounds similar to a moan. Be sure, though, that your jaw, face and back door of mouth stay relaxed, and that your jaw stays lowered so your mouth is sufficiently open. If at any time the sound is harsh or your throat feels tight, you're putting too much pressure on the vocal chords. Concentrate on relaxing and producing a more pleasant sound.

**Getting Resonance into Your Voice:** These exercises will help you transfer the "ng" quality to actual words and therefore, bring a richer, more resonant quality to your voice. First do a few counts of "ng" on one pitch, then the "ng" moan, to get your voice into position. Now pick any short sentence—"Mary had a little lamb" is good for this purpose—and say the "ng" before the sentence. Establish a rhythm—take a breath, say the "ng," holding for a count of about five, say the sentence, take a breath and start all over. As you're saying the words, try to keep the position of the back door of your mouth as close as possible to what it was when you were saying the "ng." Again, feel the lift of the sound going up through the inner space, and make sure your entire throat area feels relaxed. Doing this exercise several times a day will help get your speaking voice into the correct position almost automatically.

**Whisper Exercises for More Distinct Speech:** As you work on making the *sound* of your voice more lovely, you'll also want to practice making the actual words you say more clear and distinct. These tongue-twisters, preceded by the "ng" sound, will bring a clarity to your consonants and make your mouth and tongue more flexible, so that you speak more easily. Once more, make sure your chest is up, ribs are expanded, and breaths are deep. Now *whisper* the "ng"—it should sound like a stage whisper—and then whisper the following sentences, doing each several times before going to the next. As you're whispering, try to exaggerate or "explode" the initial consonants of each word. You should feel a push and pull in your abdomen, which is a sign that you're doing this exercise correctly:

• Tall Teddy Tommy Tinker told a

tattling tale to Tiny Tim.
• Calling all cars from cool Ketchikan to Caracas.
• The busy buzzing bumble bee bit the back of Bob's britches.
• The daring deadly Don Durke of Dowdee dashed daringly down to Dundee.

These may sound comical (you don't, however, have to practice them while anyone is listening) but they're excellent for helping your diction. You may do them slowly at first, but you'll be able to say them faster once you begin mastering them. And the faster you can go—while still saying them clearly—the more distinct your speech will become. ∎

### THE PERFECT TAN
*(Continued from page 52)*

• Teen-agers expose themselves to the sun more than any group, and the most suitable screens for them are those that contain PABA (para-aminobenzoic acid). Nearly all contain alcohol and are somewhat drying, but this is more an asset than a liability in this age group.
• If lips are dry, use a lip pomade containing amyl-dimethyl, PABA or digalloyl trioleate. Lipstick and lip gloss also give some protection.
SYNTHETIC TANS. These are perfectly safe. The chemical used to produce the tanning effect is dihydroxyacetone. It imparts a stain to the surface cells of the skin's outer layer. Many products of this type also contain chemical sunscreens and will provide some protection if applied generously before exposure. ∎

### MAKEUP TRICKS
*(Continued from page 28)*

appear somewhat fuller. Brighter colors also help the mouth appear fuller.

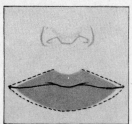

**For a wide mouth:** If the mouth is too wide, do not extend the lip color all the way to the corners.

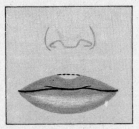

**Straight upper lip:** This is not unat-

tractive, but it can look "hard." If you create a slight—not deep—and wide dip in the middle of the upper lip by not going all the way to the outline there, the shape will be softer.

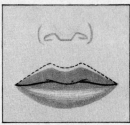

**Cupid's bow too strong:** If the tips of the Cupid's bow are too exaggerated, just cover the top edge with foundation and powder; don't fill color all the way up; even up the middle a little and don't dip down too sharply. If the strong Cupid's bow is on a small, pouty mouth, be sure that you bring the color all the way into the corners of the mouth.

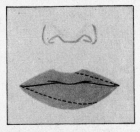

**Uneven mouth:** Try to color both sides alike and to match tips of Cupid's bow with nostrils. This brings nose and mouth into harmony.

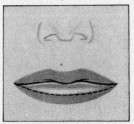

**Thin upper or lower lip:** Try to color both lips so they have the same degree of fullness. Use a brighter color on the smaller lip to bring it out. Lip gloss on a small lower lip will make it appear fuller.

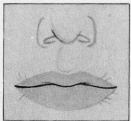

**Tiny lines:** If you have tiny lines around the mouth, use a soft color and translucent lipstick and make a perfect shape—but not a hard outline. Bring the foundation down to lip line so that the color will not spread. Never use frosted or glossy lipstick. ∎

# FACE AND BODY HAIR— WHAT TO DO ABOUT IT

The face and body are normally covered with fine, usually unnoticeable, hairs that don't become a beauty problem unless they are extra dark, long or thick. If you lightly brush down on your face with a powder brush after putting on makeup, the hairs will be less visible.

If hair on the face or other parts of the body is fine and not very thick, but dark (and for this reason a problem), *bleaching* can make it less visible. A special bleach for facial hair should be used on the face; read the label and follow package directions. If facial hair is long, bristly or thick, it tends to pick up light after bleaching (this is often the case on the upper lip), and might be better removed.

The only permanent method of hair removal is *electrolysis*. A battery-operated instrument for home use is, according to recent reports, "safe and effective if you have a steady hand and steady nerves." It can be used for hair anywhere on the face or body.

*Wax removal*—there are both hot and cold waxes—jerks the hair out of the follicle (with a little ouchiness!). It isn't permanent removal but is effective—and some women say, though this is as yet unsubstantiated, that it discourages regrowth. Hair is removed within the follicle so it grows out to become noticeable again more slowly than hair that is shaved. Do not use on underarm area; use a special facial wax for the face.

*Chemical hair removers* also dissolve hair slightly below the skin surface so stubble is less visible and resurfacing is again slower than if hair is shaved. Don't use on underarms; use facial products on face.

*Shaving*, either with an electric shaver or safety razor, is quick and effective for many women. If hair is dark, stubble often shows quickly. To get a closer shave with an electric shaver, the skin must be dry. Powder helps keep the area dry and works better on thin, fine hair than lotions.

Safety razors—many of which are designed for women's needs—work best after (or in) the bath when the hair has been softened. Shaving cream, soap or baby lotion help the razor glide easily for a close, abrasion-free shave. Shave against the direction of hair growth—moving the razor up.

Either electric shaving or razoring is safe for underarm hair. ∎

## GLOWING SKIN

*(Continued from page 16*

Soap does no harm at all if you rinse it off well.

For oily or troubled skin you may want to use a medicated cleanser; for especially dry skin it's okay to use a cleansing cream, but think of it as a makeup remover only—film left from the cream should be washed off.

• Use a facial buffer or a rough washcloth to work the soap lather over your face. One minute a day of buffing clears away surface scale and leaves "new" skin for a smoother appearance. Start slowly—a full minute of buffing can be somewhat irritating at first.

• Rinse well. The ritual of splashing the face thoroughly 30 times—or rinsing for a full minute—insures that you've removed all the soap.

• Restore skin acidity. Skin is slightly acid (almost neutral) and soap—to be an effective cleanser—is usually alkaline. Skin acidity restores itself in four to five hours, but you may want to use a low pH (slightly acid) cleanser, or, as a final rinse, splash the skin with fresh water laced with a few drops of vinegar or lemon juice.

• Astringents are refreshing for oily or normal skin but should not be used on dry skin. Instead, a face-firming lotion can be worn under makeup for a smoother appearance.

**MOISTURIZING.** Cosmetic moisturizers form a barrier between your skin and the drying air and help hold in natural moisture. Petroleum jelly is probably one of the best for dry skin, especially in windy weather, because it's very effective in preventing the loss of moisture.

Most cosmetic moisturizers, however, work well. Find one that agrees with your skin and use it *under* your foundation. For dry skin, apply the moisturizer while skin is still damp from rinsing. Apply over the whole face, including eyelids and throat, but keep in mind that moisturizers should be light in texture.

The eye skin and throat can often be dry even when the rest of the skin is normal or oily. Use a light eye oil on these areas, day and night. Pat it on gently in a circular motion, starting near the nose on the upper lid and working around and then under the eye, with the pads of the fingertips.

Another moisturizing idea that you might try was prescribed by the late Dr. Erno Lazlo, skin specialist to celebrities and founder of the cosmetic firm that bears his name. He recommended frequent splashing of tepid water onto the face during the day (without removing makeup). Many of his "beautiful faces" swear by this ritual—30 splashes and then let the skin dry naturally.

**TREATMENTS.** In addition to your regular cleansing and moisturizing routines, you may want to try some additional helps:

*Steaming* helps unclog pores in oily skin but most skin care experts are against it for dry skin. Some suggest ice-cube rubs for tightening pores or cold packs for face-firming.

*Firming masks* tighten the skin and make it feel and look smoother. Choose a peel-off mask for dry skin and use no more than once a week. For oily skin, detergent, or cleansing, masks can be used twice a week or more to keep skin refreshed. Normal skin doesn't usually need this kind of stimulation.

A complete *at-home facial,* done occasionally, can be refreshing. Here's the method recommended by the Hillhigh Spa in Horseshoe Bend, Arkansas:

• Remove makeup with a cream or liquid cleanser and soft cloth.

• Apply a mask (an astringent mask shrinks pores, removes blackheads and whiteheads in oily skin).

• Leave mask on for 10 to 15 minutes while you lie back and relax in a semi-darkened room.

• Apply hot towels to face and remove mask with the towels.

• Apply an astringent.

• With fingers, work cream up from the throat and over chin, up and over cheeks and around eyes. Use three fingers in a half-moon motion from above nose to the hairline, going over the forehead three times. Work cream over whole face twice.

• Press deep on pressure points at sides of eyes and nostrils. Slide fingers to temples and press; press in front of ear lobes, behind ear lobes.

• Remove cream with soft towel.

• Reapply astringent.

• Follow with a moisturizer.

**SPECIAL PROBLEMS.** Acne, along with enlarged pores, is sometimes a problem of oily skin. Minor outbreaks can be handled by medications and cover-ups you can buy at the drugstore.

Chronic acne has to be treated by a physician. A combination of vitamin-A acid (used at night) and benzoylperoxide (used in the daytime) has been helpful to many. A report from a Swedish physician suggests that zinc tablets may also be helpful in acne treatment. In any case, if this is your problem, don't just suffer. Seek the care of a dermatologist.

Another kind of acne sometimes develops around the lips and on the chin of those who have used face creams and cream foundations for a long time. It usually disappears when the victim switches to other cleansing methods and lighter makeup.

**DELAYING WRINKLES.** You're never too young to think about wrinkles. When our first wrinkle appears, dermatologists tell us, it has already been in the making for 20 to 30 years.

Wrinkles are of two kinds—those that form in the natural expression lines of the face (even teen-agers can have forehead lines) and those that appear as a tiny fretwork of lines on usually smooth skin surfaces.

Both are partly due to the aging process—loss of moisture in skin cells (skin can begin to feel dry in the late 20's and 30's) and the breakdown of collagen (skin fibers) and elastin (a protein of elastic tissues) in underlying skin layers.

How soon these wrinkles appear has much to do with heredity, lifestyle and how we take care of our skin.

Perhaps the most important skin-saving measure is to be sensible about sunlight. All skin specialists today agree that sunlight is the great wrinkle-maker. It's the total accumulation of exposure to sunlight—winter and summer—over the years that determines when wrinkles will appear. Enjoy yourself—ski, swim, play tennis, bike, hike—but cut down as much as possible on exposure time to your face. And take the following precautions when in the sun:

• Wear a hat. This is common-sense protection, particularly for those who enjoy outdoor sports in summer.

• Wear sunglasses. Crow's feet are often our first wrinkles, and usually appear at the corners of our eyes where the skin is thin and vulnerable. Sunglasses protect from both light and glare and if wraparound, protect eye skin from side light.

• Wear a sunscreen year round. For fair-skinned blondes and freckly redheads, skin protection should begin in infancy. Brunettes with oily skin are less in danger, but even a good tan doesn't sufficiently protect against sun damage. PABA (para-aminobenzoic acid) sunscreens come in a clear lotion that you can wear under makeup. Apply an hour before going out for best results.

• Any makeup protects a little from sunlight and some makeup contains a sunscreen. This may be adequate for brunettes with oily skin.

• Wind dries (chaps) the surface skin and also increases the effect of the sun's ultraviolet rays. In rough weather, a thin film of petroleum jelly provides a barrier against wind, but does not act as a sunscreen.

• Lip balm protects against chapping. Applied before lipstick, and wiped away, it removes flakiness and gives your lips a smooth surface. ■

# HAVE A PROFESSIONAL-LOOKING MANICURE AND PEDICURE

Your manicure and pedicure will be great-looking only if you have well cared for hands and feet to work with. Always protect your hands with gloves when you're working in the kitchen or garden or doing anything else that's hard on the cuticles and skin. Cream your hands often, massaging the lubricant well into the cuticles, and protect them with a sunscreen when outdoors. Be sure that every time you use nail polish remover you wash your hands after, since remover dries the skin.

Other hand and manicure savers: Dial the phone with a pencil instead of your finger; use a handled dish mop; avoid rummaging for things in boxes or your handbag; occasionally give your hands an overnight treatment with petroleum jelly and cotton gloves. Diet is also important—protein-rich foods are nail builders.

The same special care should be given to your feet. Don't walk barefoot in the garden or on surfaces where your feet may get cut or contract infections; smooth away rough spots and calluses with a pumice stone; moisturize every day after your bath or shower, and from time to time enjoy the luxury of a relaxing, softening, foot bath.

**MANICURE.** These simple steps to a professional-looking manicure will complete your hand-care program:

• After removing old nail polish, soak your hands in warm soapy water to soften cuticles.

• Push back cuticles very gently with the flat edge of an orange stick wrapped in cotton. Avoid cutting.

• Shape your nails with the *fine* side of an emery board—this is easier on the nails than the rougher side. If nails are thin and flexible, round them into an oval shape, working lightly from side to the tip on one side, then the other—not back and forth. Hard, brittle nails should be allowed to grow out straight for an eighth of an inch at the side, and the tip should be rounded only slightly—this produces a somewhat oblong, rather than oval, shape. *Never* file too deeply at the sides of the nails—this weakens them and can also lead to hangnails. Also avoid filing to a pointed shape, which makes nails break more easily.

• Apply a base coat, using a nail strengthener if your nails tend to be weak. This forms a kind of "elastic splint" and prevents breaking.

• Apply polish slowly starting in the middle of the nail (to avoid coating the cuticle) and work down to the base, then to the tip, rolling the side of the thumb along the tip so that the edge is beveled. Allow first coat to dry at least a minute before applying second coat.

• Apply a sealer or again, the nail strengthener, as a cover coat.

• Use the sharp end of an orange stick wrapped in a little cotton and moistened with polish remover to clear a hairline space around the base of the nail. This is really the *living* part of the nail and should not be coated.

• Wait for nails to dry until smooth to a light touch, then apply a manicure setting spray or run fingers under cold water (turn the faucet on slightly) to "set" the polish. Let your hands dry in the open air.

• Wait at least a half hour before using hands—it takes about that long for the polish to dry completely.

**PEDICURE.** Having a prettier, longer-lasting toenail polish job is as easy as the following:

• Clip toenails straight across with a nail clipper and smooth tips with an emery board.

• Work around nails of one foot with cuticle cream or oil; let this foot soak in warm soapy water while you do the other foot.

• Rinse and dry both feet and separate toes with cotton.

• Apply a base coat or strengthener.

• Apply polish in three strokes—first in the middle of the nail, then on one side, then on the other. Let dry and apply a second coat.

• Finish with two coats of sealer or nail strengthener. ∎

# NEW FOR SPRING

We all have our favorite beauty-makers—but every now and then a new product comes along that fills our own very special needs. Here is a group of new beauty aids that make grooming and makeup easier and more effective.

## HAIR-CARE HELPS
**Spray-on detangler:** *No More Tangles* (Johnson and Johnson) in spray-on form. Use after shampoos—and between—to condition hair. Gets rid of static electricity that causes flyaway hair. Body builder, too.

**Hot-oil treatment:** A classic hair-beautifier in one-minute form—*Alberto VO5 Hot Oil Treatment* in one-half-ounce measured tube. Heat oil, wet hair, apply; massage for one minute; rinse and shampoo.

**Fuller hair:** *Hair Fattener* (Love) is a conditioner you leave in your hair to give it more body, greater volume.

**Conditioning shampoo for oily hair:** *Wella Balsam Conditioning Shampoo for Oily Hair* gets rid of excess oil, but leaves hair shiny.

**Blow-dryer aids:** *The Heat Solution* (Pantene) protects hair against appliance heat, helps maintain natural moisture balance. *Power Pal* (Clairol) is a non-aerosol conditioning styling mist to use with blow-dryer, curling wand or bonnet hair dryers for control and manageability.

**Stand-up hair dryer:** *Mini-Pro* (Conair) is a blow-dryer in a dramatically different shape. Stands on table so you can use both hands to brush and shape, or can be hand held. Good for travel as it weighs only 13 ounces. 1200 watts for power; two-speed. (Available July.)

## MAKEUP AIDS
**Crease-proof eye shadow:** *Natural Wonder* (Revlon) goes on smooth, doesn't smudge, waterproof; in creams and frosteds. *Automatic Cream-On Shadow* (Maybelline) has sponge applicator. Frosted shades.

**Water-base makeups for oily skin:** Cover Girl's *Oil Control* (Noxzema) has water-base formula that diminishes shine. *Glowing Finish "Oil Free" Makeup* (Coty) contains astringent, no moisturizer. *Ultralucent Pure Moisture Oil-Free Fluid Make-Up* (Max Factor) for oily and combination skin is pH balanced.

**Clear makeup:** Sheer, moist makeup that enhances your skin tone without adding color is *Face Quencher Clearwater Natural* (Chap Stick). *Face Quencher* in tinted makeups is also available.

**Blemish cover:** *Bio-Clear Medicated Makeup* (Helena Rubinstein) contains no oil, covers blemishes with no medicated odor. In five natural-looking shades.

**Lash fattener:** *Long 'N Lush* by Cover Girl (Noxzema) coats lashes to make them thicker, as well as longer. No smudge or smear.

**Lip shaper:** *Super Shiny Lip Color* (Maybelline)—automatic with sponge applicator for lip shaping; in six shades.

## SKIN AIDS
**Masks:** *Sweet Earth Mask-Arades* (Coty)—clay mask in foam form. One is moisturizing for normal to dry skin; one is oil-absorbent for oily skin. Both contain vitamins A, D and E. *Orange Peel Masque* (Bonne Bell) stimulates

and removes flaky skin. Peels off.

**Lecithin cleanser:** Designed for skin that has both dry and oily areas, *Pure Magic Super Clear Cleanser with Lecithin* (Max Factor) splashes off with water and is companioned with a *Super Clear Makeup with Lecithin* that moisturizes without greasiness; pH balanced.

**Protein moisturizer:** *Raintree* (Noxzema) with Natural Protein Complex comes in moisture cream or lotion for normal to extra-dry skin.

**Eye cream:** Light, unscented night (or day) cream for sensitive eye skin is *Clean Skin Simply Eye Cream* (Borghese).

## BODY SOOTHERS

**Silky skin:** Soothing for body before or after sun—*Very Silky Body Lotion, Extra Silky Bath Oil* and *Silky Bubble Bath* in *Aviance* fragrance (Prince Matchabelli).

**Body scrub:** *Buf-Puf Body Scrub* (Riker Laboratories), a plastic body buffer, now comes with a handle so you can reach back and shoulders.

**Scented splash:** *Wind Song Light Perfume* (Prince Matchabelli) has "the lift of cologne; the life of perfume." A fresh spring way to scent skin.

**Non-aerosol antiperspirant:** *Ban Basic* (Bristol Myers) lets you spray-dry your underarms without endangering the environment. Scented or unscented.

**Tanning aids:** Now you can select suntan aids by tanning index number, graded from high (most protection) to low (least protection). *Coppertone Shade* (6) permits gradual tanning, great to start a tan; *Coppertone Suntan Lotion* (4) for moderate protection and all-season use. *Coppertone Suntan Oil* (2) and *Coppertone Tanning Butter* (2) are for those who tan easily and rarely burn. *Sun Science* by "Ultima II" (Charles Revson) adds to other grades *Sun-Bloc Stick* (8) for even greater protection. New for sun-sensitive skins are *Block Out Gel* and *Block Out Cream Lotion* (Sea & Ski). The cream lotion is alcohol-free.

## HAND-CARE HELPS

**Cream for problem hands:** *Extra Strength Vaseline Intensive Care Hand Lotion* goes even further than previous versions in protecting problem hands; contains zinc oxide and glycerin, as well as petroleum jelly.

**Nail-builder kit:** *Lee Nails* lets you repair a broken nail or build long nails with a special form and brush-on nail builder. *Andrea Nail Wrap & Repair Kit* helps you wrap and repair nails as it is done in expensive salons.

**Manicure kit:** *The Nail Works* (Clairol) is a battery-powered system that lets you shape and buff finger and toenails. ∎

## HEALTHIER HAIR
*(Continued from page 31)*

sage your scalp gently with back-and-forth motions, not circular ones, since these will tangle the hair. Then rinse thoroughly and apply the creme rinse. A final rinse with cold water gives hair extra bounce and shine.

When combing out your hair after the shampoo (and whenever it's tangled), start with the ends first and work upward until you can run the comb easily the entire length of your hair. *Never* tear the comb through the hair from top to bottom, Michael warns, or you'll break the hair.

**DRYING AND SETTING.** The ideal way to dry hair is the natural way—in the open air, Michael feels. If you don't have time for this, a hard-top, bouffant style dryer is safest and should be set at medium heat if it does not have an automatic temperature control. For setting, use smooth plastic or mesh rollers, *not* the kind that have teeth on the surface or brushes in the center—they're very hard on the hair. He also advises never to sleep in rollers—the tossing and turning of your head while you sleep makes them pull on the hair, resulting in breakage.

Michael doesn't advocate blow-drying, because this method tends to distribute heat unevenly. He compares the outer layer of the hair (the cuticle) to the gills of a fish. Blow-drying in different directions raises these gills which can break off once you start to comb. But, if you must blow-dry, here's the safest way to do it: Pin up the crown portion of your hair, away from the rest. Then take individual sections of hair, starting with the sides, and blow from top to bottom, *not* up and down. Do this slowly and rhythmically. When the rest of your hair is dry, let down the top portion and follow the same procedure. The idea is to avoid applying heat to already dry hair; this can make it split. He doesn't recommend the use of electric curlers for the same reason. They overheat the hair, making it susceptible to breakage.

**SUMMER AND WINTER CARE.** Hair needs special protection in both hot and cold weather, since it's sensitive to changes in temperature.

Conditioning is vital. In summer, when the hair swells, Michael recommends Flex by Revlon, a cream-type, beauty-pack conditioner that you leave on the hair about 20 minutes. In the winter, when hair contracts, an emulsion-type conditioner—one that you leave on the hair about a minute-is more effective. Wella Balsam is the one Michael uses. Getting a professional heat treatment about twice

a year is also a good idea, for the results are long-lasting.

It's important not to overdo conditioning, Michael feels, since this can result in a build-up of residue which can make your hair brittle. Once a month is about right for home conditioning. Very curly hair, however, needs more help, since this type of hair is extremely porous and absorbs too much moisture. (It's for this reason that naturally curly hair tends to "frizz" in rainy or humid weather.) Conditioning gives it an outer layer of protection for greater resiliency.

Besides conditioning, it's important to protect your hair when you're outdoors, Michael says. Always wear a white scarf when out in the sun (white reflects the sun's rays) and a hat in extreme cold. If you dislike wearing a bathing cap when swimming, you can protect your hair from chlorine and salt water damage by drenching it with creme rinse or conditioner *before* you swim. This will prevent the water from penetrating through to your hair. After, just rinse it off—shampooing isn't necessary.

**IF YOU BLEACH.** Michael favors the one-process method of bleaching, because it leaves the hair with enough resiliency to resist harmful elements in the atmosphere. The double-process method, he feels, strips the hair far too much, leaving it without protection.

It's always safer to have your hair bleached professionally, but you can get good results at home, too, if you follow these simple rules: First, your hair must be soiled when you bleach. The build-up of oils protects your hair and scalp, minimizing damage from the chemicals and preventing them from being absorbed into your system. Next, do your touch-ups every four weeks and *only* on the regrowth. The reason for this has to do with the reaction of the bleach to your body temperature, Michael claims. If you retouch your roots, say, three weeks after the initial bleaching process, there won't be much regrowth and there's a danger that the warmth from your body will make the bleach rise to the already bleached portion of your hair, and overbleach it. If you retouch at five weeks, there may be too much regrowth to touch up just the roots, and your body temperature will not raise the bleach high enough to reach all of it. "Dabbing at these areas yourself is hit-and-miss, and may result in an uneven color and a bead-like texture which can make your hair brittle," Michael explains. "Touching up every four weeks should give you an even color without these problems." ∎

# HERBS FOR BEAUTY & HEALTH

Herbs have long been used in the healing arts and in the making of cosmetics and perfumes. In ancient times, before modern medication, there was an herb or combination of herbs for any ailment from indigestion to wounds. Some were taken internally as syrups, infusions or teas. Others were applied as leaves or ointments to the outside of the body.

In medieval England, most cathedrals and castles had floors of rough stone or dirt that were hard to sweep up. It became customary to spread herbs underfoot to give the place a pleasant smell.

**Basil** was one of the most popular of these "strewing herbs." Herbs were also thrown on an open fire, both for their aroma and to ward off disease. **Rosemary** was particularly well liked for this.

The leaves of herbs—**basil, rosemary, marjoram, mint** and **sage,** among them—are still used in pot-pourris and sachets; the essential oils —in cosmetics, tonics and perfume. Today, herbal baths, hair rinses and facial washes refresh and soothe us.

## HERBAL BEAUTY BATH
For a soothing bath to calm frazzled nerves at the end of a day, mix 1 tablespoon dried **lavender** flowers, 1 tablespoon dried **rosemary** leaves, 1 tablespoon dried **mint** and 1 tablespoon dried **thyme,** and tie into a cheesecloth or muslin square. Put the bag under the faucet in a stoppered tub and turn on the hot water; let bag soak in the hot water for 10 minutes. Now fill the tub with water of bath temperature and relax in this for 15 minutes.

## HERBAL VINEGAR
Steep 1 ounce dried **rosemary, sage** or **mint**—or a combination of these—in 4 ounces of white vinegar for 2 weeks in the refrigerator; strain and use the herbal vinegar as a facial wash, skin refresher or hair rinse. The herbs are mildly astringent and the vinegar helps restore the natural skin acidity.

## HAIR RINSE
Put ½ ounce of **sage** in 1 pint of boiling water and let stand for ½ hour for a rinse to darken your hair. To restore brightness to dull hair, substitute **rosemary** for **sage.**

## HUNGARY WATER
Soak 1 ounce of dried **rosemary** leaves, **marjoram** and **lavender** flowers in 4 ounces of 90 proof vodka. To bring up the scent it may be necessary to drain out the herbs after three weeks and replace with a fresh herbal mixture. Use as a cologne or skin freshener or sprinkle a few drops in your bath or face-rinse water as a soothing and fragrant touch. This "water" was claimed to have kept a medieval Empress of Hungary young-looking into old age.

## HERBAL TEAS
Herbal teas were long used as calmatives, stimulants and as digestive aids. Brew like ordinary tea from the dried herb: 1 teaspoonful of dried herb per cup and an extra for the pot. Pour on boiling water and let steep for 3 minutes. Do not leave standing. **Basil** tea is supposed to make you more alert; **sage** and **marjoram** teas are calmatives; **savory** tea aids digestion. **Mint** tea is said to arouse passions.

## LOVE POTIONS
The fragrance of aromatic herbs, like that of perfume, makes you breathe deeper—and perhaps this is why herbs are believed to arouse the passions. **Rosemary, savory, sage** and **mint** were traditionally considered aphrodisiacs and usually included in love potions.

**Rosemary** is often used at weddings —a sprig for the bride to wear, or as a dried herb sprinkled on the bridal bed. In the language of flowers, **rosemary** means "fidelity in love."

## HICCUP HELP
Chewing **dill seed** or a sprig of fresh **tarragon** is a traditional remedy for the hiccups.

## HERBAL SKIN OIL
Add 1 tablespoon dried **rosemary, sage** or **mint** to 4 ounces safflower or wheatgerm oil. Keep in refrigerator and let stand 24 hours or longer, then use for cleansing or lubricating the skin. It is believed that the mild oils and aromatic herbs help soothe facial nerves.

## HAND WASH
**Thyme, rosemary** and **sage** steeped in vinegar was once used as an antiseptic hand wash. Today it is a soothing hand wash after using soaps and detergents or ill-smelling substances.

## HERB LORE
Through the centuries **basil** was used as a headache remedy, a fly repellent and a symbol of fidelity. The plant was revered by the ancient Hindus and is thought by some to be good, in the form of an infusion, for wasp and hornet stings. Its name comes from the Greek *basilikos,* meaning "royal."

**Sage** is called the "sacred herb" or the "herb that saves," referring to its medicinal properties that are supposed to help make you healthy and feel "purified."

**Rosemary,** as well as garlic, has a reputation for "strengthening the memory."

**Parsley** is rich in vitamin C—and, if a sprig is chewed, removes the smell of onion from the breath.

The ancients believed **mint** and **thyme** to be ruled by Venus, the planet of love and beauty. **Rosemary** and **bay** are under the rulership of the sun. **Savory, marjoram, parsley** and **dill** are herbs of Mercury, the mental planet. And **basil** and **tarragon,** because of stimulant effects, are under the fiery planet Mars.

Sprinkle **basil** water—water in which **basil** has been soaked—around your home or place of business as a good-luck charm. . .or so say those who believe in lucky charms. ■

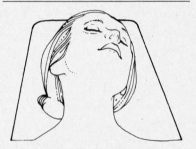

**POTPOURRIS** are a delightful way to scent a room. Make your own from dried flowers, oils, fixatives, herbs and spices, all of which can　　　　be bought in herb shops (look in your directory under *Herbs* or *Candles*).

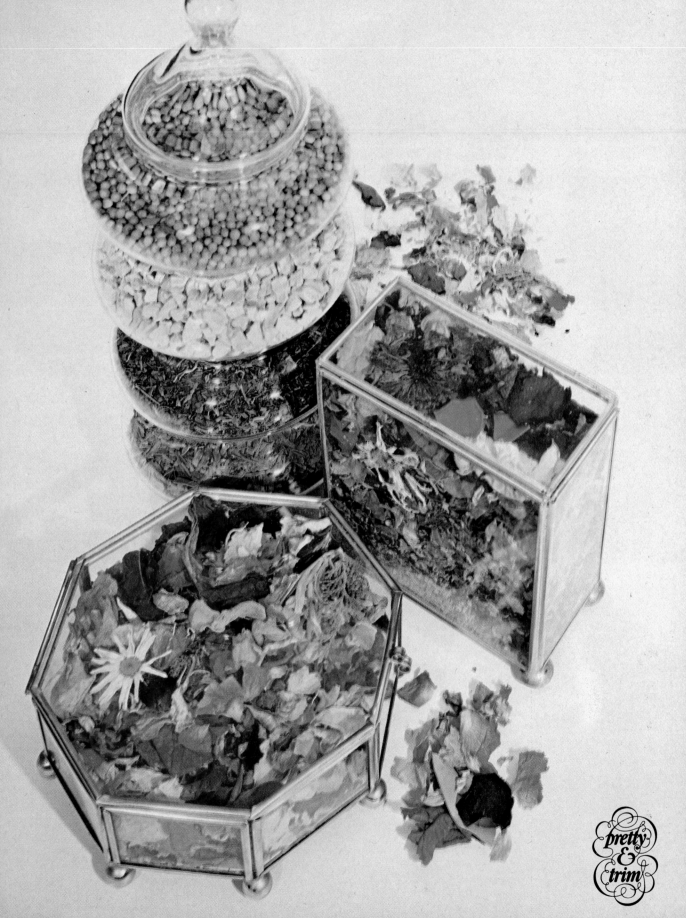

*pretty & trim*

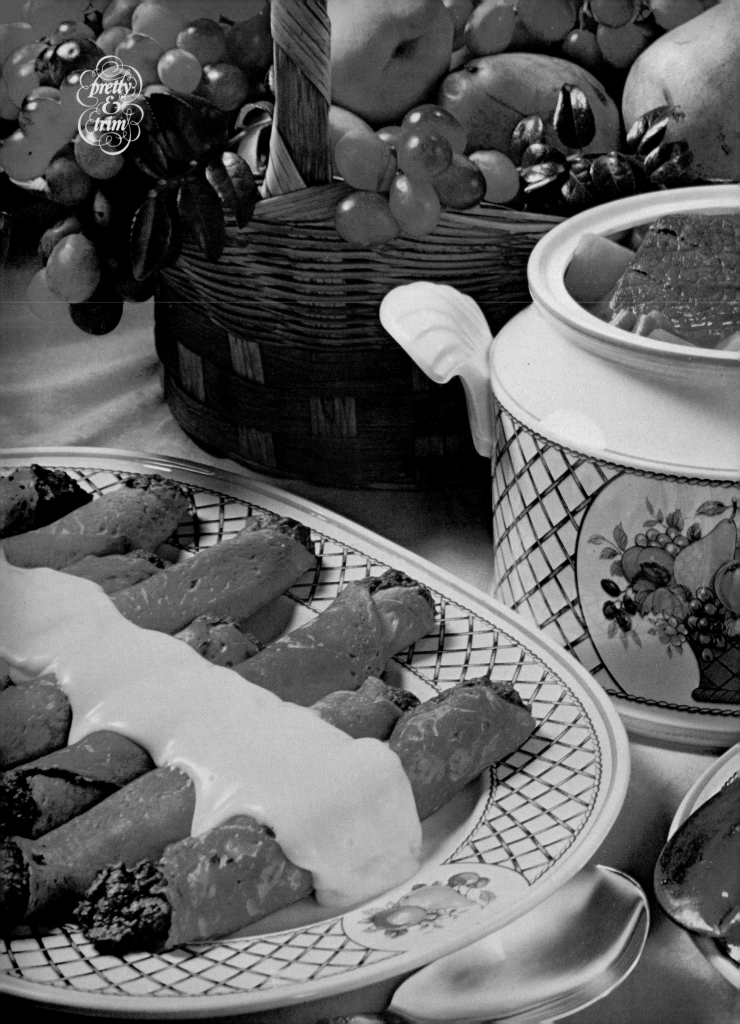

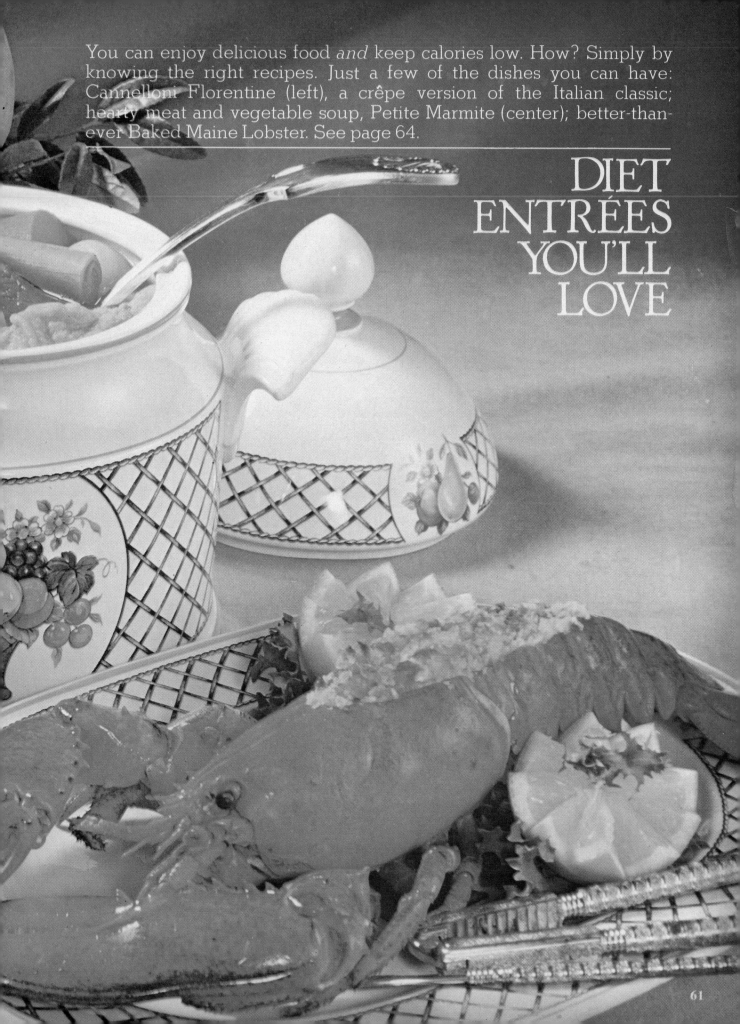

You can enjoy delicious food *and* keep calories low. How? Simply by knowing the right recipes. Just a few of the dishes you can have: Cannelloni Florentine (left), a crêpe version of the Italian classic; hearty meat and vegetable soup, Petite Marmite (center); better-than-ever Baked Maine Lobster. See page 64.

# DIET ENTRÉES YOU'LL LOVE

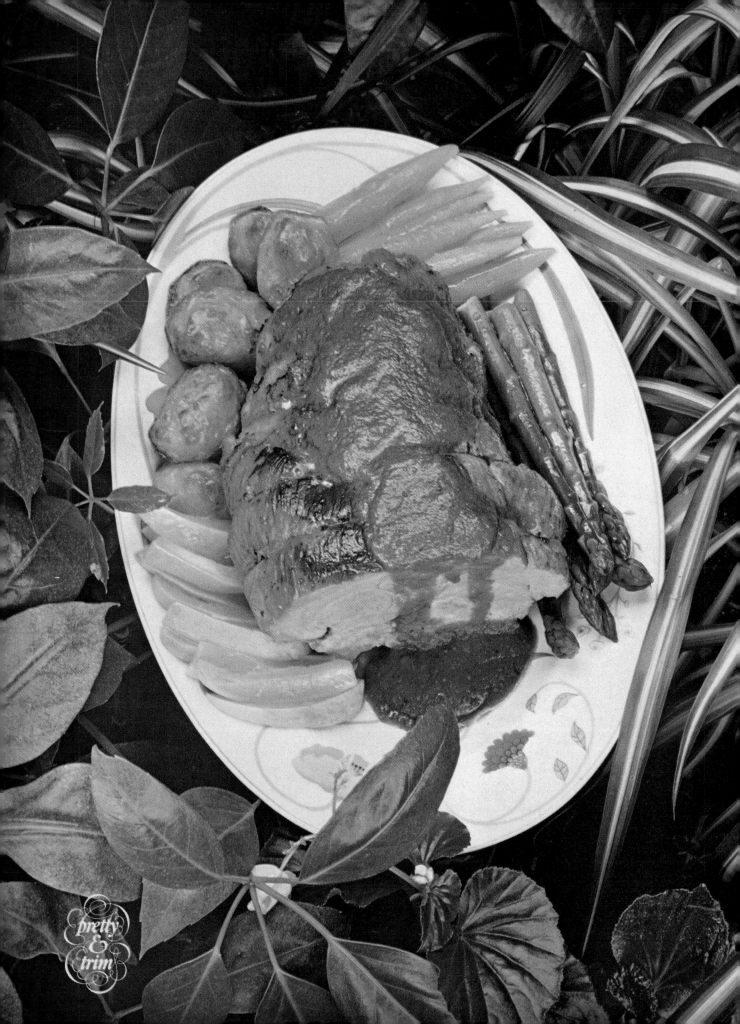

**VEAL À LA FRANÇAIS** can easily be on your diet menu when you make it our way: We've simmered the veal in a chicken broth with vegetables, then puréed the mixture for a tasty gravy that's practically calorie-free. Spring Vegetable Bouquet and Oven Roast Potatoes round out the meal. Recipes are on page 65.

Choose your own diet plan. The top menus for dinner (pages 63 & 72), lunch (pages 77 & 84) and breakfast (pages 89 & 94) total 1,200 calories a day; the middle row additions make a 1,350 calorie diet and the bottom row comes to 1,500 calories a day.

| 1 | 2 | 3 |
|---|---|---|
| **487 CALORIES** | **500 CALORIES** | **499 CALORIES** |
| Marinated Artichokes* <br> Petite Marmite* <br> 1 thin slice French Bread <br> Triple Vegetable Bowl* <br> Thin Cucumber Slices <br> Parsley Coated Tomato Slices <br> Sherry Spanish Cream* <br> Tea with Lemon | Mushroom Bouillon* <br> Veal à la Français* <br> Spring Vegetable Bouquet* <br> Oven Roast Potatoes* <br> Boston Lettuce with <br> Low Calorie French Dressing <br> Raspberry Parfait* <br> Demitasse | Parfait Verdi* <br> San Francisco Chioppino* <br> Antipasto Salad Plate of <br> Romaine Leaves, Roasted <br> Red Pepper, Artichoke Hearts <br> Low Calorie Italian Dressing <br> Fruit Tarts* <br> Espresso |
| **547 CALORIES** | **550 CALORIES** | **544 CALORIES** |
| Add: <br> 2 tablespoons grated <br> Parmesan Cheese to the <br> Triple Vegetable Bowl | Sprinkle: <br> 2 tablespoons toasted <br> Wheat Germ over <br> Raspberry Parfait | Add: <br> Steamed Broccoli Spears <br> sprinkled with <br> Toasted Sesame Seeds |
| **597 CALORIES** | **595 CALORIES** | **579 CALORIES** |
| Also Serve: <br> ½ cup Fresh Blueberries <br> with Sherry Spanish Cream | Also Serve: <br> 3 Deviled Egg Slices* <br> with Mushroom Bouillon | Instead of Broccoli serve: <br> 3 ounce glass <br> Dry Italian White Wine |
| 4 | 5 | 6 |
| **493 CALORIES** | **500 CALORIES** | **493 CALORIES** |
| 1/6 wedge Cantaloupe with <br> Lemon Wedge <br> Lamb Chops en Brochette* <br> Steamed Spinach Leaves <br> Iceberg Lettuce Wedge with <br> Curry Tomato Dressing* <br> Mocha Bavarian* <br> Spiced Tea | "Cream" of Mushroom Soup* <br> Corned Beef and Slaw Mold* <br> Ripe Tomato and Asparagus <br> with Low Calorie <br> Blue Cheese Dressing <br> 1 thin slice Italian Bread <br> Berry Floating Island* <br> Ice Tea with Mint | Minestroni* <br> Cannelloni Florentine* <br> (2 Crêpes) <br> Steamed Green Beans <br> Mixed Salad Greens with <br> Wine Salad Dressing* <br> Jeweled Melon Wedges* <br> Coffee |
| **543 CALORIES** | **550 CALORIES** | **556 CALORIES** |
| Serve Lamb with: <br> ⅓ cup cooked Brown Rice <br> sprinkled with <br> Fresh Chopped Chives | Serve: <br> 1½ teaspoons <br> Butter or Margarine with <br> Italian Bread | Serve: <br> Cooked Yellow Squash Sticks <br> with 1 teaspoon <br> Butter or Margarine |
| **593 CALORIES** | **595 CALORIES** | **600 CALORIES** |
| Increase: <br> Cooked Brown Rice to <br> ⅔ cup | Float: <br> 15 Oyster Crackers on <br> "Cream" of Mushroom Soup | Serve: <br> Jeweled Melon Wedge with <br> 3 Vanilla Wafers |

*See Recipe Index for page number.

# MAIN DISHES

## CANNELLONI FLORENTINE

*This Italian version of stuffed crêpes makes a perfect party dish, yet no one will guess it's diet fare. Photo is on page 60.*

Bake at 350° for 30 minutes.
Makes 10 crêpes/**170 calories each.**

 Diet Crêpes (recipe follows)
2 chicken breasts, split (12 ounces each)
1 cup water
1 small onion, peeled and sliced
1 teaspoon salt
¼ teaspoon seasoned pepper
2 packages (10 ounces each) frozen chopped spinach, thawed
 Dash ground nutmeg
 Creamy Cheese Sauce (recipe follows)

1. Prepare DIET CRÊPES and roll up. (This can be done ahead, if you wish.)
2. Place chicken breasts in a large saucepan; add water, onion, salt and pepper; cover saucepan.
3. Bring to boiling; lower heat; simmer 20 minutes, or until breasts are tender; remove chicken from broth; cool. Pour broth into a metal bowl; place in freezer 20 minutes, or until all fat rises to surface; skim off all fat.
4. Skin chicken; remove meat from bones and cut into small pieces.
5. Make filling: Combine ½ cup reserved broth and half of chicken and spinach in container of an electric blender; cover. Process at high speed until smooth; spoon into a medium-size bowl; repeat with ½ cup broth and remaining chicken and spinach. Add nutmeg; taste and add additional salt and pepper, if needed. (If you do not have a blender, chop chicken and spinach as fine as possible, then stir in enough chicken broth to make a smooth paste.)
6. Fill crêpes: Unroll one crêpe at a time on a wooden board; spread with ¼ cup chicken mixture; roll up; place in a shallow 10-cup baking dish or heat-proof platter; repeat with remaining crêpes and filling. Spoon CREAMY CHEESE SAUCE down center of crêpes; cover dish with aluminum foil. (This much can be done ahead. If not to be baked immediately, refrigerate until serving time. Add 15 minutes to baking time.)
7. Bake in moderate oven (350°) 30 minutes, or until bubbly hot.
COOK'S TIP: Serving-size portions of crêpes can be packaged in aluminum pans. Divide sauce evenly; cover pans with heavy-duty aluminum foil. Label, date and freeze. To serve: Heat in covered pan in moderate oven (350°) 30 minutes, or until bubbly hot.

## DIET CRÊPES

*Use for main dishes, desserts or even breakfast filled with fresh fruit.*

Makes ten 8-inch crêpes/**64 calories each.**

1 whole egg
1 egg white
1¼ cups skim milk
¾ cup all purpose flour
½ teaspoon salt
1 tablespoon vegetable oil
 Vegetable spray on (see Cook's Guide, page 127)

1. Place egg, egg white and skim milk in container of electric blender; add flour, salt and vegetable oil; cover container; process at high speed 30 seconds, or until smooth. (Or place egg, egg white, milk, flour, salt and vegetable oil in a small deep bowl; beat at high speed with electric mixer 1 minute.) Chill batter at least 2 hours, or overnight.
2. With electric crêpe maker: Season baking surface and heat pan, following manufacturer's directions.
3. Pour crêpe batter into a 9-inch pie plate; dip heated crêpe maker, baking surface down, into batter; lift up and turn over.
4. Bake until batter no longer steams or bubbles and underside is a golden brown. Remove crêpe by running a small spatula around outer edge; invert onto a large cookie sheet; roll up. Continue, to make 10 crêpes.
5. With crêpe pan or skillet: Spray an 8-inch crêpe pan or skillet with vegetable oil spray on, following label directions.
6. Heat pan until very hot over moderate heat; pour in batter, a scant ¼ cup at a time; quickly tilt pan so batter spreads and covers bottom.
7. Cook until edge of crêpe browns; loosen crêpe around edge with small spatula; turn; cook 1 minute longer; turn out onto large cookie sheet; roll up. Keep warm until ready to fill.
COOK'S TIP: Crêpes can be made ahead of time. Cool completely; wrap in serving-size portions in heavy-duty aluminum foil; label, date and freeze. Thaw 1 hour at room temperature before using or place in moderate oven (350°) for 10 minutes.

CREAMY CHEESE SAUCE:
Makes 2 cups/**10 calories per tablespoon.** Melt ¼ cup diet margarine in a medium-size saucepan; stir in ¼ cup all purpose flour and 1 teaspoon salt; cook, stirring constantly, until bubbly. Stir in 1 small can evaporated skim milk (⅔ cup) and 1⅓ cups water. Cook, stirring constantly, until sauce thickens and bubbles 3 minutes. Stir in 2 tablespoons grated Parmesan cheese until well blended.

## PETITE MARMITE

*This classic Parisian specialty was created about ninety years ago as the perfect way to serve consommé with all the meats and vegetables in a festive tureen. The photograph is on page 60.*

Makes 8 servings/**188 calories each.**

1 boneless round steak (about 1½ pounds)
1 whole chicken breast, split (about 12 ounces)
1 soup bone
1 large onion, studded with 2 whole cloves
8 cups water
1 tablespoon salt
¼ teaspoon freshly ground pepper
1 clove garlic, crushed
 Few sprigs parsley
1 bay leaf
1 teaspoon leaf thyme
4 large carrots
1 bunch leeks
1 small yellow turnip

1. Trim all fat from beef; place in a large kettle or stock pot with chicken breast, soup bone and onion; cover with water.
2. Bring slowly to boiling; skim surface until clear; stir in salt and pepper. Tie garlic, parsley, bay leaf and thyme in a piece of cheesecloth; push under liquid; cover kettle; lower heat. Simmer 2 hours, or until beef is almost tender when pierced with a two-tined fork; skim surface of liquid until clear.
3. While broth simmers, pare carrots and cut into 2-inch pieces. Trim leeks and cut into 2-inch pieces; wash well. Pare turnip; cut into 1-inch cubes.
4. Add vegetables to broth; simmer 1 hour, or until meat and vegetables are tender. Remove cheesecloth and soup bone from kettle.
5. Transfer beef, chicken and vegetables to a heated soup tureen with a slotted spoon; keep warm. Allow all fat in kettle to rise to surface of broth; skim off. Taste and season broth with additional salt, if needed. Ladle broth into tureen.
6. Present tureen, then remove beef and chicken to a small heated platter; cut into thin slices. Ladle consommé and vegetables into deep soup bowls and pass platter of beef and chicken. A small amount of prepared horseradish can be served with the meat.
COOK'S TIP: This is a perfect recipe to make ahead and freeze. Divide mixture among 8 freezing-cooking bags (10x8 inches). Close and label bags and freeze, following manufacturer's directions. To serve, place frozen bags into a large saucepan of boiling water. Allow water to return to a boil, then boil 20 minutes. Open bag and pour into a deep soup bowl.

## BAKED MAINE LOBSTER

*You deserve to splurge once in a while, and baked lobster is one of the best treats ever! Shown on page 61.*

Bake at 450° for 10 minutes.
Makes 4 servings/**286 calories each.**

- 4 small live lobsters (about 1 pound each)
- 2 teaspoons grated onion
- 1 tablespoon butter or margarine
- ¼ cup all purpose flour
- 1 envelope or teaspoon instant chicken broth
- 1 cup sliced mushrooms
- 2 cups skim milk
- 4 teaspoons lemon juice
- ⅓ cup unsalted cracker crumbs
- ¼ cup grated Parmesan cheese

1. Drop live lobsters into a very large kettle of rapidly boiling salted water; cover; lower heat; cook 8 to 10 minutes. (Lobsters will turn a bright red.) Remove at once with tongs; drain until cool enough to handle.
2. Remove meat from each lobster, saving shell for restuffing, this way: Place lobster on its stomach; cut through hard shell down middle, from below head to near tail, with a sharp knife; cut a 1-inch opening with kitchen shears. Lift out the meat and pink coral (roe), if any. Discard the stomach sac or "lady" from back of the head, black vein running from head to tail, and spongy gray tissue. Dice all meat. Set shells on a large cookie sheet.
3. Sauté lobster meat and onion in butter or margarine in a medium-size skillet 2 minutes; stir in flour, instant chicken broth, mushrooms and milk. Cook, stirring constantly, until mixture thickens and bubbles 3 minutes; remove from heat. Stir in lemon juice; spoon into lobster shells.
4. Mix cracker crumbs and cheese; sprinkle over lobster mixture; dust lightly with paprika, if you wish.
5. Bake in very hot oven (450°) 10 minutes, or until bubbly hot and crumbs are toasted.
COOK'S TIP: Frozen Rock lobster tails can be substituted for the live lobsters in this recipe. Cook, following label directions; cut through shells and proceed as in recipe above.

## SAUTÉED CHICKEN BREASTS

*Rosemary, dry red or white wine and chicken make a delicious team.*

Makes 4 servings/**161 calories each.**

- 2 whole chicken breasts, split (12 ounces each)
- 4 shallots, chopped
  OR: 1 small onion, chopped (¼ cup)
- 1 clove garlic, minced
- ¼ cup dry red or white wine
- ¾ cup water
- 1 teaspoon salt
- 1 teaspoon leaf rosemary, crumbled
- ¼ teaspoon seasoned pepper

1. Place chicken breasts, skin-side down, in a large skillet; brown slowly until red appears around riblet bones; turn and brown 5 minutes on second side; remove and reserve. Pour off all but 1 tablespoon pan drippings.
2. Sauté shallots or onion and garlic until soft in pan; pour in wine; stir up all cooked-on bits; bring to boiling; add water, salt, rosemary and seasoned pepper. Return chicken breasts to pan, skin-side up; cover.
3. Simmer 20 minutes, or until chicken breasts are tender when pierced with a two-tined fork.

## VEAL À LA FRANÇAIS

*Delicate spring veal is simmered in a mirepoix of onion, garlic, carrots and broth that makes the almost calorie-free gravy— no fat and no flour. Lamb can be substituted for the veal in this recipe. The photograph is on page 62.*

Bake at 350° for 1 hour, 30 minutes.
Makes 8 servings/**274 calories each.**

- 1 veal roast (3 pounds), boned and rolled
- 1 tablespoon olive or vegetable oil
- 1 large onion, chopped (1 cup)
- 1 clove garlic, minced
- 2 large carrots, pared and chopped
- 1 cup chopped celery
- ¼ cup chopped parsley
- 1 can condensed chicken broth
- 2 teaspoons salt
- ¼ teaspoon freshly ground pepper
- 1 teaspoon leaf rosemary, crumbled
  Gravy coloring
  Spring Vegetable Bouquet (recipe follows)
  Oven Roasted Potatoes (recipe follows)

1. Have butcher trim all fat from veal before rolling.
2. Brown veal all over in oil in a large oval flame-proof casserole or kettle; remove and reserve.
3. Sauté onion and garlic until soft in pan drippings; stir in carrots, celery and parsley; sauté 2 minutes; stir in chicken broth, salt, pepper and rosemary; return meat to casserole; cover. (If using a kettle, cover meat with aluminum foil.)
4. Bake in moderate oven (350°) 1 hour, 30 minutes, or until a meat thermometer inserted into meat reads 170°. Place veal on a heated platter and keep warm.
5. Pour liquid and vegetables from casserole into a metal bowl; place bowl in freezer 15 minutes to bring all fat to the top; skim off fat.

6. Place liquid and vegetables into the container of an electric blender; cover container; process at high speed 30 seconds, or until smooth; pour into a saucepan.
7. Stir gravy coloring into sauce to give a rich brown color; bring slowly to bubbling.
8. Arrange SPRING VEGETABLE BOUQUET and OVEN ROASTED POTATOES around veal on platter; spoon part of the sauce over meat; pass remainder in a heated gravy bowl.
DIETER'S TIP: With boned and rolled leg of lamb, this recipe is 267 calories per serving.

## SPRING VEGETABLE BOUQUET

Makes 8 servings/**49 calories each.**

- 2 pounds asparagus
  OR: 2 packages (10 ounces each) frozen asparagus spears
- 1 package (1 pound) frozen baby carrots
- 2 large yellow squash, tipped and cut into sticks
- 1 cup boiling water
- 2 envelopes or teaspoons instant chicken broth
- 1 teaspoon chopped chives
- ¼ teaspoon freshly ground pepper

1. Break woody base off each stalk of asparagus; soak asparagus in salted warm water 5 minutes to remove sand; lift asparagus out of water.
2. Arrange asparagus spears, baby carrots and yellow squash sticks in separate piles in a large skillet; add boiling water, instant broth, chives and pepper; cover skillet.
3. Bring to boiling; lower heat; separate frozen asparagus spears, if used, with two forks. Simmer 15 minutes, or until vegetables are crisply tender. Arrange around VEAL À LA FRANÇAIS and save cooking liquid for another recipe.

## OVEN ROASTED POTATOES

Bake at 350° for 1 hour.
Makes 8 servings/**61 calories each.**

- 4 medium-size potatoes
- 1 tablespoon vegetable oil
  Seasoned salt
  Freshly ground pepper

1. Pare potatoes; halve. Parboil in lightly salted boiling water 15 minutes, or until almost tender; remove with slotted spoon.
2. Place potatoes, rounded-side up, in a shallow baking pan. Brush potatoes with oil; sprinkle with seasoned salt and pepper.
3. Bake in moderate oven (350°) 1 hour, brushing several times with oil, or until golden brown.

## STEAK WITH MUSHROOMS

*Steak can be low in calories—less expensive, too—when you choose ground round.*

Makes 4 servings/**162 calories each.**

- 2 tablespoons diet margarine
- 2 teaspoons fine dry bread crumbs
- ¼ teaspoon garlic salt
- ¼ cup finely chopped parsley
- ¼ teaspoon grated lemon rind
- 1 teaspoon lemon juice
- 1 pound ground round
- 1 teaspoon garlic salt
- ⅛ teaspoon lemon pepper
- 1 can (2 ounces) sliced mushrooms, drained (save liquid for another recipe)

1. Combine diet margarine, bread crumbs, the ¼ teaspoon garlic salt, parsley, lemon rind and lemon juice in a cup; reserve.
2. Mix together ground round, the 1 teaspoon garlic salt and pepper in a medium-size bowl; shape lightly into 4 patties. Place on broiler pan.
3. Broil patties, 4 inches from heat, 4 minutes, or until lightly browned; turn and broil 5 minutes longer.
4. Top each patty with sliced mushrooms and 2 teaspoons of topping mixture. Continue broiling 3 minutes, or until topping is bubbly and browned.

## EASY VEAL PARMIGIANA

*This version of a popular Italian veal dish needs no baking.*

Makes 6 servings/**270 calories each.**

- 2 tablespoons diet margarine
- 6 frozen veal patties (1 package, about 1¼ pounds)
- 1 can (1 pound, 1 ounce) Italian tomatoes
- 1 tablespoon instant minced onion
- 1 teaspoon leaf oregano, crumbled
- ½ teaspoon leaf basil, crumbled
- 1 teaspoon salt
- ¼ teaspoon seasoned pepper
- 1 cup shredded low-fat mozzarella cheese (4 ounces)
- 3 tablespoons grated Parmesan cheese

1. Heat margarine in large nonstick skillet; brown veal patties, about 3 minutes on each side; remove as they brown. Cut each patty in half and set aside on paper towels.
2. Add tomatoes to same skillet, mashing with a fork. Stir in onion, oregano, basil, salt and pepper. Cook, uncovered, stirring often, 5 minutes, or until slightly thickened.
3. Arrange veal, in sauce in skillet; sprinkle with mozzarella cheese, then with Parmesan cheese.
4. Cover; cook over medium heat 10 minutes, or until cheese is melted.

## BOUILLABAISSE SALAD

*The famous French soup turns into salad when scallops, tuna and haddock combine with assorted vegetables.*

Makes 8 servings/**225 calories each.**

- 1 pound fresh or frozen sea scallops
- 1 slice onion
- 1 slice lemon
- 1 teaspoon salt
- 1 package (1 pound) frozen haddock fillets
  - Piquant Tomato Dressing (recipe follows)
- 2 packages (9 ounces each) frozen artichoke hearts
- 2 packages (9 ounces each) frozen Italian green beans
- 8 cups broken salad greens
- 1 can (about 8 ounces) waterpacked tuna, drained and cut into chunks
- 4 small ripe tomatoes, peeled and cut into wedges
- 1 lemon, cut into 8 wedges

1. Wash fresh scallops in cold water; drain. (No need to thaw frozen ones.)
2. Fill a large skillet to a 1-inch depth of water; add onion, lemon and salt; bring to boiling. Add scallops; cover; remove from heat. Let stand 5 minutes for fresh scallops and 10 minutes for frozen ones; lift out with a slotted spoon and place in a large shallow dish.
3. Bring same pan of water to boiling again; add frozen haddock; cover. Simmer 5 minutes; remove from heat; let stand 5 minutes. Lift out with a wide spatula and place in dish beside scallops. Drizzle each with ¼ cup PIQUANT TOMATO DRESSING; cover dish with plastic wrap; chill.
4. Cook artichoke hearts and green beans in separate saucepans, following label directions; drain. Place in mounds in a large shallow dish. Drizzle each with ¼ cup PIQUANT TOMATO DRESSING; cover; chill.
5. When ready to serve, place 1 cup of the greens in each of 8 soup plates or individual salad bowls. Cut haddock into ½-inch cubes; place with scallops, artichoke hearts and green beans in separate mounds in each plate; pile tuna in centers. Tuck tomato wedges between fish and vegetables. Sprinkle scallops with chopped parsley, and haddock with paprika, if you wish. Serve with lemon wedges and PIQUANT TOMATO DRESSING.

PIQUANT TOMATO DRESSING:
Makes 1¼ cups/**22 calories per tablespoon.** Combine ¼ cup olive or vegetable oil, ½ cup wine vinegar or cider vinegar, ½ cup tomato juice, 1 crushed garlic clove, 2 teaspoons salt, 2 teaspoons sugar and 1 teaspoon crushed fennel seeds or rosemary in a screw top jar; shake well to mix.

## MARINATED BEEF ROLLS

*The flavor magic of this steak, which is served cold, is its double marination—before and after broiling.*

Makes 4 servings/**311 calories each.**

- 1 boneless round steak (about 2 pounds)
- ¾ cup dry red wine
- 1 tablespoon olive or vegetable oil
- 1 clove garlic, crushed
- 1 teaspoon leaf basil, crumbled
- 1 teaspoon salt
- ¼ teaspoon pepper
- 1 can (5¾ ounces) pitted ripe olives

1. Trim all fat from steak and place in a shallow glass dish. Combine wine, oil, garlic, basil, salt and pepper in a cup; pour over steak; cover.
2. Marinate steak in refrigerator for at least 2 hours. Remove steak from marinade and pat dry with paper towels. Reserve marinade.
3. Broil steak, 4 inches from heat, 5 minutes on each side for rare, 7 minutes for medium.
4. Return steak to marinade; cover. Refrigerate 2 hours, or until steak is cold (overnight is even better).
5. To serve: Cut steak into ⅛-inch-thick slices and wrap each slice around a pitted ripe olive. Secure each with a wooden pick.

## BRAISED LAMB CHOPS

*The flavor will be even better and you can remove that last bit of fat from the sauce, if you chill this dish overnight.*

Makes 6 servings/**269 calories each.**

- 6 shoulder lamb chops (about 2 pounds)
- 1 medium-size onion, chopped (½ cup)
- 1 teaspoon salt
- 1 teaspoon ground allspice
- ½ teaspoon garlic salt
- ½ teaspoon ground ginger
- ¾ cup water
- ¼ cup lemon juice
- 1 tablespoon bottled steak sauce
- 1 jar (about 8 ounces) junior applesauce and apricots

1. Trim all fat from lamb chops; brown very slowly in kettle or skillet; remove and reserve. Pour off all but 1 tablespoon pan drippings.
2. Sauté onion in kettle until brown; stir in salt, allspice, garlic salt, ginger, water, lemon juice and steak sauce until well blended.
3. Bring to boiling; stir in junior fruits, then return browned meat; cover kettle; lower heat.
4. Simmer, stirring several times, 1 hour, or until meat is tender. Cool, then chill; remove any fat from sauce; Reheat in same pan.

## FRENCH VEAL RAGOÛT

*Dry vermouth adds a gourmet touch to succulent veal and mushrooms.*

Makes 6 servings/**237 calories each.**

- 1½ pounds cubed veal shoulder
- 1 teaspoon salt
- 1 large onion, chopped (1 cup)
- 1 clove garlic, minced
- ½ cup dry vermouth
- 1 cup water
- 1 envelope or teaspoon instant beef broth
- ¼ teaspoon pepper
- ½ pound fresh mushrooms, sliced OR: 1 can (6 ounces) sliced mushrooms
- 3 tablespoons all purpose flour
- ⅓ cup cold water

1. Trim any remaining fat from veal. Sprinkle salt in bottom of a large heavy skillet; heat skillet. Add veal, part at a time; brown 5 minutes on each side; remove and reserve.
2. Sauté chopped onion and minced garlic in drippings in pan until soft; pour in vermouth; stir up all cooked-on bits from pan; bring to boiling; add the 1 cup water, instant beef broth and pepper; return browned meat to skillet; cover.
3. Simmer 45 minutes, or until veal is tender when pierced with a two-tined fork. Add mushrooms and liquid, if canned ones are used; cook 10 minutes longer.
4. Blend flour and the ⅓ cup cold water in a 1-cup measure until smooth; stir into bubbling liquid; cook, stirring constantly, 3 minutes, or until sauce thickens and bubbles. Top with chopped parsley, if you wish.

## SUPPER HAM SALAD

*It's invitingly cool-looking, with cubed ham, grapes and cucumber in a creamy dressing.*

Makes 6 servings/**275 calories each.**

- 2 cups cubed cooked ham
- 1 cup cubed cooked chicken
- 1 cup halved seedless green grapes
- 1 small cucumber, quartered, lengthwise and thinly sliced
- 4 radishes, trimmed and sliced
- ¼ cup imitation mayonnaise
- ¼ cup plain yogurt (from an 8-ounce container)
- 1 head romaine

1. Combine ham, chicken, grapes, cucumber and radishes lightly in a large bowl.
2. Blend mayonnaise and yogurt in a cup; fold into ham mixture; chill at least an hour to season.
3. Just before serving, line a salad bowl with romaine leaves; shred remaining into bottom. Spoon ham mixture into center.

## SPRING CHEESE SALAD

*Diced vegetables give creamy cottage cheese added flavor, color and crunch!*

Makes 4 servings/**131 calories each.**

- 1 medium-size carrot, pared and finely diced (½ cup)
- 1 medium-size green pepper, seeded and finely diced (½ cup)
- 4 large radishes, trimmed and finely diced (½ cup)
- 1 tablespoon dillweed
- 1 container (1 pound) cream-style cottage cheese

Mix diced carrot, pepper and radish with dillweed in small bowl until well blended; stir in cottage cheese lightly until well blended. Refrigerate until serving time.

## JELLIED CHICKEN

*A perfect make-ahead for a hot summer day.*

Makes 8 servings/**223 calories each.**

- 2 broiler-fryers (about 2 pounds each)
- 1 medium-size onion, sliced
- 2 teaspoons salt
- 1 teaspoon peppercorns Handful celery tops
- 2½ cups water
- 1 envelope unflavored gelatin
- 2 hard-cooked eggs, shelled and sliced Parsley
- 1 tablespoon prepared mustard
- ½ cup plain yogurt (from an 8-ounce container)

1. Simmer chickens with onion, salt, peppercorns, celery tops and water in large covered kettle 1 hour, or until meat begins to fall off bones.
2. Strain broth into a 4-cup measure; skim off all fat that rises to top, then add water, if needed, to make 3 cups; cool broth in refrigerator.
3. Pull all chicken from bones; trim off any fat and skin; chop meat finely. (You should have about 4 cups.) Spoon into a 6-cup loaf pan.
4. Soften gelatin in 1 cup of the cooled broth in small saucepan; heat, stirring constantly, just until dissolved. Stir back into remaining broth; pour over chicken in loaf pan, pressing chicken down with a fork until completely covered (mixture should just fill pan).
5. Chill 5 to 6 hours or overnight, until the loaf is firm enough to cut into neat slices.
6. To unmold, run a thin bladed knife around edge, then dip pan *quickly* in and out of a pan of hot water; invert onto serving plate. Garnish with sliced hard-cooked eggs and parsley. Slice and serve with prepared mustard blended into the yogurt.

## EGGPLANT PROVENÇALE

*Slices of tender eggplant alternate with hamburger patties in this flavorful casserole.*

Bake at 350° for 30 minutes.
Makes 8 servings/**288 calories each.**

- 2 pounds ground round
- 2 envelopes or teaspoons instant onion broth
- 1 eggplant, about 1½ to 2 pounds All purpose flour
- 2 cans (1 pound each) tomatoes
- 2 teaspoons seasoned salt
- ¼ teaspoon pepper
- 1 teaspoon leaf basil, crumbled
- 1 pound zucchini, tipped, cut into ½-inch slices and cooked

1. Mix beef and instant onion broth lightly; divide and shape into 8 patties.
2. Heat a large nonstick skillet; sprinkle bottom of pan with salt. Brown patties 2 minutes on each side; remove and drain on paper towels.
3. Wash eggplant and cut into ½-inch slices. Spread flour on wax paper. Dip eggplant into flour to coat very lightly. Pour off all but 1 tablespoon of drippings from pan. Sauté eggplant, a few slices at a time, adding more drippings, if needed; remove slices as they brown and keep warm.
4. Add tomatoes, salt, pepper and basil to skillet; bring to boiling.
5. Reserve 8 slices eggplant; place remaining slices with half the sauce and half the zucchini in a 12-cup shallow casserole. Arrange reserved eggplant slices alternately with beef patties over bottom layer in dish. Top with remaining zucchini and sauce.
6. Bake in moderate oven (350°) 30 minutes, or until bubbly hot.

## BRAISED PORK STEAK

*Pork chops can be substituted for the pork steak in this super skillet dish.*

Makes 6 servings/**218 calories each.**

- 1 thick pork steak, trimmed (about 1½ pounds)
- 1 can (1 pound, 11 ounces) sauerkraut, drained and rinsed
- 1 large onion, chopped (1 cup)
- 1 large apple, pared, cored and sliced
- 2 teaspoons caraway seeds
- 1 teaspoon salt
- ½ teaspoon ground cinnamon
- ⅛ teaspoon pepper

1. Brown pork steak in a large nonstick skillet over moderate heat; drain off excess fat; remove meat from pan and reserve.
2. Combine sauerkraut, onion, apple, caraway seeds, salt, cinnamon and pepper in skillet; add meat.
3. Cover; cook over low heat 1 hour, or until pork is tender.

## CONTINENTAL VEAL BAKE

*A hearty dish with Old World flavor.*

Bake at 350° for 1 hour, 30 minutes.
Makes 6 servings/**204 calories each.**

- 1½ pounds veal shoulder, cut into 1-inch cubes
- 2 tablespoons all purpose flour
- 1 hot Italian sausage, sliced ½-inch thick
- 12 small white onions, peeled
- 1 can (8 ounces) tomato sauce
- 2 cups dry red wine or water
- 12 small carrots, pared and cut into sticks
- 6 medium-size zucchini, tipped and cut into sticks
- 1 can (3 or 4 ounces) sliced mushrooms
- 2 teaspoons seasoned salt
- ¼ teaspoon seasoned pepper
- 1 teaspoon mixed Italian herbs, crumbled

1. Shake veal with flour in a plastic bag to coat evenly.
2. Brown sausage slices in a large skillet; push to one side; add onions; sauté until soft; push to one side; brown veal in skillet.
3. Spoon meat and onions into an 8-cup casserole; stir tomato sauce and wine into skillet; heat to boiling, stirring up baked-on pieces from bottom and side of pan; pour over meat and onions in casserole.
4. Add carrots, zucchini, mushrooms, salt, pepper and Italian herbs to casserole; stir; cover.
5. Bake in moderate oven (350°) 1 hour, 30 minutes, or until veal and vegetables are tender.
*Suggested Variation:* Makes 8 servings/**152 calories each** for CONTINENTAL CHICKEN BAKE, substitute 1½ pounds chicken breast for the veal, 1 pound green beans for carrots and 6 yellow squash for the zucchini. Use leaf basil for mixed Italian herbs.

## TURKEY HAWAIIAN

*Pineapple, water chestnuts and crisp vegetables make cooked turkey special.*

Makes 6 servings/**334 calories each.**

- 1 large onion, chopped (1 cup)
- 1 tablespoon vegetable oil
- 1 package (10 ounces) frozen Italian green beans
- 1½ cups sliced celery
- 2 envelopes or teaspoons instant chicken broth
- 2 tablespoons cornstarch
- 1 tablespoon soy sauce
- 1 can (13¼ ounces) pineapple tidbits packed in pineapple juice
- 1 can (3 or 4 ounces) sliced mushrooms
- 1 can (5 ounces) water chestnuts, drained and sliced
- 3 cups julienne strips cooked turkey
- 3 cups fluffy hot rice

1. Sauté onion in vegetable oil just until soft in a large skillet.
2. Stir in frozen Italian green beans, celery, instant chicken broth and 1 cup water. Cover; bring to boiling; simmer 5 minutes.
3. Blend cornstarch and soy sauce until smooth in 2-cup measure. Drain and stir in juice from pineapple and liquid from mushrooms. Stir into vegetable mixture. Cook, stirring constantly, until sauce thickens and bubbles 1 minute.
4. Stir in pineapple, mushrooms, water chestnuts and turkey. Cover; heat slowly until hot.
5. Spoon hot rice in a ring on heated serving plate; mound turkey mixture in center.

## PAELLA GRANADA

*This Spanish meal-in-a-dish has all the flavor of the original.*

Bake at 350° for 1 hour.
Makes 8 servings/**295 calories each.**

- 1 broiler-fryer, cut up (about 2 pounds)
- 1 large onion, chopped (1 cup)
- 1 clove garlic, minced
- 1 cup uncooked rice
- 6 small slices salami, diced (about 2 ounces)
- 2 teaspoons salt
- ¼ teaspoon seasoned pepper
- ⅛ teaspoon crushed saffron
- 1 can (1 pound) tomatoes
- 1½ cups water
- 1 envelope or teaspoon instant chicken broth
- 1 pound fresh shrimp, shelled and deveined
  OR: 1 package (12 ounces) frozen deveined shelled raw shrimp
- 1 can (4 ounces) pimiento, drained and cut into large pieces

1. Place chicken, skin-side down, in a single layer on rack of broiler pan.
2. Broil, 4 inches from heat, 10 minutes; turn. Broil 10 minutes longer, or until lightly browned.
3. Pour 1 tablespoon drippings from broiler pan into a medium-size skillet; stir in onion and garlic. Sauté until soft; spoon into a 12-cup paella pan or shallow casserole with rice, salami, salt, pepper and saffron.
4. Combine tomatoes with water and instant chicken broth in same pan; bring to boiling. Stir into rice mixture with shrimp. Arrange chicken and pimiento over top; cover.
5. Bake in moderate oven (350°) 1 hour, or until liquid is absorbed and chicken, shrimp and rice are tender. Garnish PAELLA with fresh chopped parsley, if you wish.

## SUKIYAKI TRAY

*Dieting isn't difficult when you're allowed this sort of dish.*

Makes 4 servings/**349 calories each.**

- 1 round steak, cut ½-inch thick (about 1 pound)
- ¼ cup soy sauce
- 1 tablespoon peanut or vegetable oil
- ½ pound green beans, tipped and cut into 1-inch lengths
- 2 medium-size yellow squash, trimmed and sliced
- 1 envelope or teaspoon instant chicken broth
- ¼ cup water
- 1 package (10 ounces) fresh spinach, washed and stemmed
- 2 cups hot cooked rice

1. Cut steak diagonally into thin strips; place in a pie plate. Pour soy sauce over; let stand 15 minutes.
2. Lift beef strips from marinade and dry on paper towels; sauté quickly in oil in a large skillet; remove and keep hot. Reserve soy sauce.
3. Place green beans and squash in separate piles in skillet; sauté, stirring gently 2 to 3 minutes, or just until shiny and moist.
4. Combine instant chicken broth, water and reserved soy sauce in a cup. Pour over vegetables; cover; steam 5 minutes.
5. Lay spinach over vegetables; cover again; steam 5 minutes longer, or just until vegetables are crisply tender.
6. Spoon vegetables and beef over rice in a heated serving platter. Spoon broth from pan over. Pass additional soy sauce, if you wish.
COOK'S TIP: Beef will slice more easily if placed in freezer for 30 minutes before cutting to firm up.

## PORK IN WINE

*Pork cutlets make this a quick cooking skillet dish.*

Makes 8 servings/**223 calories each.**

- 8 pork cutlets, ⅛-inch thick (about 1½ pounds)
- ½ teaspoon salt
- ⅛ teaspoon pepper
- 2 cloves garlic, minced
- ½ cup dry white wine
- 8 thin slices boiled ham (¼ pound)

1. Trim fat from the cutlets; pound thin with meat mallet. Season with salt and pepper.
2. Place cutlets and garlic in nonstick skillet. Sauté 5 minutes on each side. Drain off excess fat.
3. Stir in wine. Cover; simmer 10 minutes. Top each cutlet with a slice of ham. Cover; simmer 5 minutes longer; or until ham is heated.

## SAN FRANCISCO CHIOPPINO

*Castagnola, one of the finest fish restaurants on Fisherman's Wharf, serves this delicious dish of King crab, prawns or shrimp and clams in a rich tomato sauce—San Francisco's answer to the Bouillabaisse of Marseilles. Photo is on page 73.*

Makes 6 servings/**226 calories each.**

- 1 large onion, chopped (1 cup)
- 1 clove garlic, minced
- 1 tablespoon olive or vegetable oil
- 1 can (1 pound, 12 ounces) tomatoes in tomato purée
- 2 tablespoons chopped fresh basil OR: 2 teaspoons leaf basil, crumbled
- 2 teaspoons salt
- 1 bottle (8 ounces) clam juice
- 2 pounds fresh or frozen King crab, in the shell
- 2 dozen clams OR: 1 can (10 ounces) whole clams
- ½ pound prawns or shrimp
- 1 pound halibut fillet OR: 1 package (1 pound) frozen halibut

1. Sauté onion and garlic in oil in a large saucepan until soft; stir in tomatoes in tomato purée, basil, salt and clam juice; bring to boiling; lower heat; simmer 30 minutes.
2. While sauce simmers, cut crab legs into 3-inch pieces (no need to thaw frozen crab); scrub clam shells well; shell and devein prawns or shrimp; cut halibut into small pieces.
3. Layer crab legs, then clams, then prawns or shrimp and finally halibut in a deep kettle; pour sauce over.
4. Bring slowly to bubbling; lower heat; simmer 15 minutes. Serve in deep soup bowls. Garnish with chopped parsley, if you wish.
COOK'S TIP: The tomato sauce in this recipe can be made up to a week ahead of serving time; refrigerate until ready to cook fish.

## BEEF STROGANOFF

*Buttermilk takes the place of sour cream in our diet version of this Continental treat.*

Makes 8 servings/**182 calories each.**

- 2 pounds ground round
- 2 tablespoons instant minced onion
- 1 teaspoon salt
- ½ cup cracked ice
- ½ cup water
- 1 tablespoon all purpose flour
- 1 envelope or teaspoon instant beef broth
- ¼ teaspoon salt
- ⅛ teaspoon pepper
- 2 tablespoons catsup
- 1 teaspoon prepared mustard
- 2 teaspoons parsley flakes
- 1 can (8 ounces) mushroom stems and pieces
- 1 cup buttermilk

1. Combine ground beef, onion, the 1 teaspoon salt and cracked ice in a large bowl. Shape into 16 balls; arrange in a single layer on broiler rack.
2. Broil, 4 inches from heat, 5 minutes, turning once.
3. Combine water, flour and beef broth in a large saucepan. Cook over medium heat, stirring constantly, until sauce thickens and bubbles 1 minute. Add the ¼ teaspoon salt, pepper, catsup, mustard and parsley; drain liquid from mushrooms into pan. Reduce heat; drop in meatballs, a few at a time. Bring to boiling; lower heat; cover and simmer 15 minutes.
4. Uncover; add mushrooms; return to boiling. Stir 1 cup hot sauce into buttermilk in a small bowl; return to saucepan; reduce heat. Cook until warmed through (do not boil), about 3 minutes.

## YELLOW SQUASH BOATS

*The perfect hot dish to serve with a tossed salad for a satisfying meal.*

Bake at 350° for 15 minutes.
Makes 4 servings/**213 calories each.**

- 2 medium-size yellow squash (about 1 pound)
- 2 ears corn
- 1 medium-size onion, chopped (½ cup)
- 1 small red pepper, halved, seeded and chopped
- 1 tablespoon butter or margarine
- 1 teaspoon leaf tarragon, crumbled
- 1 teaspoon salt
  Dash pepper
- ½ cup water
- 1 cup soft white bread crumbs (2 slices)
- 1 egg, beaten
- 1 cup shredded low fat mozzarella cheese (4 ounces)

1. Halve squash lengthwise and trim. Cook in boiling salted water, in a large skillet just until tender, about 5 minutes. Drain on paper towels.
2. Husk corn and remove silks. Holding corn upright on a cutting board, slice downward in rows to cut kernels from corn. (You should have ½ cup. Or, use ½ cup canned whole-kernel corn.)
3. Sauté onion and red pepper in butter or margarine until soft in pan.
4. Stir in cut corn, tarragon, salt, pepper and water. Cover skillet and simmer 10 minutes, or until corn is tender. Stir in bread crumbs, egg and mozzarella cheese.
5. Scoop out seeds from squash halves. Arrange in a 13x9x2-inch casserole. Divide corn mixture among squash boats.
6. Bake in moderate oven (350°) 15 minutes, or until stuffing is golden.

## BELGIAN POT ROAST

*Lower calorie light beer replaces the more fattening brew in this hearty dish.*

Makes 8 servings/**305 calories each.**

- 1 boneless round roast, well trimmed (3½ pounds)
- 2 teaspoons garlic salt
- ¼ teaspoon pepper
- 1 tablespoon vegetable oil
- 2 medium-size onions, sliced
- 1 teaspoon leaf thyme, crumbled
- 1 bay leaf
- 1 bottle or can (12 ounces) light beer
- 1 teaspoon brown sugar
- 2 tablespoons all purpose flour
- ¼ cup cold water
- 2 tablespoons chopped parsley

1. Season meat on all sides with garlic salt and pepper.
2. Heat oil in a large heavy nonstick pan or Dutch oven; brown the meat on all sides; remove and reserve. Drain off all but 1 tablespoon fat. Sauté onion slices until soft; return meat to pan.
3. Add thyme, bay leaf, beer and brown sugar; cover; simmer over very low heat 2 hours, or until meat is tender. Remove from heat; remove bay leaf and refrigerate several hours or overnight.
4. About 30 minutes before serving time, remove pot roast from refrigerator. Carefully remove hardened fat. Simmer, covered, 20 minutes, or until meat is heated through.
5. Remove meat to serving platter; keep warm. Combine flour and cold water in a 1-cup measure; stir into liquid in pan. Cook, stirring constantly, until sauce thickens and bubbles 3 minutes; add parsley. Serve sauce in heated gravy bowl with meat.

# DIET DO'S

## YOU AND YOUR FAMILY

It's possible to stay on your diet, even if you're preparing food for the rest of the family.

- Trim all fat from your portion of meat. When cooking your serving with the family meal, wrap it tightly in aluminum foil to protect it from the cooking fat or oil.
- To cook meat without fat or oil, use one of the new vegetable spray ons. Or, simmer or bake it in a sauce made of canned tomatoes, green pepper and spices or herbs for extra flavor and nutrition.
- Remove your diet portion before adding butter or cream sauces to vegetables, making gravy or thickening sauces for the family's servings.
- Never take second helpings of food.
- Remember—no gravy for the dieter, unless you use our recipes.

## DIET CHICKEN CACCIATORE

*Spaghetti sauce mix in an envelope gives a zesty flavor to baked chicken breasts.*

Bake at 350° for 1 hour.
Makes 6 servings at 177 calories each.

- **3 whole chicken breasts, split (about 12 ounces each)**
- **1 Bermuda onion, cut in 6 slices**
- **1 envelope (1½ ounces) spaghetti sauce mix**
- **1 can (1 pound) tomatoes**

1. Brown chicken breasts in a large nonstick skillet; arrange in single layer in an 8-cup shallow casserole. Top each breast with an onion slice.
2. Blend spaghetti sauce mix into drippings in skillet; stir in tomatoes; bring to boiling, stirring constantly. Spoon around chicken breasts and onions; cover casserole.
3. Bake in moderate oven (350°) 1 hour, or until chicken breasts are tender. Serve with Italian green beans, if you wish.

## SWEET AND SOUR CHICKEN

*The Oriental way to diet—delicious.*

Makes 4 servings at 306 calories each.

- **2 whole chicken breasts (about 12 ounces each)**
- **3 tablespoons teriyaki sauce or soy sauce**
- **1 tablespoon vegetable oil**
- **2 medium-size yellow squash, trimmed and sliced**
- **1 package (9 ounces) frozen cut green beans**
- **2 cups water**
- **2 tablespoons lemon juice**
- **1 can (8½ ounces) pineapple chunks in pineapple juice**
- **2 tablespoons cornstarch**
- **1 can (5 ounces) water chestnuts, sliced**
- **Granulated or liquid low-calorie sweetener**

1. Pull skin from chicken breasts; cut meat from bones; cut into thin strips.
2. Marinate chicken with teriyaki sauce or soy sauce in a bowl for 15 minutes.
3. Heat oil in a wok or large skillet; remove chicken from sauce; brown quickly in hot oil. Add yellow squash and green beans. Sauté, stirring gently, 3 minutes, or just until shiny-moist. Add remaining teriyaki sauce or soy sauce, water, lemon juice; cover; steam 5 minutes.
4. While vegetables steam, drain liquid from pineapple into small cup; stir in cornstarch to make a smooth paste.

5. Add pineapple and sliced water chestnuts to skillet; bring just to boiling. Stir in cornstarch mixture; cook, stirring constantly, until mixture thickens and bubbles 1 minute. Stir in your favorite low-calorie sweetener, using the equivalent of 1 tablespoon sugar. Serve with Chinese noodles, if you wish (70 calories per ⅓ cup for noodles).

## BARBECUE CHICKEN

*Broiled chicken with a flavorful tomato basting sauce.*

Makes 4 servings at 259 calories each.

- **1 broiler-fryer, cut up (2½ pounds)**
- **¾ cup tomato juice**
- **1 small onion, grated**
- **2 tablespoons tarragon vinegar**
- **1 tablespoon prepared mustard**
- **1 tablespoon Worcestershire sauce**
- **½ teaspoon salt**
- **¼ teaspoon pepper**

1. Place chicken, skin-side down, in a single layer on rack in broiler pan.
2. Combine tomato juice, onion, vinegar, mustard, Worcestershire sauce, salt and pepper in a small bowl. Brush some over chicken.
3. Broil, 8 inches from heat, basting often with sauce, 20 minutes; turn skin-side up. Continue broiling, basting often with sauce, 20 minutes longer, or until chicken is richly browned and tender when pierced with a fork.
4. Serve with cooked rice, if you wish (92 calories per ½ cup serving).

## CORN CRISPED FRIED CHICKEN

*Who says you can't have fried chicken on a diet?*

Bake at 375° for 1 hour.
Makes 6 servings at 251 calories each.

- **2 broiler-fryers, cut up (about 2 pounds each)**
- **½ cup skim milk**
- **1 cup packaged corn flake crumbs**
- **1½ teaspoons onion salt**
- **¼ teaspoon pepper**
- **1 teaspoon paprika**

1. Wash chicken pieces; pat dry. Pour milk into a shallow dish. Combine the corn flake crumbs, onion salt, pepper and paprika in a plastic bag.
2. Dip chicken pieces in the milk; shake pieces, a few at a time, in crumb mixture in bag to coat well.
3. Arrange chicken, skin-side up, in a single layer on a nonstick pan.
4. Bake in moderate oven (375°) 1 hour, or until tender.

## CHICKEN MARENGO, DIET STYLE

*Mushrooms and herbs add the gourmet touch without extra calories.*

Makes 8 servings at 252 calories each.

- **2 broiler-fryers, cut up (about 2½ pounds each)**
- **1 can condensed tomato soup**
- **½ pound mushrooms**
- **Instant garlic powder**
- **1 teaspoon salt**
- **½ teaspoon leaf thyme, crumbled**
- **1 can (1 pound) small boiled onions**

1. Place chicken pieces, skin-side down, in a nonstick skillet. Brown slowly over moderate heat. (Chicken will brown in its own fat.) Turn; brown other side; drain fat.
2. Add the soup, mushrooms, garlic powder, salt, thyme, and onion liquid.
3. Cover; simmer over low heat for 45 minutes, or until chicken is tender. Add onions. Uncover; continue cooking until sauce thickens, about 10 minutes.

## FRENCH CHICKEN IN SHERRY SAUCE

*Chicken breasts are a dieter's delight! No need to strip the skin if you follow our fat-reducing technique for oven-browning. Add wine sauce for a quick main course that's quite Continental!*

Bake at 375° for 45 minutes.
Makes 6 servings at 217 calories each.

- **3 whole chicken breasts, split (about 10 ounces each)**
- **½ teaspoon salt**
- **1 medium-size onion, sliced**
- **¼ cup chopped green pepper**
- **1 cup sliced mushrooms**
- **Sauce**
- **1 cup orange juice**
- **¼ cup dry sherry**
- **½ cup water**
- **1 tablespoon firmly packed brown sugar**
- **1 teaspoon salt**
- **¼ teaspoon pepper**
- **1 teaspoon grated orange rind**
- **1 tablespoon all-purpose flour**
- **2 teaspoons chopped parsley**
- **Paprika**
- **1 California orange, peeled and sliced**

1. Place chicken breasts, skin-side up, on rack of broiler pan. Broil 2 inches from heat for 10 minutes, or until skin is brown and crackly. Do not turn.
2. Place browned chicken breasts in a shallow 8-cup casserole. Sprinkle with ½ teaspoon salt. Add onion, green pepper and mushrooms.
3. Make sauce. Combine orange juice, sherry, water, brown sugar, 1

teaspoon salt, pepper, orange rind and flour in small saucepan. Blend well. Cook over medium heat, stirring constantly, until sauce thickens and bubbles; add parsley. Pour over chicken breasts.

4. Bake in moderate oven (375°) 45 minutes, or until chicken is tender. Baste several times. Sprinkle with paprika; garnish with orange slices.

## NO-FAT FRIED CHICKEN

*This magic chicken cooks golden brown with no fat, no turning.*

Makes 4 servings at 221 calories each.

- 1 broiler-fryer, cut up (about 2 pounds)
- 1 teaspoon salt
- ⅛ teaspoon pepper
- 2 large onions, sliced
- ½ cup water

1. Place chicken, skin-side down, in a single layer in a large skillet.
2. Sprinkle with salt and pepper; place onion slices on top; cover tightly. (No need to add any fat.)
3. Cook over low heat 20 minutes. Tilt lid slightly so liquid will evaporate; continue cooking 20 minutes longer, or until chicken is tender and golden.
4. Place chicken on a heated serving platter, pushing onions back into pan; stir in water, mixing with browned bits from bottom of pan; cook until liquid evaporates. Spoon pan juices over chicken.

## WEIGHT WORRIER'S FRICASSEE

*A happy combination of rich tasting gravy and sensible calorie count.*

Makes 6 servings at 200 calories each.

- 3 whole chicken breasts, split (about 12 ounces each)
- 1 small onion, chopped (¼ cup)
- ½ cup finely chopped celery
- 2 teaspoons salt
- ⅛ teaspoon pepper
- 1 cup water
- 2 tablespoons all-purpose flour
- ½ cup skim milk

1. Simmer the chicken, covered, with onion, celery, salt , pepper and water in a medium-size skillet 30 minutes, or until tender; remove to a heated serving platter and keep warm.
2. Mix flour and skim milk in a cup; stir into hot broth in pan. Cook, stirring constantly, until gravy thickens and bubbles 3 minutes. Serve in a separate bowl.

## ORANGE CHICKEN

*A taste of honey...and much more.*

Bake at 375° for 50 minutes.
Makes 4 servings at 216 calories each.

- 4 drumsticks with thighs (about 2 pounds)
- 1 teaspoon salt
- ¼ teaspoon pepper
- ¼ cup orange juice
- 1 tablespoon honey
- 1 teaspoon Worcestershire sauce
- ¼ teaspoon dry mustard

1. Place chicken, skin-side up, in a single layer in a shallow baking pan; sprinkle with salt and pepper.
2. Bake in moderate oven (375°) 30 minutes.
3. Blend orange juice, honey, Worcestershire sauce and mustard in a cup; brush part over chicken.
4. Continue baking, brushing again with remaining orange mixture, 20 minutes, or until chicken is tender and richly glazed.

## SLICK CHICK

*Each dieter rates a half golden-glazed chicken plus spicy apple stuffing in this too-good-to-be-true roast.*

Roast at 375° for 1 hour, 10 minutes.
Makes 4 servings at 321 calories each.

- 2 small broiler-fryers (about 1½ pounds each)
- 1½ teaspoons salt
- 1 large onion, chopped (1 cup)
- ¼ cup water
- ¼ teaspoon ground coriander
- ¼ teaspoon curry powder
- 3 medium-size apples, pared, quartered, cored and chopped
- 1 teaspoon paprika
- ½ cup chicken broth

1. Sprinkle chicken insides with ½ teaspoon of the salt.
2. Simmer onion in water in a medium-size skillet 5 minutes, or until soft; stir in coriander, curry powder, apples and ½ teaspoon of salt.
3. Cook, stirring often, over medium heat 10 minutes, or until apples are slightly soft. Remove from heat.
4. Stuff neck and body cavities of chickens lightly with apple mixture. Smooth neck skin over stuffing and skewer to back; tie legs to tail with string. Place chickens, side by side, in a roasting pan.
5. Mix remaining ½ teaspoon salt and paprika in cup; sprinkle over chickens.
6. Roast in moderate oven (375°), basting several times with chicken

broth, 1 hour, 10 minutes, or until drumsticks move easily and meaty part of a thigh feels soft.
7. Remove chickens to a heated serving platter; cut away strings and remove skewers. Garnish platter with parsley and a few thin apple slices, if you wish. Cut chickens in half; divide stuffing evenly.

# DIET DO'S

• Because of the fat in chicken skin, broiler-fryers can be broiled without additional fat. Simply sprinkle with salt, pepper, monosodium glutamate, lemon juice and an herb such as tarragon, thyme or basil. Broiled chicken may also be basted with a barbecue sauce.

• A savory, richly flavored broth is essential for good soup. It can be the base for cream soups, stews, chowders and appetizer soups. Whenever your soup recipe calls for broth use canned if you don't plan to make one from scratch.

• Line a freezer-to-oven casserole with heavy-duty foil, add the ingredients and freeze. When frozen, remove the food wrapped in the foil, relieving the dish for duty. To serve, remove foil, return food to the same dish and bake.

• Chicken in Parts: In most markets today, it is possible to buy only those parts of the chicken you want—all breasts, for example, or all drumsticks, wings, thighs or backs.

## DIETER'S HAWAIIAN CHICKEN

*Cooked to a turn in a soy and onion sauce.*

Bake at 350° for 1 hour.
Makes 6 servings at 287 calories each.

- 3 broiler-fryers (about 1½ pounds each)
- 1 small onion, chopped (¼ cup)
- ¼ cup soy sauce
- 1½ cups water
- 6 slices pineapple in pineapple juice (from a 1-pound, 4-ounce can)
- 2 tablespoons chopped parsley

1. Arrange split chickens, skin-side down, in a large shallow baking pan. Mix onion, soy sauce and water in a small bowl; pour over chicken.
2. Bake in moderate oven (350°) 30 minutes; turn chicken; bake, basting several times with soy mixture in pan, 30 minutes longer, or until tender.
3. Drain pineapple slices well on paper towels; roll edge of each in chopped parsley. Serve with chicken.

**KING CRAB,** prawns, halibut and clams make San Francisco Chioppino, the West Coast's answer to the Bouillibaisse of Marseilles. It's served in the finest restaurants in California, and now you can enjoy it, too, because with our recipe the dish comes out to only 226 calories a serving. See page 69 for details.

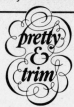

pretty & trim

## 7
### 500 CALORIES

Double Cheese Parfait*
Spaghetti with Seafood*
Steamed Broccoli and
Cauliflower Flowerets
seasoned with
Mixed Italian Herbs
Wine Jelly with Fruits*
Tea with Mint

### 540 CALORIES

Serve:
2 Zucchini Pizzas*
with the
Double Cheese Parfait

### 602 CALORIES

Serve:
Barbecued Eggplant Slices*
with Broccoli

## 8
### 480 CALORIES

Tomato Consommé*
Sukiyaki Tray*
Shredded Chinese Cabbage
and Sliced Celery Crescents
tossed with
Citrus Dressing*
Double Fruit Coupe*
Green Tea

### 545 CALORIES

Serve:
Tomato Consommé
with 1 slice
Toasted Whole Wheat Bread

### 595 CALORIES

Spread:
1½ teaspoons
Butter or Margarine on Toast

## 9
### 497 CALORIES

Mushrooms en Aspic*
Fruited Ham Steak*
Apple and Kraut Bake*
Leaf Lettuce with cooked
Italian Green Beans and
Low Calorie Russian Dressing
Chocolate Eclairs*
Hot Tea

### 547 CALORIES

Serve:
½ cup
Riced Sweet Potato with
Fruited Ham Steak

### 597 CALORIES

Increase:
Sweet Potato to
1 cup

## 10
### 479 CALORIES

Coleslaw Relish Mold*
Scandinavian Lamb Kabobs*
Bitters Baked Vegetables*
Fresh Fruit Cup made with
¼ cup each:
Sliced Peaches, Cantaloupe and
Fresh Blueberries
Café au Lait

### 549 CALORIES

Serve:
1 Small Boiled Potato
sprinkled with
Chopped Fresh Dill

### 579 CALORIES

Add:
2 tablespoons
Plain Yogurt to Potato

## 11
### 495 CALORIES

Parfait Française*
Eggplant Provençale*
Steamed Fresh Spinach with
Leaf Marjoram and
Lemon Juice
1 slice toasted French Bread
Wine Jelly with Fruits*
Coffee or Tea

### 548 CALORIES

Serve:
Low Calorie Sangria* with
Dilly Beans and Carrots*
as an appetizer

### 598 CALORIES

Add:
1½ teaspoons
Butter or Margarine

## 12
### 480 CALORIES

Yankee Clam Broth*
Marinated Beef Rolls*
Zucchini Slices poached
in Broth
Shredded Romaine with
Thousand Island Dressing*
Apricot Mold*
Hot Tea

### 520 CALORIES

Serve:
4 Blue Cheese Stuffed Celery*
with
Yankee Clam Broth

### 590 CALORIES

Add:
½ cup Whole Kernel Corn
to Zucchini

*See Recipe Index for page number.

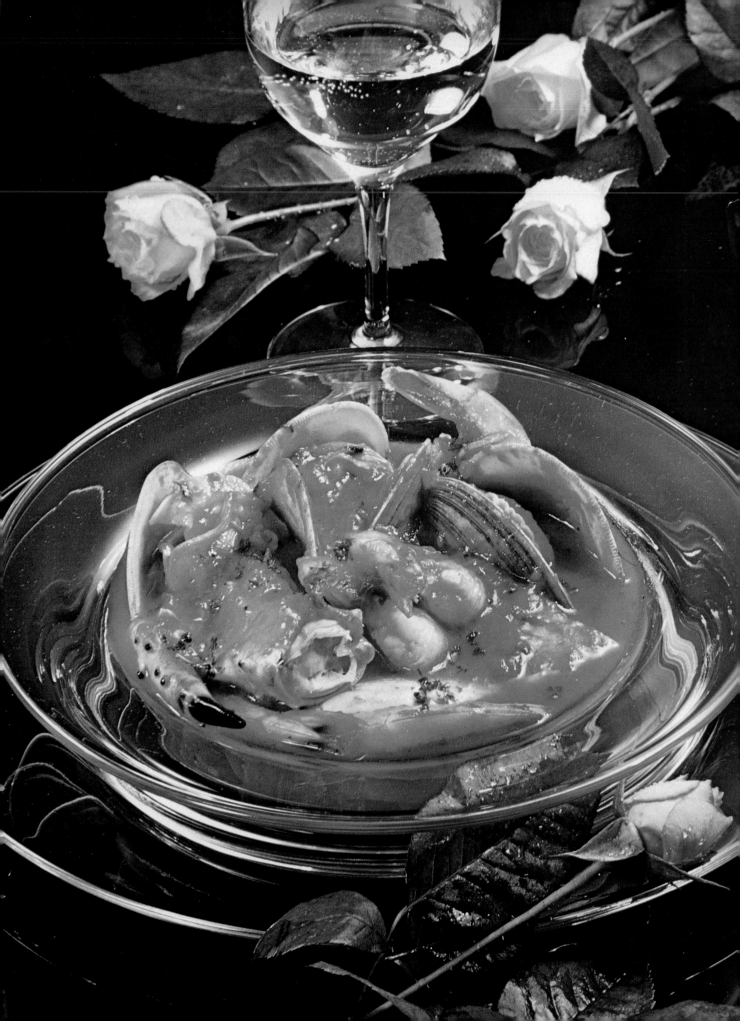

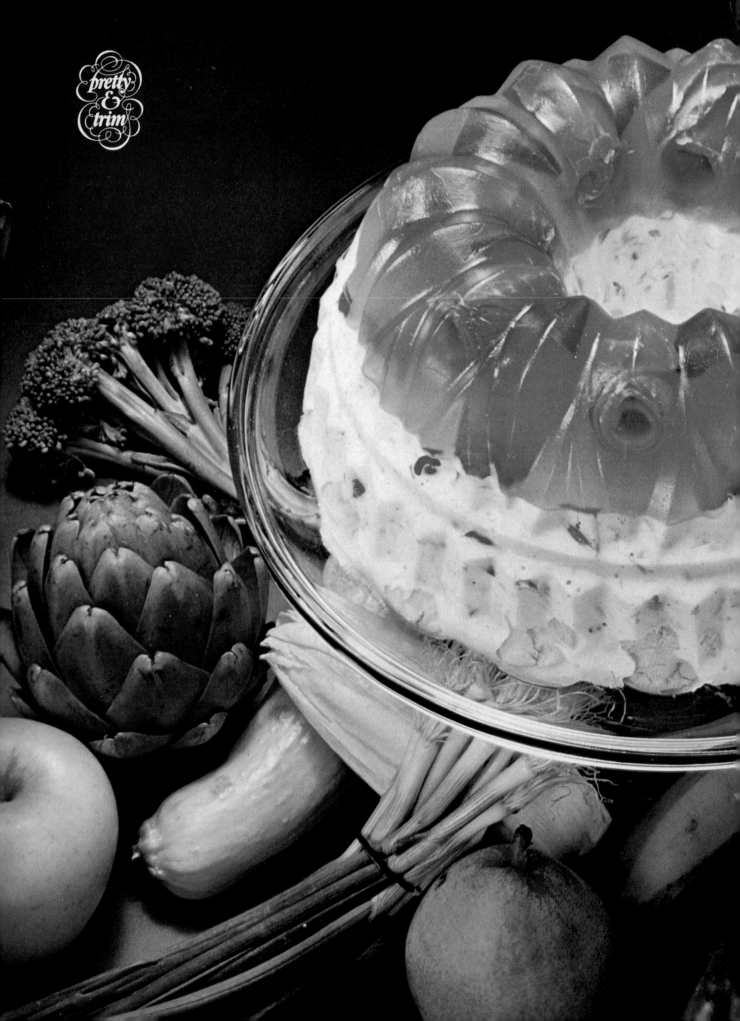

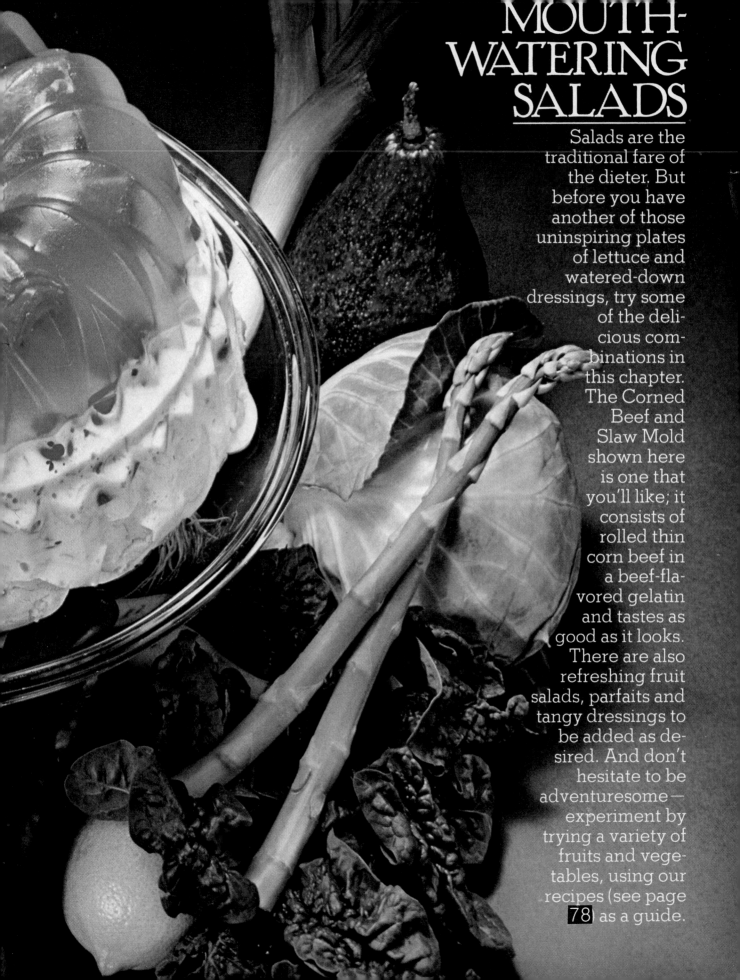

# MOUTH-WATERING SALADS

Salads are the traditional fare of the dieter. But before you have another of those uninspiring plates of lettuce and watered-down dressings, try some of the delicious combinations in this chapter. The Corned Beef and Slaw Mold shown here is one that you'll like; it consists of rolled thin corn beef in a beef-flavored gelatin and tastes as good as it looks. There are also refreshing fruit salads, parfaits and tangy dressings to be added as desired. And don't hesitate to be adventuresome— experiment by trying a variety of fruits and vegetables, using our recipes (see page 78) as a guide.

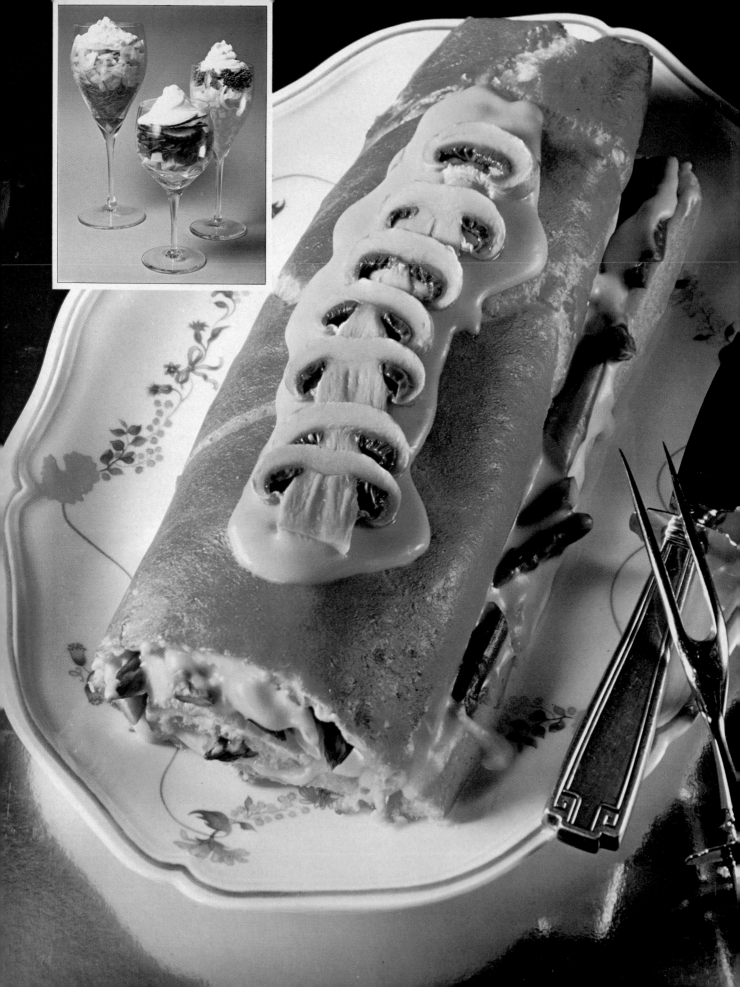

**ASPARAGUS ROULADE** is an appetizing combination of cheese sauce and vegetable rolled in a light soufflé; the dish can be varied by substituting flaked crab meat or diced chicken for asparagus. Either way it's a dieter's delight, especially when served with one of our tasty parfaits (inset photo). See page 79.

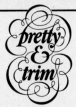

*pretty & trim*

## 1

### 368 CALORIES

Clear Chicken Broth
(Made with instant
chicken broth.)
Fish in Spinach Nests*
Red Cabbage Slaw*
½ cup Calories Reduced
Sliced Pears
1 cup Skim Milk

### 438 CALORIES

Serve:
1 slice toasted
Enriched White Bread with
Fish in Spinach Nests

### 480 CALORIES

Spread:
1½ teaspoons
Butter or Margarine on Toast

## 2

### 394 CALORIES

Asparagus Roulade*
Radish Roses
Carrot Curls
Cucumber Slices
Celery Sticks
Harlequin Parfait*
¾ cup Skim Milk
Tea with Lemon

### 427 CALORIES

Serve:
Yogurt Slaw*
with
Asparagus Roulade

### 491 CALORIES

Start with:
Gazpacho* in
chilled soup bowls

## 3

### 400 CALORIES

Greek Chicken Livers*
Shredded Iceberg Lettuce,
Fresh Spinach Leaves and
Green Pepper Strips with
¼ cup Cucumber Crisps*
½ cup Calories Reduced Plums
1 cup Skim Milk
Spiced Tea

### 436 CALORIES

Start with:
Egg Drop Soup*
served in
delicate China bowls

### 506 CALORIES

Serve:
⅓ cup Boiled Rice with
Greek Chicken Livers

## 4

### 386 CALORIES

Ham and Potato Boats*
Fresh Spinach Salad with
Sliced Radishes and
Cucumber Cartwheels
Lemon Dressing*
Spiced Fruits*
1 cup Skim Milk
Ice Tea

### 441 CALORIES

Start with:
Consommé Madrilène* with
Lemon or Lime Slices
as a garnish

### 491 CALORIES

Serve:
2 Soda Crackers with
Consommé Madrilène

## 5

### 396 CALORIES

Spring Cheese Salad* on
Shredded Lettuce
1 slice Pumpernickel Bread
Tomato Wedges with
Chopped Chives
½ cup Calories
Reduced Peaches
1 cup Skim Milk

### 466 CALORIES

Spread:
1½ teaspoons
Butter or Margarine onto
Pumpernickel Bread

### 500 CALORIES

Add:
4 Zucchini Antipasto Rounds*
to salad plate

## 6

### 384 CALORIES

Onion Broth
(Made with instant onion broth.)
Tuna Stuffed Squash*
Cucumber Sticks
Red and Green Pepper Rings
½ cup Fresh Blueberries
1 cup Skim Milk
Mint Tea

### 414 CALORIES

Top:
Blueberries with
¼ cup Plain Yogurt and
sprinkle with Nutmeg

### 484 CALORIES

Serve:
1 Small Dinner Roll with
Tuna Stuffed Squash

*See Recipe Index for page number.

## TANGY COOKED DRESSING

*A pungent dressing, sure to liven up any diet meal.*

*Makes 2 cups/***10 calories per tablespoon.**

- 1½ teaspoons (from 1 envelope) unflavored gelatin
- 1½ cups skim milk
- 1 tablespoon sugar
- 1 teaspoon salt
- 2 egg yolks
- 2 teaspoons dry mustard
- 2 tablespoons cider vinegar
- 2 tablespoons lemon juice

1. Sprinkle gelatin over milk in a small saucepan; stir in sugar and salt. Heat, stirring constantly, until gelatin, sugar and salt dissolve. (Do not allow liquid to boil.)
2. Beat egg yolks slightly in a small bowl; stir in a generous ½ cup of the hot mixture, then stir back into remaining mixture in saucepan. Cook, stirring constantly, 5 minutes, or until thick; remove from heat.
3. Stir in mustard until completely blended, then *very slowly* stir in vinegar and lemon juice; cover; chill. Store dressing in a jar with a screw top in the refrigerator. Serve over sliced tomatoes or a raw spinach and mushroom salad, topped with freshly grated carrot.

## CORNED BEEF & SLAW MOLD

*Three favorites—corned beef, cabbage and potatoes—can be part of your diet plan. Photo is on page 74.*

*Makes 8 servings/***276 calories each.**

- 2 envelopes unflavored gelatin
- 2 envelopes or teaspoons instant beef broth
- 3 cups water
- ½ cup cider vinegar
- ½ pound sliced cooked corned beef
- 1 small green pepper, halved, seeded and cut into large pieces
- 1 tablespoon prepared horseradish
- 4 cups finely shredded cabbage
- 2 cups peeled, diced, cooked potatoes
- 1 small red pepper, halved, seeded and diced
- 1 small onion, chopped (¼ cup)
- ¼ cup chopped parsley
- ½ cup imitation mayonnaise
- ½ cup plain yogurt (from an 8-ounce container)
- 1 teaspoon prepared mustard
- 1 teaspoon salt
- 1 hard-cooked egg, shelled and sliced

1. Combine gelatin and instant beef broth in a medium-size saucepan; stir in 1 cup of the water. Heat, stirring constantly, until gelatin dissolves. Remove from heat; stir in remaining 2 cups water and vinegar to mix well.
2. Measure ¾ cup gelatin mixture into a small bowl; let stand at room temperature. Pour remaining mixture into a large bowl; chill 30 minutes, or until as thick as unbeaten egg white.
3. Pour ½ cup syrupy gelatin mixture into a 10-cup tube mold; place mold in a large bowl of ice and water; swirl gelatin in pan to coat side of mold with ½-inch layer gelatin. Roll up corned beef slices and arrange in gelatin, alternately with green pepper pieces, to make a pretty pattern. Stir horseradish into remaining gelatin; gradually add to mold and keep mold in ice and water until clear gelatin is sticky and firm.
4. Combine cabbage, potatoes, red pepper, onion and parsley in a large bowl. Blend mayonnaise, yogurt, mustard and salt into the reserved ¾ cup gelatin; fold into potato mixture.
5. Press egg slices into top edge of mold. Spoon cabbage and potato mixture over sticky firm corned beef layer in mold; chill 4 hours, or until firm.
6. Just before serving, run a thin bladed knife around top of mold, then dip mold very quickly in and out of a pan of hot water. Invert onto serving plate; carefully lift off mold.

## MUSHROOMS EN ASPIC

*Savory tomato aspic filled with slices of mushroom means gourmet eating.*

*Makes 6 servings/***25 calories each.**

- 1 can (3 or 4 ounces) sliced mushrooms
- 1 envelope unflavored gelatin
- 1½ cups tomato juice
- 1 tablespoon lemon juice
- 1 teaspoon Worcestershire sauce
- ½ teaspoon celery salt
- ½ teaspoon leaf basil, crumbled
  Watercress
  Cucumber slices

1. Pour mushrooms and liquid into a medium-size bowl; sprinkle gelatin over to soften.
2. Simmer tomato juice, lemon juice, Worcestershire sauce, celery salt and basil in a small saucepan 5 minutes; stir into mushroom mixture until gelatin dissolves.
3. Chill 20 minutes, or until mixture starts to thicken; stir to evenly distribute mushrooms, then spoon into 6 individual molds or custard cups. Chill molds several hours, or overnight, until gelatin is firm.
4. When ready to serve, run a small knife around tops of salads, then dip molds, one at a time, *very quickly*, in and out of a pan of hot water; invert onto centers of 6 salad plates; lift off molds; serve garnished with watercress and sliced cucumbers.

## CHINATOWN SPECIAL

*From San Francisco's Chinatown comes the inspiration for a delightfully different, yet low in calories, vegetable dish.*

*Makes 6 servings/***39 calories each.**

- 1 medium-size onion, sliced
- 3 tablespoons water
- 1 package (10 ounces) frozen San Francisco-style vegetable combination (see Cook's Guide, page 127)
- 2 tablespoons soy sauce
- 1 package (10 ounces) fresh, not frozen, spinach, washed and trimmed

1. Combine onion slices and water in a large saucepan; bring to boiling; cover saucepan; simmer 3 minutes.
2. Remove packet of topping from frozen vegetables. Pour frozen vegetables into saucepan; bring to full boil; separate vegetables with a fork as they begin to thaw.
3. Lower heat; cover saucepan; simmer 2 minutes; add soy sauce and spinach; stir to blend well; cover saucepan.
4. Simmer 3 minutes longer, or until vegetables are crisply tender; spoon into a heated vegetable dish; sprinkle with topping from packet.

## DOUBLE CHEESE PARFAIT

*Top layers of red cabbage, yellow squash and celery with a blend of whipped blue and cottage cheeses. It is pictured on left in inset photo, page 76.*

*Makes 4 servings/***51 calories each.**

- ½ medium-size red cabbage
- 2 medium-size yellow squash
- 3 large stalks celery
  Double Cheese Topping (recipe follows)

1. Wash, quarter and core red cabbage; thinly slice with a sharp knife on a wooden board. Wash and tip squash and shred on largest hole of grater. Wash celery and thinly slice.
2. Evenly divide shredded cabbage in the bottoms of 4 large wine glasses; cover with layer of grated squash; top with sliced celery. Refrigerate until serving time.
3. When ready to serve, top each parfait with 1 tablespoon DOUBLE CHEESE TOPPING.

DOUBLE CHEESE TOPPING: Makes about ¼ cup/**28 calories per tablespoon.** Place ¼ cup cream-style cottage cheese and 1 tablespoon blue cheese in container of electric blender; cover; process at high speed 30 seconds, or until smooth. Refrigerate until serving time.

## PARFAIT FRANÇAISE

*Layered vegetables are an elegant way to open that special meat. Pictured right, inset photo, page 76.*

Makes 4 servings/**47 calories each.**

- 2 stalks Belgian endive
  OR: ¼ medium-size iceberg lettuce
- 4 medium-size carrots
- 2 medium-size spears broccoli
  French Topping (recipe follows)

1. Wash endive and slice thinly, crosswise; place shredded endive in bowl of ice water; set aside. Or, shred lettuce thinly and place in bowl of ice water; set aside.
2. Wash and pare carrots; dice finely, using sharp knife. Wash and stalk broccoli; separate into tiny flowerets.
3. Drain endive or lettuce on paper towels. Divide carrot cubes evenly in the bottoms of 4 large wine glasses; place shredded endive or lettuce over carrots in glasses; place broccoli flowerets over endive. Cover and refrigerate until serving time.
4. When ready to serve, top each parfait with 1 tablespoon FRENCH TOPPING.

FRENCH TOPPING: Makes about ¼ cup/**19 calories per tablespoon.** Place ¼ cup cream-style cottage cheese and 2 tablespoons bottled low calorie French dressing in container of electric blender; cover; process at high speed 30 seconds, or until smooth. Refrigerate until serving time.

## ASPARAGUS ROULADE

*Star of a luncheon. Who would guess it's so low in calories? Photo is on page 76.*

Bake at 325° for 35 minutes.
Makes 8 servings/**253 calories each.**

- ⅓ cup butter or margarine
- ¾ cup all purpose flour
- 1 teaspoon dry mustard
- ½ teaspoon salt
- 3½ cups skim milk
- 4 eggs, separated
- 1 pound fresh asparagus
  OR: 1 package (10 ounces) frozen cut asparagus
- 1 cup boiling water
- 2 teaspoons salt
- 4 wedges process Gruyere cheese, diced

1. Grease a 15x10x1-inch jelly roll pan; line with wax paper; grease paper and dust lightly with flour.
2. Melt butter or margarine in a medium-size saucepan; blend in flour, mustard and salt; cook, stirring constantly, until mixture bubbles; stir in 3 cups of the milk. Cook, stirring constantly, until mixture bubbles 3 minutes and is very thick. Measure 1 cup sauce into a small saucepan; stir in remaining ½ cup milk and reserve.
3. Beat egg whites until they form soft peaks in a medium-size bowl with electric mixer at high speed. Beat egg yolks slightly in a large bowl; beat in remaining hot sauce, a spoonful at a time, until thoroughly blended. Fold in beaten egg whites until no streaks of white remain with a wire whip.
4. Bake in slow oven (325°) 35 minutes, or until golden and top springs back when lightly pressed with fingertip.
5. While omelet bakes, prepare asparagus: Break woody base off each stalk; soak asparagus in salted warm water 5 minutes to remove sand; lift asparagus out of water. Cut fresh or frozen asparagus into 2-inch pieces. Arrange in a large skillet; add boiling water and salt; cover skillet. Bring to boiling; lower heat. Simmer 15 minutes, or until crisply tender; drain.
6. Blend cheese into the 1½ cups sauce in saucepan; heat slowly, stirring constantly, until cheese melts and sauce is smooth.
7. Remove baked omelet from pan this way: Loosen around edges with a spatula; cover with aluminum foil, then place a large cookie sheet or tray on top and quickly turn upside down. Lift off pan; peel off wax paper.
8. Spoon cooked asparagus in a single layer over omelet; drizzle with about 1 cup of the hot cheese sauce. Starting at a short end, roll up, jelly roll fashion, lifting foil as you go to steady and guide roll. Place on heated serving platter.
9. Top with remaining cheese sauce; garnish with mushroom slices poached in water and lemon juice, if you wish.

## OUR FRENCH DRESSING

*Tart and tangy, it makes your salad more distinctive, yet keeps calories under control.*

Makes 1 cup/**18 calories per tablespoon.**

- 1 tablespoon cornstarch
- 1 cup water
- ¼ cup wine vinegar
- 2 tablespoons vegetable or olive oil
- 1 clove garlic, minced
- ¾ teaspoon salt
- ¾ teaspoon paprika
- ¼ teaspoon pepper

1. Mix cornstarch, water, vinegar, oil, garlic, salt, paprika and pepper in a small saucepan.
2. Bring to boiling over low heat, stirring constantly; cook 5 minutes longer, or until dressing thickens. Pour into a glass bowl; cover with plastic wrap; chill at least 2 hours to blend flavors before serving.

## PARFAIT VERDI

*Avocado gives this dish rich taste and texture; spiced yogurt topping adds tang. It's pictured middle, inset photo, page 76.*

Makes 4 servings/**74 calories each.**

- 3 medium-size beets
- 1 medium-size cucumber
  Lemon juice
- ¼ medium-size avocado
  Spicy Yogurt Topping (recipe follows)

1. Pare and trim beets; shred on largest hole of grater into medium-size bowl; cover with cold water; set aside.
2. Wash cucumber and remove ends; score with fork, to give a "cartwheel" effect; slice thinly.
3. Place lemon juice in saucer to cover bottom. Pare avocado section and cut into ½-inch cubes; toss cubes gently with lemon juice in saucer to prevent darkening.
4. Drain beets on paper towels; drain avocado. Divide avocado evenly in bottoms of 4 small wine glasses; cover with layer of shredded beets; top with sliced cucumber. Refrigerate until serving time.
5. When ready to serve, top each parfait with 1 tablespoon SPICY YOGURT TOPPING.

SPICY YOGURT TOPPING: Makes ¼ cup/**8 calories per tablespoon.** Combine ¼ cup plain yogurt, ¼ teaspoon salt and ¼ teaspoon curry powder in small bowl; beat with fork until well blended.

## RATATOUILLE NIÇOISE

*Eggplant and zucchini bubble in an herb-rich tomato sauce—incredible!*

Makes 8 servings/**51 calories each.**

- 1 large onion, chopped (1 cup)
- 1 clove garlic, minced
- 1 tablespoon olive or vegetable oil
- 1 medium-size eggplant, sliced, pared and diced
- 3 medium-size zucchini, tipped and sliced
- 1 can (1 pound) stewed tomatoes
- 2 teaspoons salt
- 1 teaspoon leaf oregano, crumbled
- ½ teaspoon leaf rosemary, crumbled
- ¼ teaspoon lemon pepper
- 1 bay leaf

1. Sauté onion and garlic in oil in a large saucepan until soft. Stir in eggplant, zucchini, tomatoes and liquid, salt, oregano, rosemary, lemon pepper and bay leaf until well blended.
2. Bring to boiling; lower heat; simmer 45 minutes to blend flavors.
COOK'S TIP: Serve hot or cold. It is even more delicious if made ahead and refrigerated overnight.

## STEAMED CELERY CABBAGE

*Celery seeds add a gourmet touch to steamed Chinese cabbage.*

Makes 6 servings/**15 calories each.**

- 1 medium-size head Chinese cabbage
- 1 teaspoon salt
- 1 teaspoon celery seeds

1. Shred cabbage finely; wash; drain.
2. Place in a large skillet. (No need to add water; there is enough clinging to the cabbage.) Sprinkle with salt and celery seeds; cover.
3. Steam 5 minutes, or just until crisply tender. Drain well before serving.

## BITTERS BAKED VEGETABLES

*An exotic ingredient from the West Indies, aromatic bitters, adds flavor to vegetables.*

Bake at 350° for 30 minutes.
Makes 6 servings/**67 calories each.**

- 1 medium-size onion, sliced
- 1 medium-size green pepper, halved, seeded and cut into strips
- 1 tablespoon vegetable oil
- 1 small eggplant, pared and cut into 1½-inch strips
- 1 can (4 ounces) sliced mushrooms
- 1 can (1 pound) tomatoes
- ¼ teaspoon pepper
- ½ teaspoon leaf basil, crumbled
- 1 teaspoon leaf oregano, crumbled
- 1 teaspoon aromatic bitters
- 2 tablespoons grated Parmesan cheese

1. Sauté onion and pepper in oil until soft in large skillet; add eggplant and mushrooms and sauté for 3 minutes.
2. Add tomatoes, pepper, basil, oregano, aromatic bitters and grated cheese; mix thoroughly. Spoon into a 6-cup casserole.
3. Bake in moderate oven (350°) 30 minutes, or until bubbly hot.

## BLUE CHEESE DRESSING

*Spoon on cold poached fish or tuna salad.*

Makes 1 ⅓ cups/**20 calories per tablespoon.**

- 1 container (8 ounces) small curd dry cottage cheese
- 1 envelope blue cheese salad dressing mix
- ½ cup skim milk

1. Place cottage cheese, salad dressing mix and skim milk in container of electric blender; cover. Process at low speed until smooth, scraping sides frequently with rubber scraper.
2. Transfer dressing to covered container; chill 2 hours to blend flavors. Serve on top of mixed salad greens with red onion rings, if you wish.

## MARINATED BEAN BOWL

*Water chestnuts are an oriental contribution to the battle of the bulge. Here they add crunch to canned beans.*

Makes 4 servings/**64 calories each.**

- 1 can (1 pound) sliced green beans, drained
- ½ cup halved cherry tomatoes
- ¼ cup sliced water chestnuts
- ¼ cup bottled low calorie Italian salad dressing
- 2 teaspoons minced onion
- 1 teaspoon dried parsley flakes
- ½ teaspoon leaf basil, crumbled
- 1 small head iceberg lettuce

1. Combine beans, tomatoes and water chestnuts in a medium-size bowl.
2. Combine dressing, onion, parsley and basil in a jar with a tight lid; cover; shake until well blended. Pour dressing over vegetables; cover. Marinate in refrigerator 3 hours.
3. Break lettuce into a salad bowl. Drain vegetables; spoon into bowl.

## COLESLAW RELISH MOLD

*Coleslaw is layered in lemon gelatin with shredded carrots and green peppers.*

Makes 6 servings/**88 calories each.**

- 1 package (3 ounces) lemon flavored gelatin
- 1 envelope unflavored gelatin
- 2 cups boiling water
- 1½ cups cold water
- ½ cup finely shredded green pepper
- 1 cup finely shredded carrot
- ¼ cup imitation mayonnaise
- ¼ teaspoon salt
- 3 tablespoons skim milk
- 4 teaspoons cider vinegar
- 3 cups coarsely shredded cabbage Chicory (curly endive)

1. Dissolve both gelatins in boiling water in a medium-size bowl; stir in cold water. Measure ½ cup gelatin into a 6-cup mold. Place in a pan of ice and water to speed setting. Chill 10 minutes; stir in green pepper. Chill just until sticky and firm.

2. Measure 1 cup of remaining gelatin mixture into a second small bowl; chill until as thick as unbeaten egg white; stir in carrot; spoon over pepper layer. Chill just until sticky and firm.
3. While carrot layer chills, beat mayonnaise, salt, milk and vinegar into remaining gelatin in medium-size bowl; fold in cabbage; spoon over sticky and firm layer in mold. Chill in refrigerator 6 hours, or until firm.
4. To unmold, run a thin bladed sharp tipped knife around edge to loosen, then dip *quickly* in and out of a pan of hot water. Invert onto serving plate; garnish with chicory.

## CITRUS SALAD DRESSING

*Grapefruit juice in the dressing adds tang to a fruit or fish salad.*

Makes 1 ⅓ cups/**21 calories per tablespoon.**

- 2 teaspoons cornstarch
- 1 teaspoon sugar
- ¾ teaspoon salt
- ½ teaspoon paprika
- ½ teaspoon dry mustard
- 1 cup unsweetened grapefruit juice
- 2 tablespoons vegetable oil
- ⅛ teaspoon liquid red pepper seasoning
- ¼ cup catsup

1. Combine cornstarch, sugar, salt, paprika and dry mustard in a small saucepan; stir in grapefruit juice. Bring to boiling over medium heat, stirring constantly. Boil 1 minute; remove from heat.
2. Add oil, red pepper seasoning and catsup; mix well. Chill several hours.

## WINE SALAD DRESSING

*Treat tossed salads to this California-style dieter's dressing.*

Makes 1 ½ cups/**28 calories per tablespoon.**

- ¾ cup dry white or red wine
- ¼ cup olive or vegetable oil
- 2 tablespoons tarragon vinegar
- 1 small onion, finely chopped (¼ cup)
- 1 clove garlic, minced
- 1 teaspoon salt
- ¼ teaspoon lemon pepper

1. Combine wine, oil, vinegar, onion, garlic, salt and pepper in a jar with a screw top; cover tightly; shake until thoroughly mixed.
2. Refrigerate at least 2 hours to blend flavors.

## WEST COAST SALAD BOWL

*It's amazing how fast a salad goes together with a few convenience foods.*

Makes 6 servings/**56 calories each.**

- 4 cups broken iceberg lettuce
- 1 can (1 pound) tomato wedges in tomato juice
- 1 package (9 ounces) frozen artichoke hearts, cooked, drained and chilled
- ½ teaspoon seasoned salt
- ¼ cup packaged rye croutons
- ⅓ cup bottled low calorie Italian salad dressing

1. Place lettuce in a salad bowl. Drain tomatoes, saving juice for another meal. Arrange artichoke hearts and tomato wedges on lettuce. Sprinkle with seasoned salt.
2. Sprinkle salad with croutons; pour dressing over; toss gently.

## SAN FRANCISCO CRAB SALAD

*Serve as an appetizer, California style, or spoon into lettuce cups for a main dish salad.*

Makes 4 appetizer servings/**70 calories each**, OR:
Makes 2 main dish servings/**139 calories each**.

    1 package (6 ounces) frozen crab
      meat, thawed and drained
    ½ cup diced celery
    2 tablespoons bottled low calorie
      Italian dressing
      Dash liquid red pepper seasoning
      Parsley
    4 lemon wedges

1. Cut crab meat into medium-size chunks, carefully removing any bony tissue; add to celery in a small bowl.
2. Sprinkle with salad dressing and red pepper seasoning; toss to mix well. Chill at least 1 hour to blend flavors.
3. Serve in small scallop shell-shape dishes or salad plates; garnish with parsley and lemon wedges.

## STRAWBERRY SALAD BOWL

*You can substitute blueberries, diced apple or pear for the strawberries.*

Makes 4 servings/**31 calories each**.

    6 cups broken mixed salad greens
    1 cup strawberries, washed, hulled,
      and halved
    ¼ cup Tangy Cooked Dressing
      (recipe, page 76)

1. Place greens in a large shallow salad bowl; top with strawberries.
2. Just before serving, drizzle TANGY COOKED DRESSING over; toss lightly to coat well.

## SHANGHAI DRESSING

*Your blender whips this soy flavored dressing to a creamy consistency; it's excellent over bean sprouts, chopped water chestnuts and grated carrots.*

Makes 1¼ cups/**32 calories per tablespoon**.

    ¼ cup soy sauce
    ¼ cup red wine vinegar
    ¼ cup peanut or vegetable oil
    1 clove garlic
    4 teaspoons dry Sherry
    ¼ teaspoon ground ginger
    ½ cup evaporated skim milk

1. Combine soy sauce, wine vinegar, peanut oil, garlic, Sherry and ginger in container of electric blender; cover container; process at high speed until well blended and smooth.
2. Turn off blender; add evaporated skim milk; cover container and process at high speed until smooth and well blended. Refrigerate in covered container before serving.

## MUSHROOMS AND SQUASH

*Vegetables with a Scandinavian flavor—dill gives a spark to zucchini or yellow squash plus mushrooms.*

Makes 6 servings/**33 calories each**.

    ½ pound fresh mushrooms
      OR: 1 can (6 ounces) sliced
      mushrooms
    2 large zucchini or yellow squash
    1 envelope or teaspoon instant
      chicken broth
    1 teaspoon dillweed
    ¾ cup water
    1 tablespoon cornstarch
    2 tablespoons cold water

1. Wipe mushrooms with a damp cloth; slice; place in a large skillet. Or, pour canned mushrooms and liquid into skillet. Tip and slice squash; add to skillet; sprinkle over instant chicken broth and dillweed; add water; cover skillet.
2. Bring to boiling; lower heat; steam 10 minutes, or until vegetables are crisply tender. Blend cornstarch and cold water in a cup until smooth; stir into bubbling vegetables; cook, stirring constantly, 1 minute. Garnish with fresh dill, if you wish.

## TRIPLE VEGETABLE BOWL

*This recipe makes lots, so you can keep any extra for another meal.*

Makes 8 servings/**69 calories each**.

    2 pounds green beans, tipped and
      cut into 1-inch pieces
    4 small yellow squash, trimmed and
      thinly sliced
    5 medium-size tomatoes
    1 envelope cheese-garlic salad
      dressing mix
    1 cup tomato juice
    2 tablespoons chopped parsley

1. Cook beans, covered, in boiling salted water in a medium-size saucepan 15 minutes, or until tender; drain. Place beans in a shallow dish.
2. Cook squash, covered, in small amount of boiling salted water in a medium-size saucepan 5 minutes, or until crisply tender; drain well. Place squash in a second shallow dish.
3. Peel tomatoes and cut out stem ends; cut each into ¼-inch thick slices. Place tomatoes in a third shallow dish.
4. Prepare salad dressing mix with tomato juice; add parsley and shake to mix well. Pour over vegetables, dividing evenly among dishes; cover. Chill at least an hour to season and blend flavors.
5. When ready to serve, spoon squash, then tomato slices, then beans into a shallow serving bowl.

## YOGURT COLESLAW

*Celery seeds and yogurt give crisp green cabbage a sparkling flavor.*

Makes 4 servings/**33 calories each**.

    ½ cup plain yogurt
    1 teaspoon cider vinegar
    2 teaspoons sugar
    1 teaspoon celery seeds
    ½ teaspoon salt
    ⅛ teaspoon pepper
    4 cups finely shredded
      cabbage

1. Combine yogurt, vinegar, sugar and celery seeds in a medium-size bowl; stir in salt and pepper.
2. Add the cabbage; mix until well blended. Cover with plastic wrap; chill several hours or overnight.

## BARBECUED EGGPLANT SLICES

*Crumb-coated slices of eggplant make a delicious vegetable.*

Makes 8 slices/**56 calories each**.

    1 large eggplant
    2 tablespoons vegetable or olive oil
    2 tablespoons lemon juice
    ¼ teaspoon liquid red pepper
      seasoning
    ½ teaspoon salt
    2 tablespoons fine dry bread
      crumbs

1. Cut unpared eggplant into ¾-inch slices.
2. Combine oil, lemon juice, red pepper seasoning and salt in a cup. Brush eggplant slices with mixture on rack of broiler pan.
3. Broil, 4 inches from heat, 5 to 7 minutes. Turn and brush with remaining seasoning mixture. Broil 5 minutes. Sprinkle with crumbs; cook 2 minutes, or until crumbs are golden. Keep eggplant slices warm by covering with a sheet of aluminum foil.

## BAKED CORN ON THE COB

*Fresh or frozen corn tastes butter-rich with our cooking trick.*

Bake at 350° for 20 minutes.
Makes 6 servings/**87 calories each**.

    6 ears of corn, shucked
      OR: 3 packages frozen corn on
      the cob, thawed
    6 teaspoons diet margarine
    ½ teaspoon butter flavored salt
    ⅛ teaspoon coarsely ground pepper

1. Spread 1 teaspoon margarine on each ear; place ears on double thickness of aluminum foil. Season with salt and pepper. Wrap securely.
2. Bake in moderate oven (350°) 20 minutes, or until kernels are tender.

## SHRIMP STUFFED MUSHROOMS

*If you can't find big mushrooms, simply pile mixture into smaller mushrooms. The photograph is on page 85.*

Bake at 350° for 15 minutes.
Makes 4 servings/**116 calories each.**

- 4 very large mushrooms
    OR: ½ pound mushrooms
- 1 teaspoon or envelope instant chicken broth
- 1 package (8 ounces) frozen shelled raw deveined shrimp, thawed
- 1 tablespoon diet margarine
- 1 tablespoon finely chopped onion
- 1 cup saltine cracker crumbs
- ¼ teaspoon finely chopped parsley
- ½ teaspoon salt
- ¼ teaspoon lemon pepper

1. Wipe mushrooms with a damp cloth; remove stems and save for another dish. Place mushroom caps in a medium-size skillet with instant chicken broth and 1 cup water; bring to boiling; lower heat; simmer 5 minutes, basting mushrooms with broth several times; drain mushrooms on paper towels; reserve poaching liquid.
2. Sauté shrimp in diet margarine in a large nonstick skillet; push to one side; sauté onion in same pan 2 minutes; stir in cracker crumbs, parsley, salt and pepper until well blended.
3. Arrange mushrooms, hollow-side up, in a 6-cup baking dish. Spoon mixture into poached mushrooms, dividing evenly. Pour a thin layer of reserved mushroom poaching liquid into baking dish.
4. Bake in moderate oven (350°) 15 minutes, basting mushrooms several times with poaching liquid, or until piping hot.

## HAM AND POTATO BOATS

*Meat and potato eaters, don't despair—even on a diet you can enjoy these favorites, when you follow this recipe. Photo is on page 85.*

Bake at 400° for 1 hour,
then at 350° for 15 minutes.
Makes 4 servings/**225 calories each.**

- 2 large potatoes (12 ounces each)
    Creamed Curry Sauce (recipe follows)
- 1 cup diced cooked ham
- 1 cup frozen peas (from a 1-pound bag), cooked and drained
    Paprika

1. Scrub potatoes well with a stiff brush; wipe dry with paper towel. Place on small cookie sheet.
2. Bake in hot oven (400°) 1 hour, or until potatoes are tender when pierced with a two-tined fork; split potatoes in half, lengthwise; scoop out potato

and mash or press through potato ricer into a medium-size bowl.
3. While potatoes bake, make CREAMED CURRY SAUCE.
4. Add CREAMED CURRY SAUCE, cooked ham and peas to bowl; stir to blend well. Pile mixture into potato shells, dividing evenly; sprinkle with paprika. Place on cookie sheet.
4. Bake in moderate oven (350°) 15 minutes, or until piping hot. Place on hot serving plates.

CREAMED CURRY SAUCE: Makes 1 cup/**16 calories per tablespoon.** Melt 2 tablespoons diet margarine in a small saucepan; stir in 1 teaspoon curry powder and cook 1 minute; add 1 tablespoon finely chopped onion; sauté 2 minutes; blend in 2 tablespoons all purpose flour and cook 2 minutes. Stir in 1 cup skim milk, ½ teaspoon salt and a dash of pepper. Cook, stirring constantly, until mixture thickens and bubbles 3 minutes.

## TUNA STUFFED SQUASH

*Yellow squash or zucchini work equally well in this hearty main dish. Photograph on page 83 shows yellow squash.*

Bake at 375° for 20 minutes.
Makes 4 servings/**218 calories each.**

- 2 medium-size yellow squash or zucchini
- 1 cup cooked rice
- 1 can (6½ ounces) water packed tuna, drained and flaked
- ½ cup diced red pepper
- 1 envelope (4 to a package) instant cream of chicken soup
- ¾ cup boiling water
- 1 tablespoon lemon juice
- 2 slices mozzarella cheese (from an 8-ounce package)

1. Halve squash lengthwise; place, cut-side down, in a large skillet; add water to a depth of ½ inch; cover skillet; bring to boiling; lower heat; cook 5 minutes.
2. Remove squash halves from skillet with pancake turner and drain on paper towels until cool enough to handle. Scoop out seeds with a teaspoon; drain on paper towels.
3. Combine rice, tuna and red pepper in a medium-size bowl. Prepare instant chicken soup with boiling water, following label directions; stir in lemon juice; pour over tuna mixture; stir until well blended.
4. Spoon mixture into squash shells, dividing evenly. Place in an 8-cup shallow baking dish.
5. Bake in moderate oven (350°) 15 minutes; cut mozzarella cheese into strips; arrange over shells. Bake 5 minutes longer, or until cheese melts.

## GOLDEN TOMATO CUPS

*Cream puff batter bakes on top of broccoli-stuffed tomatoes. Do plan to serve this at your next luncheon. Photo is on page 85.*

Bake at 400° for 25 minutes.
Makes 6 servings/**91 calories each.**

- 6 medium-size firm tomatoes
- 1 package (10 ounces) frozen broccoli
- ¼ cup water
- 2 tablespoons butter or margarine
- ¼ cup all purpose flour
- ⅛ teaspoon salt
- 1 egg
- ½ teaspoon salt
- ¼ teaspoon leaf oregano, crumbled

1. Cut off tops of tomatoes; scoop out insides with a teaspoon. Turn cups upside down to drain. (Use pulp to season soup or stew.)
2. Cook broccoli, following label directions; drain. Keep hot.
3. Bring water and butter or margarine to boiling in a small saucepan. Add flour and the ⅛ teaspoon salt all at once; stir vigorously with a wooden spoon about 2 minutes, or until batter forms a thick smooth ball that follows spoon around pan. Remove from heat at once; cool slightly.
4. Beat in egg until mixture is thick and shiny smooth.
5. Sprinkle tomato cups with the ½ teaspoon salt and oregano; fill with hot cooked broccoli.
6. Spread about 1 tablespoon batter over broccoli in each tomato, then spoon remaining batter, dividing evenly, in a mound on top. Place tomatoes in a shallow baking dish.
7. Bake in hot oven (400°) 25 minutes, or until topping is puffed and lightly golden.

## FISH IN SPINACH NESTS

*Savory fish fillets are surrounded with herbed spinach leaves, then crowned with carrot purée. Photo is on page 85.*

Makes 4 servings/**165 calories each.**

- Florida Baked Fillets (recipe, page 105)
- 4 large carrots, pared and sliced
- 1 teaspoon sugar
- 1 teaspoon lemon juice
    Salt and pepper
- 2 packages (10 ounces each) fresh, not frozen, spinach
- ½ teaspoon leaf marjoram, crumbled

1. Prepare FLORIDA BAKED FILLETS; keep warm.
2. Cook carrots in salted boiling water with sugar 10 minutes, or until tender; drain, reserving cooking liquid. Place carrots in container of electric blender; cover; process until

smooth, adding a little cooking liquid, if necessary. Return carrot purée to saucepan; stir in lemon juice; taste and season with salt and pepper; keep hot.

3. Wash spinach well; remove stems; place in a large kettle with water clinging to leaves. Season with marjoram, salt and pepper; cover kettle; bring to boiling over high heat; turn off heat; allow to stand *covered* for 3 minutes.

4. Place FLORIDA BAKED FILLETS in four individual serving dishes; arrange a ring of spinach leaves around fish, dividing evenly; spoon carrot purée over fish, coating fish.

## CREAMED SPINACH

*Using the vegetable cooking water to make a sauce is nutritionally wise—it's lower in calories, too.*

Makes 4 servings/**62 calories each.**

2 packages (10 ounces each) frozen chopped spinach
1 tablespoon all purpose flour
½ teaspoon salt
¼ teaspoon ground nutmeg
¼ cup water

1. Place blocks of frozen spinach, side by side, in a medium-size skillet. Sprinkle with flour, salt and nutmeg; pour in water.

2. Heat slowly, breaking up spinach with a fork, just until thawed; then cook 1 minute, or until hot.

3. Stir with wooden spoon until mixture thickens and bubbles 3 minutes.

## ORIENTAL VEGETABLE BOWL

*Start with one of the new frozen vegetable combinations and serve a sensational dish in minutes.*

Makes 4 servings/**36 calories each.**

4 green onions, cut into 1/2-inch pieces
3 tablespoons water
1 package (10 ounces) frozen Japanese-style vegetable combination (see Cook's Guide, page 127)
1 tablespoon soy sauce
1 cup shredded lettuce

1. Combine green onions and water in a medium-size saucepan; bring to boiling; cover saucepan; simmer 3 minutes.

2. Remove seasoning pouch from frozen vegetables. Pour frozen vegetables into saucepan; cover; cook 2 minutes; add seasonings from pouch and soy sauce.

3. Mix to blend well; cook, stirring constantly, 30 seconds, or until sauce thickens. Stir in shredded lettuce just before serving.

## KRAUT VEGETABLE SALAD

*Tangy sauerkraut teams with carrots, cucumber, onion and red or green pepper for a colorful supper salad.*

Makes 4 servings/**78 calories each.**

1 can (1 pound) sauerkraut, well drained
1 cup grated carrot
1 cup chopped cucumber
1 medium-size red onion, thinly sliced
½ cup chopped red or green pepper
⅓ cup bottled low calorie Italian salad dressing
1 teaspoon leaf oregano, crumbled

1. Combine sauerkraut, carrot, cucumber, onion and red or green pepper in a medium-size bowl.

2. Drizzle Italian dressing and oregano over; toss to coat evenly. Serve at room temperature or chill before serving.

## DIET DO'S

• When dining in a restaurant, order roasts, plain meats or broiled chicken or fish rather than dishes with sauce or gravy.

• Choose a low calorie white wine rather than a high calorie cocktail as your appetizer.

• For dessert, choose plain fruit or small wedge of cheese.

• Don't ask your hostess to provide special diet foods for you. Instead, eat small portions of whatever you are served.

• If you use less than the total of your calorie budget in any day, do *not* make up for it the next day. If you plan to dine out, save part of your calorie allowance from other meals to add to your dinner allowance.

## CRAB FILLED ARTICHOKES

*Whole artichokes make pretty, as well as delicious, containers for flavorful crab and crumb filling. Shown on page 85.*

Bake at 350° for 15 minutes.
Makes 4 servings/**114 calories each.**

2 slices white bread
1 tablespoon diet margarine
1 package (6 ounces) frozen King crab, thawed and broken into small pieces
½ teaspoon salt
¼ teaspoon seasoned pepper
½ teaspoon lemon rind
Marinated Artichokes (recipe, page 112)

1. Break bread into quarters; place, 4 quarters at a time, in container of electric blender; cover container; process at high speed 15 seconds, or

until crumbed. Pour into a large skillet. (Or, break bread into crumbs with a fork on a wooden board.)

2. Heat skillet slowly, stirring crumbs constantly, until golden brown; add margarine; toss until evenly blended; remove from heat.

3. Stir in crab meat, salt, pepper and lemon rind until well blended.

4. Open MARINATED ARTICHOKES and fill centers with crab mixture, dividing evenly; place in an 8-cup shallow baking dish.

5. Bake in moderate oven (350°) 15 minutes, or until piping hot. Serve with lemon wedges, if you wish.

## APPLE AND KRAUT BAKE

*Here's a fragrant side dish for broiled franks or lean pork loin.*

Bake at 350° for 40 minutes.
Makes 8 servings/**42 calories each.**

1 can (1 pound, 11 ounces) sauerkraut, drained
1 envelope or teaspoon instant beef broth
1 medium-size onion, chopped (½ cup)
1 cup unsweetened applesauce
2 teaspoons caraway seeds

1. Drain sauerkraut; rinse in cold water. Drain well.

2. Combine sauerkraut, beef broth, onion, applesauce and caraway seeds in an 8-cup baking dish. Cover.

3. Bake in a moderate oven (350°) 40 minutes, or until bubbly.

## CUCUMBER CRISPS

*Overnight chilling in ice water keeps the cucumbers crunchy.*

Makes 4 cups/**17 calories per ¼ cup.**

2 medium-size cucumbers, sliced, but not pared (about 2 cups)
2 large red onions, thinly sliced (about 2 cups)
2 teaspoons salt
½ cup white vinegar
½ cup water
2 tablespoons sugar
¼ cup chopped fresh dill

1. Mix cucumbers, onions and salt in a large glass or ceramic bowl; pour in ice water to cover; cover with plastic wrap. Let stand overnight in refrigerator.

2. Drain vegetables well.

3. Bring vinegar, water and sugar to boiling, stirring constantly, in a medium-size saucepan; stir in dill; pour over vegetables; stir to mix well. Cover bowl with plastic wrap.

4. Allow to stand in refrigerator at least 2 days to develop flavor before serving.

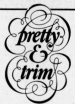

*pretty & trim*

| | | |
|---|---|---|
| **7** | **8** | **9** |
| **386 CALORIES** | **399 CALORIES** | **382 CALORIES** |
| 1 cup Beef Broth<br>Puffy Italian Omelet*<br>Steamed Frozen Artichoke<br>Hearts marinated with<br>Low Calorie Italian Dressing<br>1 cup cubed Watermelon<br>1 cup Skim Milk<br>Black Coffee | Crab Filled Artichokes*<br>Hard Cooked Egg Slices on<br>Leaf Lettuce with<br>Blue Cheese Dressing*<br>1 cup Grapefruit and<br>Orange Sections<br>1 cup Skim Milk<br>Spiced Tea | Oven Fried Fish*<br>Skillet Okra and Tomatoes*<br>Diced Red and Green Peppers,<br>Onion Rings with<br>Lemon Juice<br>1/6 Wedge Honeydew<br>1 cup Skim Milk<br>Black Coffee |
| **436 CALORIES** | **443 CALORIES** | **414 CALORIES** |
| Serve:<br>1 thin slice<br>Italian Bread with<br>Puffy Italian Omelet | Start with:<br>1 cup Tomato Juice<br>sprinkled with<br>Chopped Dill | Serve:<br>¼ cup Spicy Yogurt Topping*<br>over the<br>Oven Fried Fish |
| **486 CALORIES** | **493 CALORIES** | **480 CALORIES** |
| Spread:<br>1½ teaspoons<br>Butter or Margarine on Bread | Serve:<br>2 Seasoned Rye Wafers<br>with Crab Filled Artichokes | Start with:<br>Southern Cream Soup*<br>Topped with Chopped Parsley |
| **10** | **11** | **12** |
| **400 CALORIES** | **379 CALORIES** | **397 CALORIES** |
| Golden Tomato Cups*<br>Cold Sliced Chicken Breast<br>(4 thin slices)<br>Mixed Greens with<br>Lemon Dressing*<br>Jeweled Melon Wedges*<br>1 cup Skim Milk<br>Spiced Tea | Aloha Lamburgers*<br>Steamed Celery Cabbage*<br>Carrot Curls<br>Celery Sticks<br>Radish Roses<br>Harlequin Parfait*<br>¾ cup Skim Milk<br>Ice Coffee | Chilled Cucumber Soup*<br>Cape Cod Scallop Salad*<br>½ cup Fruit Cup that includes<br>Pineapple, Watermelon<br>and Cantaloupe with<br>2 tablespoons Orange Juice<br>1 cup Skim Milk<br>Ice Tea |
| **450 CALORIES** | **439 CALORIES** | **444 CALORIES** |
| Start with:<br>½ cup chilled Orange Juice<br>garnished with<br>Orange Slice | Serve:<br>1 Small Boiled Potato<br>with<br>Aloha Lamburgers | Serve:<br>2 Soda Crackers with<br>Chilled Cucumber Soup or<br>Cape Cod Scallop Salad |
| **490 CALORIES** | **489 CALORIES** | **489 CALORIES** |
| Add:<br>Steamed Sliced Carrots with<br>Chopped Celery Leaves | Top:<br>Potato with<br>1 tablespoon Diet Margarine | Spread:<br>1 tablespoon Cream Cheese<br>onto Crackers |

*See Recipe Index for page number.

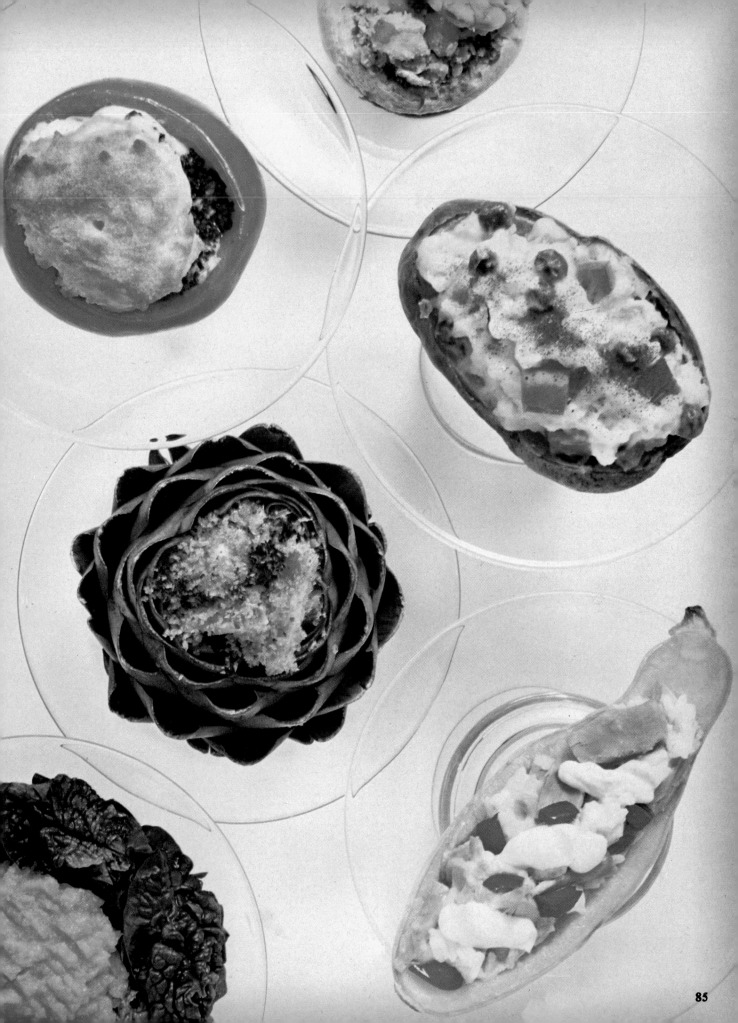

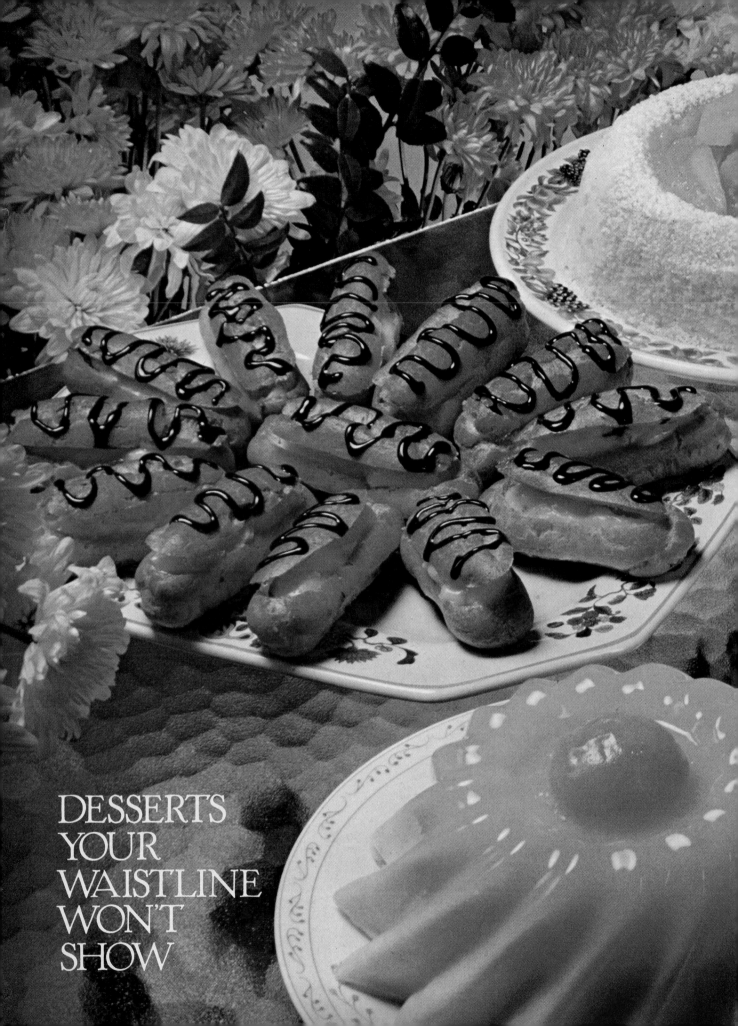

DESSERTS
YOUR
WAISTLINE
WON'T
SHOW

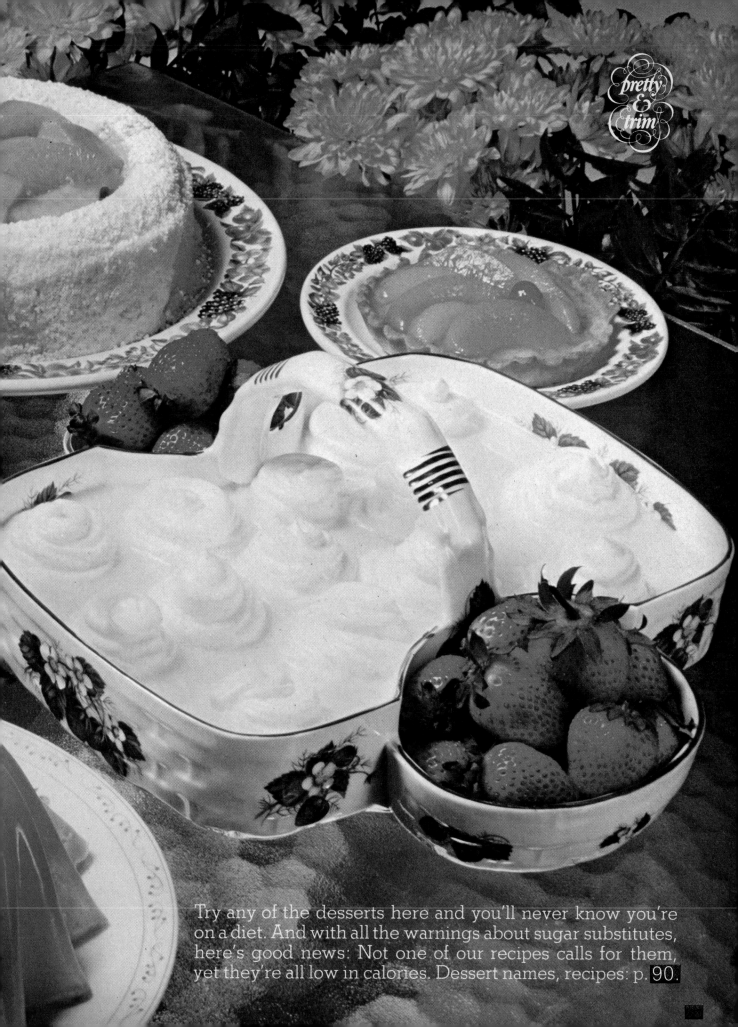

Try any of the desserts here and you'll never know you're on a diet. And with all the warnings about sugar substitutes, here's good news: Not one of our recipes calls for them, yet they're all low in calories. Dessert names, recipes: p. 90.

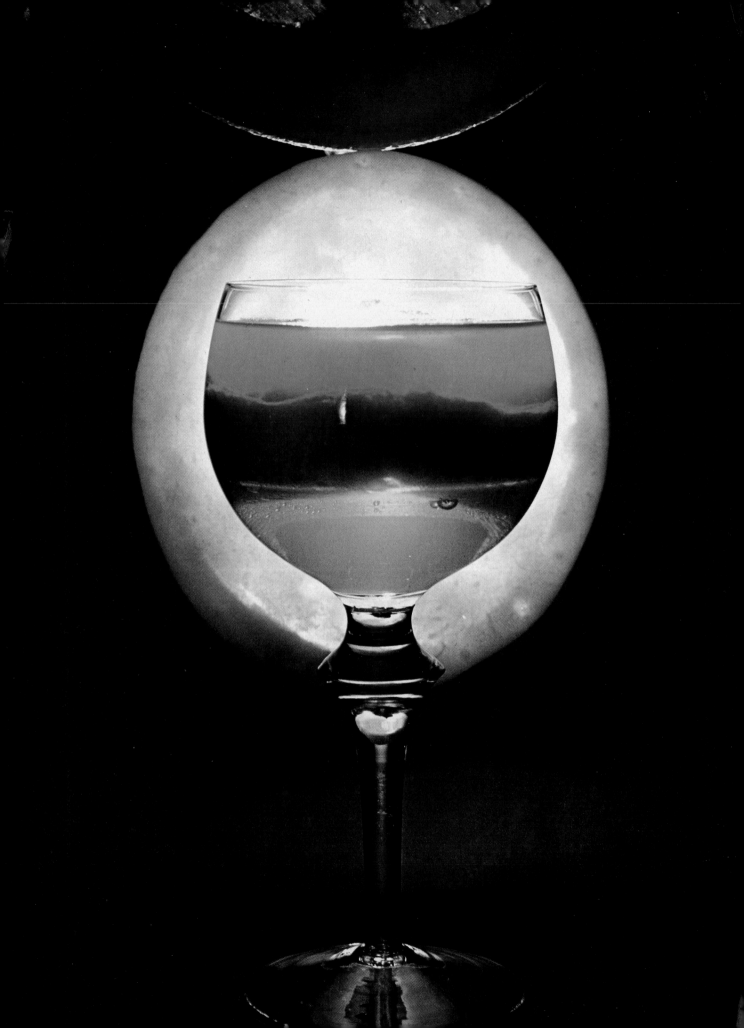

**COLORFUL** Harlequin Parfait and Jeweled Melon Wedges are musts in your collection of diet desserts. The recipes on page 91 will show you how surprisingly easy they are to put together—simply setting gelatin inside a melon gives you the wedges; mixing fruit juices with gelatin produces the parfait. See page 91

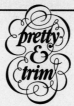

pretty & trim

| 1 | 2 | 3 |
|---|---|---|
| **301 CALORIES** | **300 CALORIES** | **263 CALORIES** |
| ½ cup Fresh Strawberries sprinkled with 10X Powdered Sugar<br>Omelet with Chives*<br>Ham "Bacon"*<br>1 slice White Toast<br>1 teaspoon Strawberry Jam<br>Tea with Lemon | ½ cup Orange Sections in own Orange Juice<br>Fluffy Coconut Pancakes*<br>(Made with cottage cheese.)<br>topped with<br>Honey Lemon Syrup*<br>Black Coffee or<br>Tea with Lemon | ¾ cup Orange Juice<br>Tropical Breakfast Blend*<br>(This is Breakfast-In-A-Glass with juice, cereal and yogurt all blended in a quick-to-fix drink.)<br>Black Coffee or<br>Tea with Lemon |
| **336 CALORIES** | **360 CALORIES** | **333 CALORIES** |
| Pour:<br>½ cup Skim Milk<br>over the<br>Fresh Strawberries | Top Orange Sections with:<br>½ cup Plain Yogurt<br>mixed with<br>¼ teaspoon Cinnamon | Add:<br>1 slice<br>Whole Wheat, Rye or<br>Pumpernickel Toast |
| **386 CALORIES** | **410 CALORIES** | **386 CALORIES** |
| Serve:<br>1½ teaspoons<br>Butter or Margarine on Toast | Serve:<br>1 slice<br>Crisp Bacon with Pancakes | Spread:<br>1½ teaspoons<br>Butter or Margarine on Toast |
| **4** | **5** | **6** |
| **324 CALORIES** | **287 CALORIES** | **309 CALORIES** |
| ¾ cup Orange Juice<br>Apple French Toast*<br>topped with<br>¼ cup Cottage Cheese<br>and served with<br>Spicy Apple Syrup*<br>Black Coffee or<br>Tea with Lemon | ½ cup Tomato Juice<br>Crunch-Topped Egg Cups*<br>1 slice Toasted Protein Bread<br>1 teaspoon Marmalade<br>or Strawberry Preserves<br>¾ cup Skim Milk<br>Black Coffee or<br>Tea with Lemon | Plums Devonshire*<br>(Calories reduced plums poached in spice and topped with a low calorie version of Devonshire Cream.)<br>1 Slice Whole Wheat Toast<br>1½ teaspoons Diet Margarine<br>Black Coffee or Tea with Lemon |
| **351 CALORIES** | **337 CALORIES** | **364 CALORIES** |
| Sprinkle:<br>1 tablespoon<br>Sugar and Honey Wheat Germ<br>over Cottage Cheese | Spread Toast with:<br>1½ teaspoons<br>Butter or Margarine or<br>2 teaspoons Cream Cheese | Add:<br>½ cup<br>freshly squeezed<br>Orange Juice |
| **401 CALORIES** | **387 CALORIES** | **399 CALORIES** |
| Serve:<br>1 slice Crisp Bacon with<br>Apple French Toast | Serve:<br>½ cup Corn Flakes with<br>part of the Skim Milk | Substitute:<br>1 cup Skim Milk<br>for Orange Juice |

*See Recipe Index for page number.

Shown clockwise on pages 86-87: Daffodil Cake Ring, filled with Spiced Fruits; Fruit Tart, made with fruit in its own natural juice; Berry Floating Island, light with little puffs of meringue swimming on custard; Apricot Mold made with apricot halves and unflavored gelatin; Chocolate Eclairs, as rich as the original version, but with half the calories. Recipes start on this page.

## DESSERT RECIPES

### DAFFODIL CAKE RING

*A dream come true for dieters, this cake is as pretty to look at as it's low in calories. Photo is on page 87.*

Bake at 325° for 30 minutes.
Makes 10 servings/**133 calories each.**

- ¾ cup cake flour
- ½ teaspoon salt
- 3 eggs, separated
- ½ teaspoon cream of tartar
- ⅔ cup granulated sugar
- 1 teaspoon vanilla
- 3 tablespoons hot water
- 1 teaspoon orange extract
- 1 tablespoon 10X (confectioners' powdered) sugar
- Spiced Fruits (recipe follows)

1. Sift cake flour and salt together onto wax paper.
2. Beat egg whites with cream of tartar until foamy white and double in volume in large bowl of electric mixer at high speed. Beat in ⅓ cup of the granulated sugar, 1 tablespoon at a time, until meringue stands in firm peaks; beat in vanilla.
3. Sprinkle 2 tablespoons of the flour mixture over meringue; fold in completely with wire whip. Repeat with 4 tablespoons more flour mixture; reserve remaining flour mixture.
4. Beat egg yolks with hot, *not* boiling, water until very thick and light lemon color in small bowl of electric mixer at high speed. Beat in remaining ⅓ cup granulated sugar, 1 tablespoon at a time, until mixture is creamy and thick; beat in orange extract.
5. Sprinkle 2 tablespoons of the remaining flour mixture over top of egg yolk mixture; fold in completely. Repeat with remaining flour mixture.
6. Spoon batters, alternating spoonfuls of white and yellow, into an ungreased 9-inch ring mold. (Do not stir batters in pan.)
7. Bake in slow oven (325°) 30 minutes, or until cake is golden and top springs back when lightly pressed

with fingertip.
8. Turn cake in pan upside down on a wire rack; cool completely. When ready to unmold, loosen around edge and center with a sharp knife; invert onto a serving plate. Sprinkle 10X sugar over top.
9. Spoon SPICED FRUITS into center just before serving.

### SPICED FRUITS

Makes 2½ cups/**37 calories for each ½ cup.**

- 1 California orange, pared and sectioned
- 1 fresh peach, pared, halved and sliced
- 1 cup diced cantaloupe
- ¼ cup orange juice
- ½ teaspoon ground ginger

Combine orange sections, peach slices and cantaloupe in a medium-size bowl; add orange juice and ground ginger; toss to coat evenly. Cover bowl with plastic wrap. Chill at least 1 hour to blend flavors.

### FRUIT TARTS

*Pretty enough for a French pâtisserie shop! Picture is on page 87.*

Bake at 400° for 10 minutes.
Makes 8 servings/**159 calories each.**

- Low Calorie Pastry (recipe follows)
- 1 package (3 ounces) Neufchâtel cheese
- 1 tablespoon lemon juice
- 1 can (16 ounces) calories reduced fruits for salad
- 1 tablespoon cornstarch
- ¼ teaspoon ground nutmeg
- 1 teaspoon grated lemon rind

1. Prepare LOW CALORIE PASTRY, following directions for tart shells. Place shells on a large cookie sheet.
2. Bake in hot oven (400°) 10 minutes, or until pastry is golden; cool in tart pans on wire rack 10 minutes; loosen pastry around edges with tip of knife; remove shells; cool completely on wire rack.
3. Blend Neufchâtel cheese and lemon juice until smooth in a small bowl; spread over bottom of tart shells, dividing evenly.
4. Drain fruits for salad, reserving syrup. Cut pear and peach slices into thinner slices; arrange fruits, in a pretty pattern, over cheese layer in tarts, dividing evenly.
5. Blend ¾ cup of the reserved fruit syrup into cornstarch until smooth in a small saucepan; stir in nutmeg and lemon rind. Cook, stirring constantly, until mixture thickens and bubbles 1 minute; spoon glaze over fruits in tarts to coat evenly. Chill tarts until serving time.

### LOW CALORIE PASTRY

*Even pie is possible, if you use our crust.*

Makes one 9-inch pie shell, or 8 servings/**100 calories each.**

- 1 cup all purpose flour
- ½ teaspoon salt
- ¼ cup (½ stick) margarine
- 2½ tablespoons ice water

1. Sift ½ cup of the flour and salt into a medium-size bowl; cut in margarine with a pastry blender until mixture is crumbly, then blend in remaining ½ cup flour until crumbly.
2. Sprinkle ice water over, 1 tablespoon at a time; mix lightly with a fork just until pastry holds together and leaves side of bowl clean.
3. Shape dough into a ball; place between two pieces of wax paper; roll dough to a 12-inch round; peel off top paper; invert dough into 9-inch pie plate; peel off wax paper.
4. Trim edge to ½-inch; turn under; flute edge.

TART SHELLS: Makes 8 three-inch tarts. Divide dough into 8 portions. Roll each portion between wax paper into a 4-inch round; press into a 3-inch tart shell. Arrange tart pans on cookie sheet for ease in handling.

### SHERRY SPANISH CREAM

*A smooth Spanish cream can be part of your diet plan, when you follow this smooth and rich-tasting recipe.*

Makes 8 servings/**90 calories each.**

- 3 eggs, separated
- 1½ cups skim milk
- 1 envelope unflavored gelatin
- ¼ cup dry Sherry
- ¼ cup sugar

1. Beat egg yolks and milk until smooth with a wire whip in a medium-size saucepan; sprinkle gelatin over.
2. Cook over low heat, stirring constantly, until mixture thickens slightly and coats a metal spoon. Pour into a large bowl; stir in Sherry. Chill until as thick as unbeaten egg white.
3. Beat egg whites until foamy white and double in volume in small bowl of electric mixer at high speed. Beat in sugar, 1 tablespoon at a time, until meringue stands in soft peaks. Fold into chilled gelatin mixture. Spoon into a 4-cup mold. Chill 4 hours, or until firm.
4. Just before serving, loosen mold around edge with a knife; dip mold *very quickly* in and out of hot water. Shake mold gently to loosen. Cover with a serving plate; turn upside down; gently lift off mold. Garnish with mint or fresh berries, if you wish.

## JEWELED MELON WEDGES

*Shimmering gelatin nestled in melon wedges —almost too pretty to be eaten. Try different melon and gelatin combinations as new varieties of melon come into season. Photo on page 88.*

Makes 8 servings/**44 calories each.**

- 1¾ cups water
- 4 whole cloves
- 4 whole allspice
- ¼ cup sugar
- 1 envelope unflavored gelatin
- 3 tablespoons lime juice
  Green food coloring

1. Cut a 1½-inch circle into stem end of melon with a sharp paring knife; remove seeds from melon by running a long thin knife around inside of melon and turning upside down and shaking; invert melon into a bowl and drain while preparing gelatin.
2. Heat water to boiling with whole cloves and allspice; simmer 5 minutes; remove spice.
3. Combine sugar and gelatin in a cup until well blended; stir into saucepan until gelatin dissolves. Pour into a medium-size metal bowl; stir in lime juice and a few drops green food coloring.
4. Chill gelatin in freezer, stirring several times, 30 minutes, or until gelatin is syrupy. Stand melon, hole-side up, in bowl; pour gelatin into melon, filling to top; replace cut-out piece of melon. Pour any remaining gelatin into a dessert dish for another dessert.
5. Chill melon 6 hours, or until firm; cut into wedges with a large sharp knife.

## CHOCOLATE ECLAIRS

*Even classic pastry tray treats can be on your diet menu, when you have the right recipe. Shown on page 86.*

Bake at 400° for 30 minutes.
Makes 20 eclairs/**81 calories each.**

- ½ cup water
- ¼ cup (½ stick) butter or margarine
- ½ cup all purpose flour
- ⅛ teaspoon salt
- 2 eggs
- ¼ cup all purpose flour
- ¼ cup sugar
- 2 cups skim milk
- 2 teaspoons vanilla
- 1 teaspoon brandy extract
- 1 tablespoon butter or margarine
- 1 tablespoon corn syrup
- 1 tablespoon water
- ¼ cup semi-sweet chocolate pieces (from a 6-ounce bag)

1. Heat the ½ cup water and the ¼ cup butter or margarine to boiling in a medium-size saucepan. Stir in the ½ cup flour and salt all at once with a wooden spoon; continue stirring vigorously about 2 minutes, or until batter forms a thick smooth ball that follows spoon around pan.
2. Remove from heat; cool slightly; beat in eggs, one at a time, until mixture is thick and shiny smooth.
3. Pack mixture into a pastry bag fitted with a #4 plain tip; pipe into 3-inch strips, about 1 inch apart, on ungreased cookie sheets.
4. Bake in hot oven (400°) 30 minutes, or until puffed and lightly golden. Remove at once from cookie sheets; cool completely on wire racks.
5. Combine the ¼ cup flour and sugar in a medium-size saucepan; stir in milk until smooth. Cook, stirring constantly, until mixture thickens and bubbles 3 minutes; stir in vanilla and brandy extract; cover surface with plastic wrap; chill.
6. Cut a slice across top of each eclair and lift off. Scoop out any bits of soft dough from bottoms with tip of teaspoon. Fill each with one rounded tablespoon pudding. Return tops to eclairs.
7. Combine the 1 tablespoon butter or margarine, corn syrup and the 1 tablespoon water in a small saucepan. Bring to boiling; remove from heat. Stir in chocolate pieces until melted; beat over a bowl of ice and water until stiff enough to drizzle over eclairs. Drizzle coating from back of teaspoon onto eclairs.

## APRICOT MOLD

*Pretty enough for a party, yet it takes so little time to make. Photo on page 87.*

Makes 8 servings/**58 calories each.**

- 1 envelope unflavored gelatin
- ½ cup cold water
- 1 can (16 ounces) calories reduced apricot halves
- 2 egg whites
- ⅛ teaspoon salt
- 2 tablespoons sugar
- ½ cup evaporated skim milk, whipped

1. Sprinkle gelatin over cold water in a small saucepan; stir until gelatin softens; heat, stirring constantly, until gelatin dissolves.
2. Drain apricots and reserve an apricot half for garnish, if you wish. Place remaining apricot halves in container of an electric blender; pour gelatin mixture over; cover blender; process at high speed until mixture is smooth, about 30 seconds.
3. Beat egg whites with salt until foamy white and double in volume in a medium-size bowl with electric mixer at high speed; gradually beat in sugar until well blended.
4. Fold in apricot mixture until smooth with a wire whip; fold in whipped evaporated milk until well blended. Spoon into a 6 cup fancy mold. Chill 4 hours, or until firm.
5. Just before serving, run a thin bladed knife around top of mold; then dip mold *very quickly* in and out of a pan of hot water. Invert onto serving plate; lift off mold. Top with apricot.
COOK'S TIP: To whip evaporated skim milk, place milk in a small deep bowl with electric mixer beaters. Freeze 15 minutes, or until milk begins to freeze around edge. Beat with electric mixer at high speed until stiff.

## HARLEQUIN PARFAITS

*Layers of whipped and clear wine-flavored gelatin are truly a dieter's delight. Photograph is on page 88.*

Makes 8 servings/**56 calories each.**

- 3⅓ cups water
- 1 3-inch piece stick cinnamon
- 6 whole cloves
- 6 allspice
- ½ cup sugar
- 2 envelopes unflavored gelatin
- ⅓ cup dry white wine
- 2 tablespoons lime juice
  Green, yellow and red food coloring
- 2 tablespoons orange juice
- 2 tablespoons lemon juice

1. Combine 2 cups of the water, cinnamon, cloves and allspice in a medium-size saucepan; bring to boiling; lower heat; simmer 5 minutes.
2. Combine sugar and gelatin in a small cup until well blended; stir into saucepan until gelatin dissolves; strain into a 4-cup measure. Stir in remaining 1⅓ cups water and white wine.
3. Measure 1¼ cups gelatin mixture into 2 separate small bowls; stir lime juice and a few drops green food coloring into one bowl; stir orange juice plus yellow and red food coloring to tint mixture a bright orange into second bowl. Stir lemon juice and a few drops yellow food coloring into remaining gelatin in 4-cup measure.
4. Place bowl with lime gelatin in a larger bowl of ice and water; stir until syrupy. Divide gelatin evenly among 8 wine glasses. Chill until layer is firm.
5. Place 4-cup measure with lemon gelatin in larger bowl of ice and water; stir until syrupy; beat with electric mixer at high speed until foamy white and triple in volume; spoon over lime layer in wine glasses, dividing evenly. Chill until firm, about 30 minutes.
6. Place remaining bowl of orange gelatin in larger bowl of ice and water; stir until syrupy. Spoon over whipped lemon layer, dividing evenly. Chill at least 2 hours before serving.

## WINE JELLY WITH FRUITS

*Always a favorite, this sparkling gelatin dessert is jeweled with fruits.*

Makes 10 servings/**80 calories each.**

- **3 cups water**
- **1 3-inch piece stick cinnamon**
- **3 whole allspice**
- **1 package (3 ounces) lemon flavored gelatin**
- **1 envelope unflavored gelatin**
- **1 cup dry white wine**
- **1 medium-size red apple, quartered, cored and chopped**
- **1 medium-size California orange, pared and sectioned**
- **1 medium-size banana, peeled and sliced**

1. Heat water with cinnamon stick and allspice to boiling in a small saucepan; strain into medium-size bowl.
2. Combine lemon gelatin and unflavored gelatin in a cup; stir into spiced water until gelatin dissolves; stir in wine.
3. Chill until as thick as unbeaten egg white; fold in apple, orange and banana until well blended.
4. Pour into an 8-cup mold. Chill 4 hours, or until firm.
5. To unmold: Loosen jelly around edge with a sharp knife; dip mold *very quickly* in and out of a pan of hot water. Cover with serving plate; turn upside down; shake gently; lift off mold. Garnish with mint leaves.
COOK'S TIP: Substitute lime gelatin for the lemon gelatin above.

## RASPBERRY PARFAIT

*Keep your refrigerator filled with colorful parfaits and you won't be tempted by caloric treats.*

Makes 8 servings/**47 calories each.**

- **1 package (3 ounces) raspberry flavored gelatin**
- **1 cup boiling water**
  **Ice cubes**
- **½ cup plain yogurt**
  **Fresh raspberries**

1. Dissolve gelatin in boiling water in a 4-cup measure. Add enough ice cubes to bring liquid to 2-cup level; stir until almost all of the ice melts and gelatin is just starting to set. (Remove any pieces of unmelted ice.)
2. Beat gelatin mixture until thick and foamy with electric mixer at high speed.
3. Spoon gelatin into 8 parfait glasses or dessert dishes, dividing evenly; top each with 1 tablespoon yogurt. (It will sink in slightly.) Chill until firm.
4. When ready to serve, place fresh berries on top of yogurt in each glass. Garnish with mint, if you wish.

## DIET DO'S

### AN APPLE A DAY

If you're interested in a simple habit that will in the long run help reduce the tendency to arteriosclerosis, eat an apple a day. So says director of nutrition Dr. James Scala of Thomas J. Lipton, Inc. Also, add a salad to your diet to get necessary fiber. This was tested by putting a group of men with high blood cholesterol on a high-fiber diet. Their cholesterol decreased significantly.

This also explains why vegetarians, who live on milk, cheese, eggs and other foods that should produce high blood cholesterol, usually have very low cholesterol levels. It's because they also eat large amounts of fiber.

## STRAWBERRY WONDER TORTE

*It's six layers high and super delicious.*

Bake at 400° for 10 minutes.
Makes 16 servings/ **92 calories each.**

- **¾ cup cake flour**
- **1 teaspoon baking powder**
- **¼ teaspoon salt**
- **4 eggs**
- **½ cup sugar**
- **1 teaspoon vanilla**
- **¼ teaspoon lemon extract**
  **Strawberry Filling (recipe follows)**
- **1 tablespoon 10X (confectioners' powdered) sugar**

1. Grease bottoms of 3 eight-inch layer cake pans; line with wax paper; grease paper.
2. Measure cake flour, baking powder and salt into sifter.
3. Beat eggs until foamy and light in large bowl of electric mixer at high speed; sprinkle in sugar, 1 tablespoon at a time, beating all the time until mixture is creamy and thick. Beat in vanilla and lemon extract.
4. Sift flour mixture over; fold in with wire whip until no streaks of white remain.
5. Measure 1 cup of batter into each of the prepared pans; spread to edges to make thin layers. (Cover remaining batter for baking 3 more layers.)
6. Bake in hot oven (400°) 10 minutes, or until centers spring back when lightly pressed with fingertip.
7. Cool on wire racks 5 minutes; loosen around edges with a knife; turn out onto racks: peel off wax paper; cool completely.
8. Wash pans; grease and line with wax paper. Bake and cool 3 more layers with remaining batter.

9. Make STRAWBERRY FILLING. Put layers together with about ⅓ cup filling between each on a serving plate. Dust top with 10X sugar. Garnish with a ring of strawberries, if you wish.

## STRAWBERRY FILLING

Makes about 2 cups/**220 calories per cup.**

- **2 cups (1 pint) strawberries, washed**
- **1 cup water**
- **2 tablespoons cornstarch**
- **¼ cup sugar**
- **1 teaspoon vanilla**

1. Set aside a few of the strawberries for garnish; hull and slice remaining berries into a small bowl.
2. Stir water, a little at a time, into cornstarch until smooth in a small saucepan. Stir in sliced berries and sugar.
3. Cook, stirring constantly and mashing berries well with back of spoon, over low heat until mixture thickens and bubbles 1 minute. Remove from heat; stir in vanilla; cool.

## CHEESECAKE MOLD

*Cheesecake fans, this is for you. We've taken out the calories, not the taste.*

Makes 16 servings/**114 calories each.**

- **2 eggs, separated**
- **1 cup water**
- **½ cup sugar**
- **¼ teaspoon salt**
- **3 envelopes unflavored gelatin**
- **⅓ cup instant nonfat dry milk powder**
- **1 teaspoon grated lemon rind**
- **3 tablespoons lemon juice**
- **1 teaspoon vanilla**
- **3 cups (1½ pounds) cream-style cottage cheese**
- **1 cup evaporated skim milk, well chilled**

1. Beat egg yolks slightly with water, sugar and salt in a small bowl.
2. Mix unflavored gelatin and dry milk powder in a small saucepan; stir in egg yolk mixture. Cook, stirring constantly, 5 minutes, or until gelatin dissolves and mixture coats a metal spoon; remove from heat.
3. Pour into a large bowl; stir in lemon rind, 2 tablespoons of the lemon juice and vanilla. Chill 30 minutes, or just until as thick as unbeaten egg white.
4. Press cottage cheese through a sieve into a medium-size bowl; stir into gelatin custard mixture.
5. Beat egg whites until foamy and white in the small bowl of an electric mixer at high speed. Beat well chilled evaporated skim milk with remaining 1 tablespoon lemon juice until stiff in a small bowl with mixer at high speed.

6. Fold beaten egg white, then whipped milk into gelatin cheese mixture; pour into an 8-cup mold. Chill at least 4 hours, or until firm.

7. To unmold, run a sharp tipped knife around top of mold, then dip mold *very quickly* in and out of a pan of hot water. Cover mold with a serving plate; turn upside down; carefully lift off mold. Garnish with a cluster of green grapes, if you wish.

## SOUTH SEAS CUP CUSTARDS

*Silky smooth and slimming. The perfect diet dessert for a hot summer day.*

Bake at 325° for 30 minutes.
Makes 6 servings/**110 calories each.**

    3  eggs
    ½  teaspoon grated lemon rind
    ⅛  teaspoon salt
    2¼ cups skim milk
    ¼  cup sugar
    ½  teaspoon vanilla
    2  tablespoons flaked coconut

1. Beat eggs slightly with lemon rind and salt in a medium-size bowl. Stir in milk, sugar and vanilla. Strain into six 6-ounce custard cups, using about ½ cup for each.
2. Set cups in a shallow pan; place on oven shelf; pour boiling water into pan to depth of about 1 inch.
3. Bake in slow oven (325°) 30 minutes, or until centers are almost set but still soft. (Custard will set as it cools.) Remove at once from pan of water; cool, then chill at least 4 hours, or until firm.
4. Loosen custards around edges with a thin bladed knife, then invert into serving dishes. Sprinkle tops with coconut just before serving.

## DOUBLE FRUIT COUPE

*Fresh fruits at their very best, with a touch of wine for the continental touch.*

Makes 6 servings/**55 calories each.**

    1  pint (2 cups) strawberries, washed
    2  tablespoons dry white wine
    1  tablespoon sugar
    2  cups diced pared fresh pineapple

1. Set aside 6 whole strawberries for garnish. Hull and slice remaining berries into a small bowl; sprinkle with half of the sugar and wine. Sprinkle remaining sugar and wine over pineapple in a second small bowl. Chill both fruits until serving time.
2. Spoon strawberries into 6 dessert dishes; top each with a mound of pineapple; garnish with reserved strawberries.

COOK'S TIP: For a summertime treat, serve DOUBLE FRUIT COUPE over plain or vanilla yogurt.

## HONEY GLAZED PEARS

*A nutritious and delicious ending to your dinner or a different fruit for breakfast.*

Bake at 400° for 45 minutes.
Makes 6 servings/**98 calories each.**

    3  large pears
    ½  cup water
    ¼  cup honey
    ½  teaspoon grated lemon rind
    ¼  teaspoon ground nutmeg

1. Pare pears, then halve and core; place, cut-side down, in a shallow baking dish.
2. Mix water, honey, lemon rind and nutmeg in a 1-cup measure; pour over pears; cover baking dish.
3. Bake in hot oven (400°), basting once or twice with syrup in dish, 30 minutes; uncover; baste pears again; bake 15 minutes longer, or until tender, but still firm enough to hold shape.
4. Cool pears in baking dish, basting once or twice to make a rich glaze. Garnish with a sprig of fresh mint, if you wish.

## MOCHA BAVARIAN

*We've taken a few calorie cuts with this coffee and chocolate gelatin dessert, but you'd never know it by the taste.*

Makes 10 servings/**88 calories each.**

    4  teaspoons instant coffee powder
       Cold water
    ½  cup sugar
    ⅓  cup cocoa powder (not a mix)
    2  envelopes unflavored gelatin
    ⅛  teaspoon salt
    2  cups skim milk
    1  teaspoon vanilla
    1  teaspoon rum extract
    1  cup evaporated skim milk,
       whipped (see page 90)

1. Dissolve instant coffee in 1½ cups water in a 2-cup measure.
2. Mix sugar, cocoa, gelatin and salt in a medium-size saucepan; stir in milk. Heat slowly, stirring constantly, until gelatin dissolves; stir in the 1½ cups coffee, vanilla and rum extract. Pour into a large bowl.
3. Place bowl in a pan of ice and water to speed setting. Chill, stirring several times, just until as thick as unbeaten egg white. Fold in whipped evaporated skim milk with a wire whip until no streaks of white remain. Spoon into a 6-cup mold. Chill several hours, or until firm.
4. When ready to serve, loosen dessert around edge with a knife; dip mold *very quickly* in and out of hot water. Cover with a serving plate; turn upside down; lift off mold. Garnish with orange sections and a sprinkling of cocoa powder, if you wish.

TRAIN YOURSELF
Remember—a diet should be a readjustment of eating habits, not a temporary change.
• Get used to the taste of less sweet, less rich food. Try taking half as much sugar in your coffee or tea, half as much butter on your bread.
• Don't taste food during cooking more than once, and then, only take a teaspoonful as your sample.
• Use a diet scale to weigh food, until you can judge portions by yourself.
• Try not to have second helpings. If you must, take only half at first; you'll feel you're eating more.

## BERRY FLOATING ISLAND

*This grand Victorian dessert is a great make-ahead dish. Photograph is on page 87.*

Makes 8 servings/**131 calories each.**

    2  eggs, separated
       Dash cream of tartar
    ¼  cup sugar
    3  cups skim milk
    ¼  cup sugar
    2  tablespoons all purpose flour
       Dash salt
    1  teaspoon vanilla
    1  teaspoon rum extract
    2  pints strawberries, washed

1. Beat egg whites until foamy and double in volume in a small bowl with electric mixer at high speed. Gradually add first ¼ cup of sugar, 1 tablespoon at a time, beating until meringue forms firm peaks.
2. Bring milk to a simmer in a large skillet. Pack meringue mixture into pastry bag fitted with a star tip; pipe into small mounds on pancake turner; slide into skim milk. Or, shape meringue mixture into small mounds with tablespoons. Poach in simmering milk 3 minutes, or until firm; remove with pancake turner to shallow plate; chill; reserve milk.
3. Combine remaining ¼ cup sugar, flour and salt in a medium-size saucepan; stir in reserved milk.
4. Cook, stirring constantly, until mixture thickens slightly and bubbles 1 minute. Beat egg yolks in a small bowl with wire whip; beat in about ½ cup hot mixture; return to saucepan; cook, stirring constantly, over *low heat* 2 minutes; pour into a medium-size bowl. Stir in vanilla and lemon or almond extract; cover; chill.
5. Spoon pudding into a shallow serving dish; float meringues on pudding; Chill until serving time.
6. At serving time, spoon strawberries into separate compartments of serving dish, to be eaten with the meringue and pudding mixture.

**BREAKFAST** is always important, even when you're dieting, because it provides you with energy for the rest of the day. Try the recipes here and you'll get the nutrition you need without having to worry about putting on weight. At right are Omelet with Chives and special Ham "Bacon" on the side. See page 98.

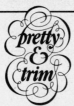

*pretty & trim*

| **7**<br>**300 CALORIES** | **8**<br>**300 CALORIES** | **9**<br>**295 CALORIES** |
|---|---|---|
| Orange Caribe*<br>1 slice Rye Toast or<br>Whole Wheat Toast with<br>¼ cup Low Fat Cottage Cheese<br>1 teaspoon Cherry Jelly<br>¾ cup Skim Milk<br>Black Coffee or<br>Tea with Lemon | ½ cup Fresh Blueberries<br>1 cup Corn Flakes or<br>1 cup Whole Wheat Flakes<br>1 cup Skim Milk<br>1 slice Toasted Protein Bread<br>1 teaspoon Grape Jelly<br>Black Coffee or<br>Tea with Lemon | ¾ cup Grapefruit Juice<br>1 Egg<br>(Baked in custard cup with<br>2 tablespoons skim milk,<br>salt and pepper at 350°<br>for 10 minutes.)<br>1 slice Rye Toast<br>1 cup Skim Milk  Coffee |
| **350 CALORIES** | **350 CALORIES** | **345 CALORIES** |
| Substitute:<br>1 ounce<br>American or Cheddar Cheese<br>for Low Fat Cottage Cheese | Spread:<br>¼ cup<br>Low Fat Cottage Cheese on<br>Toast with Jelly | Serve:<br>3 thin slices<br>Baked Canadian Bacon with<br>Baked Egg |
| **380 CALORIES** | **400 CALORIES** | **405 CALORIES** |
| Serve:<br>1 Boiled Egg with<br>300 Calorie Menu | Increase:<br>Protein Toast to<br>2 slices | Add:<br>1 cup Whole Wheat Cereal to<br>295 Calorie Menu |
| **10**<br>**298 CALORIES** | **11**<br>**297 CALORIES** | **12**<br>**305 CALORIES** |
| ½ cup Tomato Juice<br>Ready-To-Eat Cereal Mix*<br>(This includes three different<br>cereals tossed with<br>raisins and almonds.)<br>¼ cup sliced Strawberries<br>1 cup Skim Milk<br>Black Coffee or Tea with Lemon | Grapefruit Deluxe*<br>Poached Egg on<br>1 slice White Toast or<br>1 Soft Boiled Egg on<br>1 slice Pumpernickel Toast<br>1 cup Skim Milk<br>Black Coffee or<br>Tea with Lemon | ¾ cup Orange Juice<br>Make Your Own Yogurt*<br>(Flavor it with instant<br>coffee powder, ground<br>cinnamon or nutmeg.)<br>1 slice Whole Wheat Toast<br>Black Coffee or<br>Tea with Lemon |
| **352 CALORIES** | **352 CALORIES** | **345 CALORIES** |
| Serve:<br>1 slice<br>Toasted Protein or<br>Gluten Bread | Add:<br>¾ cup High Protein Rice and<br>Wheat Cereal (See Cook's<br>Guide, page 127) to menu above | Spread:<br>3 tablespoons<br>Cottage Cheese over<br>Whole Wheat Toast |
| **386 CALORIES** | **392 CALORIES** | **390 CALORIES** |
| Spread:<br>1 teaspoon Butter or Margarine<br>on Toast | Sprinkle:<br>½ cup Fresh Blueberries over<br>Cereal in bowl | Top:<br>Cottage Cheese with<br>2 tablespoons Dried Apricots |

*See Recipe Index for page number.

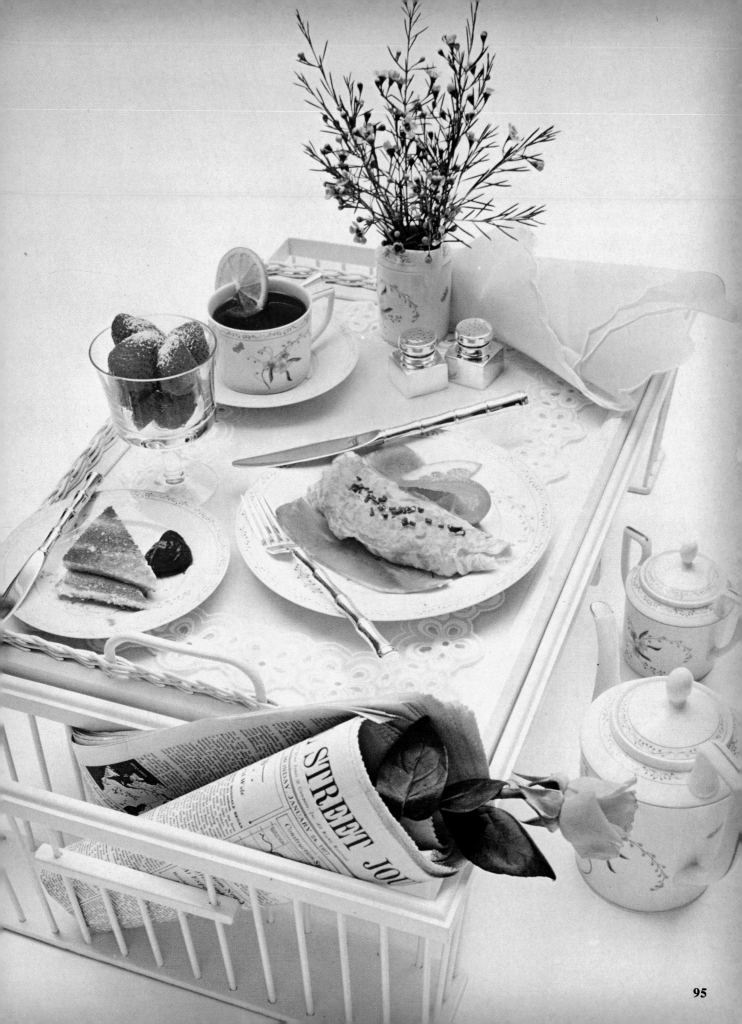

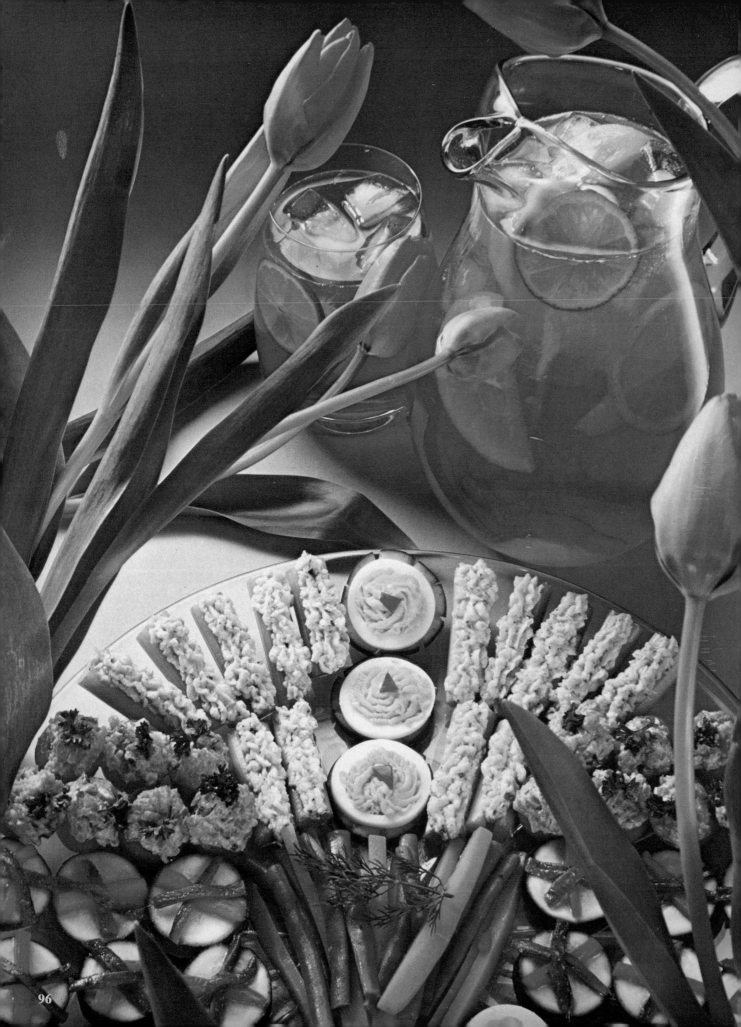

**FINGER-LICKING** snacks *can* be low in calories, and those at left prove the point: Deviled Egg Slices are surrounded by Blue Cheese Stuffed Celery; to the left of that, Ham in Cherry Tomatoes; below are Zucchini Antipasto Rounds and Dilly Beans and Carrots. Also—dieter's version of Sangria. See below.

## APPETIZER RECIPES

### ZUCCHINI PIZZAS

*Zucchini slices replace bread as the base for a healthy appetizer treat.*

Makes 36 slices/**20 calories each.**

- 3 medium-size zucchini, diagonally sliced
  Boiling salted water
- 1 can (6 ounces) tomato paste
- 3 slices part-skim mozzarella cheese (from an 8 ounce package), cut into 36 thin pieces
- ⅓ cup grated Parmesan cheese
  Garlic powder
  Leaf oregano, crumbled
  Salt

1. Parboil zucchini slices in water 1½ minutes, or until crisp and tender; drain on paper towels.
2. Place drained zucchini slices in a single layer on a heatproof dish. Top each with 1 teaspoon tomato paste, then with a piece of mozzarella cheese; sprinkle each slice with ½ teaspoon Parmesan cheese; top with garlic powder, leaf oregano and salt.
3. Broil, 4 inches from heat, 3 minutes, or until cheese is melted and zucchini is heated through.

### LOW CALORIE SANGRIA

*Cool and refreshing—just a little wine goes into this festive version of a Spanish classic. Pictured on page 96.*

Makes 10 servings/**43 calories each.**

- 1 cup dry white wine
- 1 3-inch piece stick cinnamon
- 6 whole cloves
  Ice cubes
- 1½ cups cranberry juice cocktail, chilled
- 2 bottles (32 ounces each) club soda, chilled
  Red food coloring
- 1 peach, pared, halved, pitted and sliced
- 1 orange, halved and sliced
- 1 lime, sliced
- 1 lemon, sliced

1. Combine wine, cinnamon and whole cloves in a small saucepan; heat slowly to boiling; lower heat; simmer 5 minutes; cool; remove spices.
2. Fill a tall pitcher with ice cubes; add wine, cranberry juice cocktail, club soda and red food coloring; stir until well blended. Garnish with peach, orange, lime and lemon slices.
COOK'S TIP: You can substitute melon for the sliced peach in this recipe.

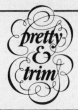
*pretty & trim*

### DILL-CARAWAY DIP

*Laura Hoefler serves this flavorful dip to participants in her "Yoga and Lunch" hour at Manhattan's Levy Shea Studio.*

Makes 4 servings/**90 calories each.**

- 1 container (8 ounces) plain yogurt
- 1 container (8 ounces) cream-style cottage cheese
- ½ cup dillweed
- ¼ cup caraway seeds

Mix yogurt, cottage cheese, dill and caraway with a fork in a medium-size bowl until well blended. Refrigerate at least 6 hours, or overnight. Serve with an assortment of raw vegetables, such as carrots, radishes, broccoli and cherry tomatoes.

### PÂTÉ INDIENNE

*Delicately flavored with curry powder and Cognac, this pâté is delicious on melba toast or celery sticks.*

Makes 10 servings/**106 calories each.**

- ½ pound chicken livers
- 1 small onion, quartered
- 6 tablespoons chicken broth (made with an instant broth cube)
- 2 tablespoons brandy or Cognac
- ½ teaspoon paprika
- ½ teaspoon curry powder
- ½ teaspoon salt
- ⅛ teaspoon white pepper
- ½ cup diet margarine (from a 4-ounce tub)
- ½ cup Neufchâtel cheese (from an 8-ounce package), softened

1. Clean chicken livers; cut in half and remove connecting tissue. Put into medium-size saucepan with onion, chicken broth and brandy or Cognac; bring to boiling; cook 5 minutes.
2. Empty mixture (including liquid) into container of electric blender; add paprika, curry powder, salt and white pepper. Cover and process at high speed until smooth. With blades spinning, remove inner cap or cover and slice in diet margarine and Neufchâtel cheese, stopping blender to stir down mixture with a thin rubber spatula, if it is no longer churning.
3. Pour into a small crock and chill at least 2 hours, or until serving time.

Serve with garnish of shredded carrots, if you wish.

### DEVILED EGG SLICES

*Perfect on a canapé tray, even better for a delicious luncheon plate. Photo on page 96.*

Makes 24 slices/**16 calories each.**

- 3 hard-cooked eggs, shelled
- 2 tablespoons imitation mayonnaise
- 2 teaspoons mustard with horseradish
- ½ teaspoon salt
- 1 large cucumber, scored
  Red pepper or pimiento

1. Cut eggs with an egg slicer or a sharp knife. Carefully remove yolks from white rings; press through a sieve into a small bowl; reserve whites.
2. Blend imitation mayonnaise, mustard with horseradish and salt into egg yolks to make a smooth paste; pack into a pastry bag fitted with a star tip.
3. Cut cucumber into thin slices; place a ring of egg white on each slice; pipe egg yolk mixture into rings, dividing evenly; garnish with tiny pieces of red pepper or pimiento. Place in single layer on cookie sheet; cover with plastic wrap. Chill until serving time.

### HAM IN CHERRY TOMATOES

*Chicken, tuna or Cheddar cheese can be substituted for the ham in this recipe. Photo is on page 96.*

Makes 24 canapes/**16 calories each.**

- 24 cherry tomatoes (from a pint box)
- ½ cup finely chopped ham
- ¼ cup finely chopped dill pickle
- ¼ cup finely chopped celery
- 2 tablespoons chopped pimiento
- 2 tablespoons imitation mayonnaise
- ½ teaspoon seasoned salt
- ¼ teaspoon lemon pepper
  Parsley

1. Hollow out cherry tomatoes with a small, sharp knife; invert onto paper towels to drain.
2. Combine ham, pickle, celery and pimiento on a wooden chopping board; chop and blend with a French knife until very smooth; place in a small bowl. Stir in imitation mayonnaise, salt and pepper until well blended.
3. Fill cherry tomatoes with mixture, dividing evenly. Garnish each with a puff of parsley. Arrange in a shallow dish; cover with plastic wrap; chill.

## DILLY BEANS AND CARROTS

*Turn these vegetable favorites into special low cal snacks. Photograph is on page 96.*

Makes 4 pint jars/**4 calories per stick.**

- 1 pound green beans
- 1 pound carrots
- 2 cups water
- 2 cups white vinegar
- 2 tablespoons kosher salt
    Few drops liquid red pepper seasoning
- 4 cloves garlic
- 4 teaspoons dillweed

1. Wash green beans and carrots well. Tip green beans and cut into 4-inch lengths. Pare carrots and cut into 4-inch sticks. Pack green beans and carrots into 4 hot sterilized pint jars.
2. Combine water, vinegar, salt and red pepper seasoning in a large saucepan; bring to boiling; lower heat; simmer 5 minutes.
3. Pour into jars to within ¼ inch of rim; add 1 clove garlic and 1 teaspoon dillweed to each jar. Seal and process in hot water bath 10 minutes, following manufacturer's directions.

## DIET DO'S

- For an outdoor party, arrange mushrooms and other raw vegetables around a table-type hibachi; dip in a mixture of soy sauce, dry white wine or Sherry, ground ginger and garlic powder; grill and serve with picks.
- Use yogurt instead of sour cream in your favorite party dip recipes; you'll cut calories in half!

## ZUCCHINI ANTIPASTO ROUNDS

*Marinated squash slices are topped with tiny slivers of anchovy and pimiento—delizioso! Shown on page 96.*

Makes 24 rounds/**13 calories each.**

- 2 large zucchini
- ¼ cup bottled low calorie Italian dressing
- 1 can (2 ounces) anchovy fillets, drained
- 1 jar (4 ounces) pimiento

1. Wash and tip zucchini; cut into thin slices; place in a medium-size bowl; drizzle Italian dressing over; toss to blend well. Allow to stand at least 2 hours.
2. Arrange zucchini in a single layer on a cookie sheet. Blot all oil from anchovy fillets with paper towels; cut into tiny strips. Drain pimiento on paper towels; cut into tiny strips.
3. Arrange anchovy and pimiento strips, spoke-fashion, over zucchini rounds; cover rounds with plastic wrap; chill until serving time.

## BLUE CHEESE STUFFED CELERY

*Keep a platter of these crisp sticks in the refrigerator to munch when you get an attack of the hungries. Shown on page 96.*

Makes 24 sticks/**10 calories each.**

- 6 large celery stalks
- ½ cup dry cottage cheese
- 2 tablespoons skim milk
- 2 tablespoons crumbled blue cheese
- 1 teaspoon blue cheese flavored seasoning for salads (see Cook's Guide, page 127)

1. Trim celery stalks; cut into 2-inch pieces.
2. Combine cottage cheese, skim milk, blue cheese and seasoning for salads in a small bowl until well blended with a fork.
3. Fill celery pieces with cheese mixture, using a fork and dividing evenly. Arrange in shallow pan; cover with plastic wrap. Chill at least 2 hours before serving to blend flavors.

## BREAKFAST RECIPES

### OMELET WITH CHIVES

*High, light and flavorful—no one would guess it's lower in calories. Just follow our cooking directions. Shown on page 95.*

Makes 1 omelet/**122 calories.**

- 1 whole egg
- 2 egg whites
    Dash salt and pepper
- 1 teaspoon chopped chives
    Vegetable spray on (see Cook's Guide, page 127)

1. Beat egg, egg whites, salt and pepper and chives until light and foamy in a small bowl.
2. Spray an 8-inch skillet with vegetable spray on, following directions.
3. Heat skillet until very hot; pour egg mixture into skillet. As soon as eggs begin to set, start lifting the edge of egg mixture all the way around with a spatula, until all liquid has cooked and omelet has puffed.
4. Turn omelet out by tipping pan and lifting edge with spatula; fold omelet over onto heated plate. Sprinkle with chopped parsley, if you wish.
*Suggested Variations:* For HAM OMELET, add ¼ cup finely chopped cooked ham to egg mixture/**227 calories.** For CHEESE OMELET, add ¼ cup shredded Cheddar cheese to cooked omelet, just before beginning to turn out of pan/**222 calories.** For SALMON OMELET, add ¼ cup flaked cooked salmon and 1 teaspoon chopped fresh dill to cooked omelet, just before beginning to turn out of pan/**232 calories.**

## TROPICAL BREAKFAST BLEND

*Good nutrition in a glass for breakfast on the run.*

Makes 1 serving/**193 calories each.**

- 1 cup high protein rice and wheat cereal (see Cook's Guide, page 127)
- ½ cup plain yogurt
- ¼ cup orange juice
- ¼ cup crushed pineapple in pineapple juice (from an 8¼-ounce can)
- 3 ice cubes

1. Combine cereal, yogurt, orange juice, crushed pineapple and ice cubes in container of an electric blender.
2. Cover; process at high speed 2 minutes, or until smooth. Pour into a tall glass and serve immediately.

## ORANGES CARIBE

*Serve as a bright eye opener in the morning or as a refreshing end to dinner.*

Makes 2 servings/**98 calories each.**

- 2 small California oranges, pared
- 2 teaspoons sugar
- 1 tablespoon lime juice
- 3 tablespoons water
- ½ teaspoon rum extract
- ½ teaspoon coconut extract
- ½ teaspoon aromatic bitters

1. Section oranges, working over a small bowl to catch juice. Sprinkle orange sections with sugar; toss lightly to coat sections.
2. Combine lime juice, water, rum and coconut extracts and bitters in a cup; pour over oranges. Toss lightly until well mixed. Chill at least 2 hours to blend flavors.

## CRUNCH TOPPED EGG CUPS

*Cheese flavored corn flakes top this easily fixed baked egg dish.*

Bake at 350° for 10 minutes.
Makes 4 servings/**130 calories each.**

- 1 cup corn flakes cereal
- 2 tablespoons shredded American cheese
- 1 tablespoon chopped parsley
- 4 eggs
- ½ teaspoon salt
    Dash pepper

1. Combine corn flakes, shredded cheese and parsley in a small bowl until well blended.
2. Break eggs into 4 individual baking dishes; season with salt and pepper; sprinkle seasoned corn flakes over, dividing evenly.
3. Bake in moderate oven (350°) 10 minutes, or until eggs are done as you like them.

## READY-TO-EAT CEREAL MIX

*Keep this combination of cereals, raisins and nuts in a glass jar, ready to serve.*

Makes 3 servings/**158 calories each.**

- 1½ cups high protein rice and wheat cereal (see Cook's Guide, page 127)
- 1 cup four-grain multi-vitamin and iron supplement cereal (see Cook's Guide, page 127)
- ¼ cup shreds of wheat bran cereal (see Cook's Guide, page 127)
- ¼ cup raisins or chopped dried fruits
- 2 tablespoons slivered almonds

1. Combine rice cereal, four-grain cereal, wheat bran cereal, raisins and slivered almonds; toss to mix well.
2. Store at room temperature.

# DIET DO'S

## BREAKFAST BRIGHTENERS

- Poach your egg in skim milk to serve on toast with the hot milk over.
- Diet-fry your egg: Pour cold water into a small frying pan just to cover the bottom; break an egg into the pan; season with salt, pepper and herbs, if you wish. Cover the pan and steam slowly till the egg is done as you like.
- Diet margarine has half the calories of regular margarine.
- Drink unsweetened juices.
- Honey, jam, jelly, molasses, or syrup can be an occasional 50-calorie treat for the calorie counter.
- Don't omit bread if you're on a diet; 1 slice of pumpernickel is only 65 calories, enriched white bread is 70 calories and whole wheat and rye bread are 65 calories per slice.

## FLUFFY COCONUT PANCAKES

*Cottage cheese gives these "silver dollars" extra tenderness.*

Makes 6 servings/**250 calories each.**

- 1 cup cream-style cottage cheese
- 3 eggs, well beaten
- 1 tablespoon sugar
- ¼ teaspoon salt
- 2 tablespoons butter or margarine, melted and cooled slightly
- ¼ cup all purpose flour
  Vegetable spray on (see Cook's Guide, page 127)
- ¼ cup flaked coconut
  Diet margarine
  Honey Lemon Syrup (recipe follows)

1. Beat together cottage cheese, eggs, sugar and salt in medium-size bowl with fork until well blended; stir in melted and cooled butter or margarine and flour gently, just until blended.

2. Spray a large heavy skillet with vegetable spray on, following label directions; heat skillet slowly over low heat. Test temperature by sprinkling in a few drops of water. When drops bounce about, temperature is right.
3. Measure 1 tablespoon batter for each pancake into skillet, letting one set before pouring the next one; immediately sprinkle each pancake with ½ teaspoon coconut.
4. Cook until edge appears dry and underside is golden; turn and brown other side. Repeat with rest of batter, to make 24 pancakes. As pancakes are baked, stack in a pie plate; cover with a colander and keep warm.
5. For each serving, top 4 pancakes with 2 teaspoons diet margarine and 1 tablespoon HONEY LEMON SYRUP.

HONEY LEMON SYRUP: Makes about ¼ cup/**66 calories per tablespoon.** Mix ¼ cup honey and 1 tablespoon lemon juice in small saucepan with spoon until well blended; cook over low heat, stirring constantly, until heated through.

## MAKE YOUR OWN YOGURT

*Eleanor Schwartz shares her recipe for a yogurt that keeps for several weeks in the refrigerator. She suggests you add your favorite fruits, nuts or flavorings for a change of pace taste.*

Preheat oven to 300°
Makes 8 servings/**165 calories each.**

- ½ teaspoon unflavored gelatin (from 1 envelope)
  Water
- 1 tablespoon sugar (optional)
- 3 cups instant nonfat dry milk powder
- 1 tall can evaporated milk (1⅔ cups)
- 3 tablespoons plain yogurt

1. Soften gelatin in 1 tablespoon cold water in a large glass or ceramic bowl; stir in 1 cup boiling water and sugar until dissolved.
2. Add dry milk, evaporated milk, yogurt and 3 cups lukewarm water; stir until well blended. Cover bowl with plastic wrap.
3. Place in preheated oven (300°); *turn off oven;* keep in oven, with door closed, 8 to 10 hours.
4. Spoon into 8 individual containers (½-pint canning jars are perfect); flavor with fresh or dried fruits, nuts, instant coffee, ground cinnamon or vanilla, if you wish; cover jars. Chill until serving time.
COOK'S TIP: For a period of time you can use yogurt from one batch to act as the "starter" for another batch, but after about 5 times, you should start afresh with 3 tablespoons commercial yogurt.

## DOLLAR PANCAKE STACKS

*Breakfast should be a nutritious meal. These pancakes make it good eating, too.*

Makes 6 servings/**150 calories each.**

- 4 eggs
- 1 cup skim milk
- ½ cup all purpose flour
- 1 tablespoon butter or margarine
- ¾ cup cream-style cottage cheese
- 1 cup fresh blueberries

1. Beat eggs until thick in a medium-size bowl with a wire whip; beat in milk, then flour, just until smooth.
2. Heat a large nonstick skillet slowly over low heat. Test temperature by sprinkling in a few drops of water. When drops bounce about, temperature is right. Grease pan with some of the butter or margarine.
3. Measure 1 tablespoon batter for each pancake into pan. (Wait until one has set before pouring the next one.) Bake until edge appears dry and underside is golden; turn; brown other side. Repeat baking, lightly greasing pan each time, to make 36 pancakes.
4. As pancakes are baked, stack in a pie plate; cover with a colander and set in a warm oven.
5. For each serving, spread 2 tablespoons cottage cheese onto 6 pancakes; stack on a serving plate. Top with about 3 tablespoons blueberries. Serve warm.
COOK'S TIP: You can freeze leftover pancakes. Cool on wire rack; stack between layers of aluminum foil; seal. Reheat, still frozen, in 350° toaster oven, or conventional oven.

## PLUMS DEVONSHIRE

*Warmed spicy plums with sweetened cheese topping—almost like being in England!*

Makes 4 servings/**229 calories each.**

- 1 can (16 ounces) calories reduced purple plums
- 1 3-inch piece stick cinnamon
  Devonshire Cream Topping (recipe follows)
- ¼ cup slivered almonds, toasted

1. Place plums and their liquid plus cinnamon stick in a small saucepan. Bring to boiling; lower heat; simmer 5 minutes, or until heated through.
2. Spoon plums into individual serving dishes; top each serving with 2 tablespoons DEVONSHIRE CREAM TOPPING and 1 tablespoon toasted almonds. Refrigerate any remaining plums with cinnamon stick and syrup in a covered container, to be eaten warm or cold.
COOK'S TIP: You can substitute calories reduced apricots for the plums in this recipe.

## DEVONSHIRE CREAM TOPPING

Makes ½ cup/**49 calories per tablespoon.**

- ½ **cup Neufchâtel cheese (from an 8-ounce package), softened**
- 1 **tablespoon honey**
- 1 **teaspoon vanilla**
- ¼ **teaspoon grated lemon rind**

Mash Neufchâtel cheese with fork in a medium-size bowl until soft and fluffy; stir in honey, vanilla and lemon rind until well blended. Refrigerate remainder in covered container.

## HAM "BACON"

*Thin strips of oven baked ham are half the calories of bacon. Photo is on page 95.*

Bake at 350° for 10 minutes.
Makes 3 servings/**66 calories each.**

- 2 **slices boiled ham (from a 4-ounce package)**

1. Cut ham slices into bacon strip-like shapes; lay in a single layer on a cookie sheet.
2. Bake in moderate oven (350°) 10 minutes, or until heated through.

## GRAPEFRUIT DELUXE

*So easy to make, you don't have to wait for the weekend to serve it.*

Bake at 350° for 5 minutes.
Makes 2 servings/**66 calories each.**

- 1 **grapefruit**
- 2 **teaspoons sugar**
- ¼ **teaspoon ground cinnamon**
- ¼ **teaspoon aromatic bitters**

1. Cut grapefruit in half. Loosen each section from skin and membrane with a sharp paring knife. Sprinkle sugar, cinnamon and bitters over halves.
2. Bake in moderate oven (350°) 5 minutes, or until heated through.

## APPLE FRENCH TOAST

*An old breakfast favorite, but with far fewer calories.*

Makes 4 servings/**165 calories each.**

- 2 **eggs**
- ⅔ **cup skim milk**
- 1 **tablespoon sugar**
- 1 **teaspoon vanilla**
  **Dash salt**
- 6 **slices enriched white bread**
  **Vegetable spray on (see Cook's Guide, page 127)**
  **Spicy Apple Syrup (recipe follows)**

1. Beat eggs slightly in deep pie dish with fork or wire whip; add milk, sugar, vanilla and salt and beat until well blended and fluffy.
2. Dip bread, a slice at a time, into milk mixture, turning to coat both sides; set dipped slices on plate.
3. Spray large heavy skillet with vegetable spray on, following label directions; heat skillet slowly over low heat. Test temperature by sprinkling in a few drops of water. When drops bounce about, temperature is right.
4. Cook bread slices, a few at a time, until browned on 1 side; turn and brown other side; remove and keep warm while preparing remaining slices.
5. For each serving, top 1½ slices French toast with 2 tablespoons SPICY APPLE SYRUP.

SPICY APPLE SYRUP: Makes about 1 cup/**10 calories per tablespoon.** Mix 1 cup apple juice and ½ teaspoon ground cinnamon in a small saucepan; bring to boiling; lower heat. Mix 1 tablespoon cornstarch with 2 tablespoons cold apple juice in a 1-cup measure; add to simmering juice. Cook, stirring constantly, until sauce thickens and bubbles, about 1 minute. COOK'S TIP: For SPICY ORANGE SYRUP, substitute 1 cup orange juice for apple juice and dash ground cardamom for cinnamon in above recipe.

# SUPER SLIM SOUPS

## CHILLED VICHYSSOISE

*Here's a lower calorie version of a French favorite created in New York at the Ritz.*

Makes 8 servings/**107 calories each.**

- 2 **pounds potatoes**
- 1 **tablespoon diet margarine**
- 2 **cups chopped leeks**
  **OR: 2 large onions, chopped (2 cups)**
- 4 **envelopes or teaspoons instant chicken broth**
- 3½ **cups boiling water**
- 3⅓ **cups skim milk**
- ½ **teaspoon salt**
  **Pinch pepper**
  **Chives**

1. Cook potatoes in boiling salted water 30 minutes, or until tender; drain; peel and mash.
2. Melt margarine in a large saucepan. Add leeks or onion; cook until tender. Dissolve chicken broth in the boiling water in a 4-cup measure; add to leeks or onions; simmer 5 minutes.
3. Add skim milk and mashed potatoes to broth; season with salt and pepper. Cook and stir over medium heat until steaming.
4. Pour 2 cups at a time into container of electric blender; cover; process at medium speed until smooth. Serve cold, sprinkled with chopped chives.

## MINESTRONE

*A low-fat vegetable soup that's easy to make, yet so delicious.*

Makes 6 servings/**26 calories each.**

- 2 **envelopes or teaspoons instant beef broth**
- 3 **cups boiling water**
- 2 **cups (½ an 8-ounce package) produce department vegetables for coleslaw**
  **OR: 2 cups shredded cabbage**
- 1 **cup sliced celery**
- 1 **tablespoon chopped parsley**
- 1 **medium-size onion, chopped (½ cup)**
- 1 **can (1 pound) Italian plum tomatoes, chopped**
- 1 **bay leaf**
- 1 **teaspoon leaf oregano, crumbled**
- 1 **teaspoon salt**
- ¼ **teaspoon pepper**

1. Dissolve instant beef broth in boiling water in a large saucepan. Add coleslaw vegetables or cabbage, celery, parsley, onion, tomatoes, bay leaf, oregano, salt and pepper.
2. Cover; simmer until vegetables are tender and flavors are blended, about 15 minutes.

## EGG DROP SOUP

*Tender bits of egg float in a rich chicken broth; so easy, yet so good.*

Makes 6 servings/**39 calories each.**

- 2 **cans (14 ounces each) chicken broth**
- 1 **egg, slightly beaten**
- 2 **tablespoons chopped parsley**

1. Bring chicken broth to boiling in a medium-size saucepan. Pour in beaten egg very slowly, stirring constantly, just until egg cooks and separates into shreds.
2. Ladle into heated cups; sprinkle with parsley.

## YANKEE CLAM BROTH

*Starting your meal with a satisfying broth makes it easier to stay on your diet.*

Makes 4 servings/**20 calories each.**

- 2 **bottles (8 ounces each) clam juice**
- 1 **cup water**
- ½ **cup finely cut celery**
- 2 **teaspoons finely cut chives**
  **Few drops liquid red pepper seasoning**

1. Combine clam juice, water, celery, 1 teaspoon of the chives, and red pepper seasoning in a small saucepan; bring to boiling; cover. Simmer 15 minutes, or until celery is tender.
2. Ladle into heated soup bowls or cups; sprinkle with remaining chives.

## MUSHROOM BOUILLON

*Lightly flavored with Sherry, this broth is sheer delight for mushroom lovers.*

Makes 8 servings/**25 calories each.**

- **8 cups water**
- **8 envelopes or teaspoons instant chicken broth**
- **1 pound fresh mushrooms, finely chopped**
- **1 green onion, trimmed and sliced crosswise**
- **2 tablespoons dry Sherry**

1. Bring water to boiling in large saucepan; add instant chicken broth, chopped mushrooms and sliced green onion. Cover.
2. Simmer 1 hour, or until mushroom pieces are cooked and broth is a rich brown color; add Sherry and stir until well blended. Serve each portion with a dollop of yogurt and additional sliced green onion, if you wish.

## CHILLED CUCUMBER SOUP

*Buttermilk is the tangy base for a refreshing summer soup.*

Makes 6 servings/**75 calories each.**

- **2 cups buttermilk**
- **1 cup (8 ounces) cream-style cottage cheese**
- **1 medium-size cucumber, diced**
- **1 clove garlic**
- **½ teaspoon salt**
- **¼ teaspoon celery seed**

1. Place buttermilk, cottage cheese, diced cucumber, garlic, salt and celery seed in container of electric blender; cover container; process at high speed until smooth.
2. Pour soup into glass or ceramic bowl; cover and chill. Serve soup in bowls, garnished with chopped red pepper, if you wish; refrigerate any remainder in covered container.

## "CREAM" OF MUSHROOM SOUP

*This soup only tastes rich!*

Makes 8 servings/**65 calories each.**

- **Mushroom Bouillon (recipe, above)**
- **2 cups evaporated skim milk**
- **Parsley**

1. Mix MUSHROOM BOUILLON and evaporated skim milk in large bowl until well blended.
2. Place mixture, a cup at a time, in container of electric blender; cover; process at high speed 30 seconds, or until smooth.
3. As mixture is blended, place in large heavy saucepan; bring almost to boiling; lower heat; simmer 5 minutes, or until heated through. Garnish with

chopped parsley.
COOK'S TIP: This soup is also delicious served chilled.

## SOUTHERN CREAM SOUP

*Frozen Southern turnip greens are the basis of this nutritious soup.*

Makes 6 servings/**66 calories each.**

- **1 package (10 ounces) frozen chopped turnip greens**
- **1 bay leaf**
- **3 thin strips lemon rind**
- **3 envelopes or teaspoons instant chicken broth**
- **3 cups boiling water**
- **1 tall can evaporated skim milk (1⅔ cups)**
- **1 teaspoon salt**
- **⅛ teaspoon white pepper**
- **Dash nutmeg**
- **½ cup plain yogurt (from an 8-ounce container)**

1. Combine turnip greens, bay leaf, lemon rind, instant chicken broth and boiling water in a large saucepan. Bring to boiling; lower heat; simmer 5 minutes. Cool a few minutes; remove bay leaf.
2. Pour into container of an electric blender; cover; process at high speed until smooth; return to saucepan. Stir in evaporated skim milk; simmer over low heat until heated through; stir in salt, white pepper, nutmeg and yogurt. Serve hot or cold with an extra dollop of yogurt, if you wish.

## COLD ZUCCHINI SOUP

*Serve with a crisp salad and a slice of protein bread for a light, yet satisfying luncheon.*

Makes 4 servings/**130 calories each.**

- **2 tablespoons butter or margarine**
- **2 large zucchini, tipped and cubed**
- **1 large onion, chopped (1 cup)**
- **1 clove garlic, minced**
- **2 cups chicken broth**
- **1 teaspoon salt**
- **¼ teaspoon pepper**
- **1 container (8 ounces) plain yogurt**
- **¼ cup chopped parsley**

1. Melt butter or margarine in a kettle; sauté zucchini, onion and garlic in butter, until soft.
2. Stir in chicken broth; simmer 10 minutes; season with salt and pepper. Chill at least 4 hours, or overnight. Stir in yogurt and sprinkle with chopped parsley, just before serving.

## DIET DO'S

- So your diet portion won't look lost on a plate, serve your food on small or medium-size plates. Choose an attractive garnish, too.

## CONSOMMÉ MADRILÈNE

*Shimmering spoonfuls of flavor-rich consommé make a delightful way to start a summer meal.*

Makes 6 servings/**55 calories each.**

- **2 cups tomato juice**
- **Celery leaves**
- **1 slice lemon**
- **1 slice onion**
- **½ cup water**
- **2 envelopes unflavored gelatin**
- **½ cup cold water**
- **2 cups chicken broth**
- **2 teaspoons lemon juice**
- **1 teaspoon aromatic bitters.**

1. Combine tomato juice, celery leaves, lemon slice, onion and first ½ cup cold water in a medium-size saucepan. Simmer over low heat 10 minutes.
2. Soften gelatin in second ½ cup cold water in a medium-size bowl; strain tomato juice into bowl; stir until gelatin dissolves; add chicken broth, lemon juice and aromatic bitters until well blended.
3. Chill 3 hours, or until set. Beat with fork and pile into chilled bouillon cups. Garnish each serving with sliced lemon, minced parsley or plain yogurt, if you wish.

## GAZPACHO

*From Granada comes this chilled tomato soup with a Spanish flavor.*

Makes 6 servings/**64 calories each.**

- **4 large ripe tomatoes**
- **1 medium-size onion, chopped (½ cup)**
- **1 clove garlic, minced**
- **1 large green pepper, halved, seeded and coarsely chopped**
- **1 large cucumber, coarsely chopped**
- **1 cup tomato juice**
- **1 tablespoon wine vinegar**
- **2 teaspoons olive oil**
- **2 teaspoons salt**
- **¼ teaspoon pepper**

1. Spear tomatoes, one at a time, with a two-tined fork and rotate over medium heat for 1 minute, or plunge tomatoes, one at a time, into boiling water for 30 seconds, then plunge into cold water. Peel off skin; chop tomato coarsely.
2. Combine tomato, onion, garlic, green pepper and cucumber with tomato juice, vinegar, oil, salt and pepper in a large ceramic or glass bowl; cover with plastic wrap.
3. Refrigerate for several hours. Serve icy cold in small bowls, topped with a dollop of plain yogurt, thinly sliced green onion, and shredded raw carrot, if you wish.

## TOMATO CONSOMMÉ

*Onion and herbs simmer in tomato juice, so refreshing and satisfying.*

Makes 8 servings/**25 calories each.**

- 2 cups water
- 4 envelopes or teaspoons instant beef broth
  Handful celery leaves
- 1 medium-size onion, peeled and sliced
- ¼ cup chopped parsley
- 1 teaspoon seasoned salt
- ½ teaspoon leaf basil, crumbled
- ¼ teaspoon seasoned pepper
- 2 bay leaves
- 1 can (46 ounces) tomato juice

1. Combine water, instant beef broth, celery leaves, onion, parsley, salt, basil, seasoned pepper and bay leaves in a large saucepan. Bring to boiling; simmer 15 minutes.
2. Stir in tomato juice; heat 5 minutes longer, or until bubbly hot. Strain into heated soup bowls or cups.

# MORE MAIN DISHES

## POTATOES AND OYSTERS

*This Victorian favorite, creamed oysters in baked potato, works well into our modern diet plan.*

Bake at 425° for 40 minutes.
Makes 4 servings/**178 calories each.**

- 4 small baking potatoes, scrubbed
- 12 shelled oysters (½ pint)
- 1 tablespoon chopped shallots
- 3 tablespoons diet margarine
- ¼ cup dry white wine
- ¼ cup evaporated skim milk
- 2 tablespoons chopped parsley
- 1 teaspoon salt
- ¼ teaspoon freshly ground pepper
  Dash nutmeg

1. Bake potatoes in hot oven (425°) 40 minutes, or until tender when pierced with a two tined fork.
2. Drain oysters, reserving liquid.
3. Sauté shallots in 1 tablespoon of the margarine in a small saucepan until soft; stir in wine; bring to boiling; add oysters; cook gently, just until edges of oysters curl; remove oysters with slotted spoon.
4. Add reserved oyster liquid to saucepan; boil liquid until reduced by half; stir in evaporated milk and cook 1 minute; add oysters and 1 tablespoon of the parsley; keep warm.
5. Split skin of baked potatoes open with a fork; scoop out potato; beat with remaining 2 tablespoons margarine, salt, pepper, and nutmeg.
6. Pile mixture back into potato shells, using the back of a spoon, keeping a hollow in center. Spoon oyster mixture into potatoes, dividing evenly. Sprinkle with parsley.

## KABOB CHICKEN LIVERS

*Tender chicken livers are threaded with fresh mushrooms and cherry tomatoes for an epicure's delight.*

Makes 4 servings/**246 calories each.**

- 1 pound chicken livers
- 1 tablespoon butter or margarine, melted
- ¼ cup dry white wine
- 1 teaspoon onion salt
- ¼ teaspoon leaf basil, crumbled
- 4 large mushrooms, quartered
- 8 cherry tomatoes
  White Wine Sauce (recipe follows)

1. Halve chicken livers; combine melted butter or margarine, wine, onion salt and basil in a medium-size bowl; add chicken livers and marinate for at least 1 hour in the refrigerator.
2. Thread chicken livers, mushrooms and cherry tomatoes alternately on 4 skewers; brush with wine mixture.
3. Broil or grill, 4 inches from heat, 10 minutes, turning once, or until liver is slightly browned. Serve with WHITE WINE SAUCE.
WHITE WINE SAUCE: Makes ½ cup/**20 calories per tablespoon.** Sauté ¼ cup chopped green onions in 1 tablespoon butter or margarine in a medium-size saucepan 5 minutes, or until tender; stir in 1 tablespoon all purpose flour, ¼ teaspoon salt and ⅛ teaspoon pepper. Cook, stirring constantly, just until bubbly. Stir in ½ cup dry white wine; continue cooking and stirring until sauce thickens and simmers 10 minutes.

## SPRING LAMB ROLL-UPS

*Thin slices of cooked lamb are wrapped around tender asparagus spears.*

Makes 4 servings/**276 calories each.**

- 8 thin slices cooked lamb
- 1 pound asparagus, cooked and drained
- ½ cup bottled low calorie Italian salad dressing
- 2 tablespoons lemon juice
- 1 teaspoon instant minced onion
- 1 teaspoon salt
- ½ teaspoon leaf thyme, crumbled
- ¼ teaspoon garlic powder

1. Wrap one slice of lamb around 2 asparagus spears for each bundle; secure with picks. Place lamb bundles in a shallow dish.
2. Combine salad dressing, lemon juice, onion, salt, thyme and garlic powder in a 1-cup measure; pour over lamb; cover dish with plastic wrap. Refrigerate several hours, or until thoroughly chilled.
3. Remove lamb from marinade and arrange on platter. Garnish with tomato and cucumber, if you wish.

## FRANKS AND KRAUT SALAD

*The All-American favorite duo, franks and kraut, makes a hearty main dish salad.*

Makes 6 servings/**317 calories each.**

- 1 can (1 pound, 12 ounces) sauerkraut, well drained
- 3 cups broken lettuce
- 1 pound heated frankfurters, sliced
- 1 can (16 ounces) cut green beans, drained
- ¾ cup grated carrot
- 1 medium-size green pepper, halved, seeded and chopped
- 1 medium-size red onion, chopped
- ¼ cup imitation mayonnaise
- ¼ cup bottled low calorie French salad dressing
- ½ teaspoon salt
- ¼ teaspoon pepper

1. Combine sauerkraut, lettuce, sliced frankfurters, green beans, carrot, pepper and onion in a large salad bowl until well blended.
2. Add imitation mayonnaise, French dressing, salt and pepper; toss to coat evenly. Serve at room temperature, or chill before serving.

## ITALIAN MEATBALLS

*Brown these spicy meatballs under your broiler. It's simpler than frying in oil.*

Makes 4 servings/**253 calories each.**

- 1 pound ground round
- 2 tablespoons instant minced onion
- ½ teaspoon garlic salt
- 1 package (10 ounces) frozen chopped spinach, thawed
- ¼ cup seasoned bread crumbs
- 1 egg
- 1 tablespoon water
- 1 can (8 ounces) tomato sauce
- 1½ cups water
- 1 large stuffed olive, chopped
- 1 teaspoon leaf oregano, crumbled

1. Combine ground beef, onion, garlic salt, spinach and bread crumbs in a large bowl. Beat egg with the 1 tablespoon water in a small bowl; blend into beef mixture. Shape into balls, using a tablespoon of beef mixture per ball; arrange in a single layer on broiler pan.
2. Broil, 4 inches from heat, 5 minutes, turning once.
3. Combine tomato sauce, the 1½ cups water, olive and oregano in a large saucepan; heat to boiling.
4. Add broiled meatballs to sauce. Bring to boiling; lower heat; cover; simmer 30 minutes. Remove cover during last 10 minutes of cooking to allow sauce to thicken slightly. Skim off fat from sauce, if necessary.
DIETER'S TIP: A ½ cup serving of tender-cooked spaghetti adds 78 calories per serving.

## GERMAN STEAK PLATTER

*With low calorie salad dressing for basting, this dish is truly a dieter's delight.*

Makes 6 servings/**235 calories** each.

- 1 small cabbage (about 1½ pounds)
- 1½ teaspoons salt
- ¾ teaspoon caraway seeds
- 1 flank steak (about 2 pounds)
  Instant unseasoned meat tenderizer
- 4 tablespoons bottled low calorie Italian salad dressing
  Parsley

1. Place cabbage in a medium-size saucepan with salt, caraway and enough water to almost cover. Cover; cook 15 minutes, or just until tender.
2. Lift out carefully; drain well, then cut out core. Place cabbage, rounded-side up, on a heated serving platter; cut into 6 wedges. Keep warm while cooking steak.
3. Moisten steak with water and sprinkle with meat tenderizer, following label directions. Brush one side with 2 tablespoons salad dressing.
4. Broil steak, 4 inches from heat, 3 to 4 minutes; turn; brush other side with remaining salad dressing. Broil 3 to 4 minutes longer for rare, 5 to 6 minutes for medium, or until steak is done as you like it.
5. Remove steak to a cutting board; carve diagonally into thin slices. Place, overlapping, over cabbage wedges. Garnish with parsley.

## FRUITED HAM STEAK

*Calories reduced pack of fruits means out-of-season fruits, without excess sugar.*

Bake at 350° for 1 hour.
Makes 4 servings/**296 calories** each.

- 1 slice ready-to-eat ham (about 1 pound)
- 1 can (1 pound) calories reduced peach halves
  Whole cloves
- 1 tablespoon prepared mustard
- ½ teaspoon pumpkin pie spice

1. Trim fat from ham; score edge so slice will lay flat during cooking; place in a large shallow baking dish.
2. Drain syrup from peaches into a cup; stud peach halves with two or three whole cloves each for a spicy flavor. Arrange peach halves around ham in baking dish.
3. Stir mustard and pumpkin pie spice into peach syrup; pour over ham and peach halves.
4. Bake in moderate oven (350°), basting often with syrup in dish, 1 hour, or until ham and peaches are glazed and heated through.

## SKILLET TURKEY SCRAMBLE

*Turkey and ham go with rice, tomatoes and seasonings in this top-of-the-range dinner.*

Makes 6 servings/**325 calories** each.

- 1 medium-size onion, chopped (½ cup)
- 1 clove garlic, minced
- 1 tablespoon butter or margarine
- 1 teaspoon salt
- 1 teaspoon chili powder
- ⅛ teaspoon pepper
  Dash cayenne pepper
- 1 bay leaf
- 2 cans (1 pound each) stewed tomatoes
- 3 cups diced cooked turkey
- ½ cup diced cooked ham
- 1 cup regular rice
- 1 tablespoon chopped parsley

1. Sauté onion and garlic in butter or margarine just until soft in large non-stick skillet. Stir in salt, chili powder, pepper, cayenne and bay leaf; cook 2 minutes; add stewed tomatoes, turkey, ham, rice and parsley; cover.
2. Simmer, stirring often, 40 minutes, or until rice is tender.

## SPAGHETTI WITH SEAFOOD

*Shrimp, clams or scallops can be used in this zesty pasta sauce.*

Makes 6 servings/**330 calories** each.

- 1 large onion, chopped (1 cup)
- 1 clove garlic, minced
- 2 tablespoons butter or margarine
- 1 bag (1 pound) frozen deveined shelled raw shrimp
  OR: 1 pound fresh or frozen sea scallops, sliced
  OR: 2 cans (10 ounces each) minced clams
- 1 can (1 pound) tomatoes
- 1 can (6 ounces) tomato paste
- 1 can (6 ounces) sliced mushrooms
- 1½ teaspoons leaf oregano, crumbled
- 1 teaspoon salt
- ¼ teaspoon lemon pepper
- 1 bay leaf
- 1 package (8 ounces) thin spaghetti

1. Sauté onion and garlic in butter or margarine until soft in a large skillet; add shrimp, scallops or clams and liquid.
2. Stir in tomatoes, tomato paste, mushrooms and liquid, oregano, salt, lemon pepper and bay leaf. Simmer 20 minutes, or until sauce is rich and flavorful.
3. While sauce cooks, prepare spaghetti, following label directions; drain; keep hot until ready to serve.
4. Spoon spaghetti onto serving plate; top with seafood sauce. Garnish plate with watercress, if you wish.

## LEMONY LAMB KABOBS

*Tart and tangy—so simple to make!*

Makes 4 servings/**236 calories** each.

- ¼ cup water
- ½ teaspoon grated lemon rind
- 3 tablespoons lemon juice
- 2 teaspoons Worcestershire sauce
- ½ teaspoon salt
- ¼ teaspoon leaf thyme, crumbled
- ½ teaspoon leaf rosemary, crumbled
- ⅛ teaspoon pepper
- 1 small clove garlic, crushed
- 1 pound lean boneless lamb, cut into 1-inch cubes
- 8 small white onions (about ½ pound)
- 1 medium-size green pepper, halved, seeded and cut into 8 wedges

1. Combine water, lemon rind, lemon juice, Worcestershire sauce, salt, leaf thyme, rosemary, pepper and crushed garlic in a 1-cup measure until well blended.
2. Place lamb cubes in a single layer in a shallow glass dish; drizzle marinade over; cover dish with plastic wrap. Chill at least 2 hours to blend flavors.
3. Peel onions and parboil in boiling salted water 5 minutes; drain.
4. Thread marinated lamb, onions, and green peppers onto 4 skewers.
5. Broil, 4 inches from heat, 5 minutes; turn; brush with marinade; broil 4 minutes longer, or until meat and vegetables are tender. Garnish with lemon wedges, if you wish.

## LEMON CHICKEN

*White wine and lemon slices add the crowning touch to microwave chicken.*

Microwave for 17 minutes.
Makes 4 servings/**308 calories** each.

- 1 broiler-fryer, cut up (2½ pounds)
- 1 teaspoon salt
- ½ teaspoon fines herbes, crumbled
- ¼ teaspoon pepper
- ¼ cup chopped shallots
  OR: 1 small onion, chopped (¼ cup)
- 1 large lemon, thinly sliced
- ½ cup dry white wine

1. Season chicken pieces with salt, fines herbes and pepper; skin-side down, arrange in a 12-cup shallow glass baking dish. (Place large pieces in corners and smaller ones in the center.) Cover dish with plastic wrap.
2. Microwave 6 minutes; turn chicken pieces, sprinkle with shallots or chopped onion and layer with lemon slices; pour wine over.
3. Microwave 6 minutes; rotate dish; microwave 5 minutes longer. Allow to stand 10 minutes before serving.

## LOBSTER AND EGGS

*Stir-fry this Oriental specialty in minutes.*

Makes 6 servings/**160 calories each.**

- 3 packages (4 ounces each) frozen Rock lobster tails
- 2 slices bacon, diced
- ½ cup chopped green onions
- ½ cup sliced celery
- 1 cup sliced fresh mushrooms OR: 1 can (3 or 4 ounces) sliced mushrooms, drained
- 1 can (5 ounces) water chestnuts, drained and sliced
- 1 can (5 ounces) bamboo shoots, drained
- 6 eggs, well beaten
- 1 tablespoon soy sauce
- 1 teaspoon salt
- ¼ teaspoon pepper

1. Thaw frozen lobster tails slightly. Remove underside membrane with scissors and pull out meat; dice meat.
2. Fry bacon until crisp in a large skillet; remove bacon with slotted spoon and drain on paper towels.
3. Add lobster pieces, green onion, celery and mushrooms and sauté quickly over high heat until lobster is white and opaque. Add water chestnuts and bamboo shoots.
4. Beat eggs with soy sauce, salt and pepper in a medium-size bowl; pour over vegetables and stir gently until eggs are firm and creamy. Top with crisp bacon. Serve over shredded iceberg lettuce, if you wish.

## GOURMET BEEF PATTIES

*Beef and gravy lovers, here's a way to have your dish, and cut calories, too.*

Makes 4 servings/**235 calories each.**

- 1 pound ground round
- ½ teaspoon salt
- ¼ cup dry vermouth or dry red wine
- ¾ cup water
- 1 teaspoon instant onion broth
- ¼ teaspoon pepper
- 1 tablespoon all purpose flour
- 2 tablespoons cold water
  Chopped chives

1. Shape beef into 4 patties lightly.
2. Sprinkle salt in bottom of a large heavy skillet; heat skillet. Brown patties 5 minutes on each side, or until beef is done as you like it; remove.
3. Pour off all fat from skillet; add wine; stir up all cooked-on bits from pan; bring to boiling; add the ¾ cup water, instant onion broth and pepper; simmer 5 minutes.
4. Blend flour and 2 tablespoons cold water in a cup; stir into bubbling liquid in pan; cook, stirring constantly, 3 minutes; return patties to skillet; spoon part of sauce over; simmer 2 minutes; sprinkle with chives.

## CAPE COD SCALLOP SALAD

*Deep sea scallops are tossed with crisp vegetables in a cool, creamy dressing.*

Makes 4 servings/**167 calories each.**

- 1 pound fresh or frozen sea scallops
- 2 tablespoons bottled low calorie Italian salad dressing
- 1 tablespoon chopped parsley
- ½ teaspoon grated lemon rind
- 1 cup chopped celery
- ½ cup sliced radishes
- ¼ cup thinly sliced cucumber
- ¼ cup imitation mayonnaise
- 1 head lettuce

1. Wash scallops; cut in thin slices.
2. Coat slices well with Italian dressing in a large skillet; cover; cook slowly 5 minutes.
3. Lift out with spoon and place in a medium-size bowl; toss with parsley and lemon rind; cover. Chill several hours to season and blend flavors.
4. Stir in celery, radishes, cucumber and imitation mayonnaise carefully until well blended.
5. Make nests of lettuce in 4 individual salad bowls or seashells. Spoon scallop salad into centers; garnish each with slices of cucumber, radish and ripe olive, if you wish.

## SCANDINAVIAN LAMB KABOBS

*The Scandinavians have a different way of flavoring lamb—they use brewed coffee!*

Makes 6 servings/**244 calories each.**

- ¼ cup hot strong coffee
- 1 tablespoon vegetable oil
- 1 teaspoon lemon juice
- 2 cloves garlic, crushed
- 1 teaspoon salt
- ⅛ teaspoon pepper
- 1½ pounds boneless lamb shoulder, cut into 1½-inch cubes
- 2 medium-size zucchini, cut into 1-inch cubes
- 12 small white onions, peeled

1. Combine coffee, oil, lemon juice, garlic, salt and pepper in a medium-size bowl; add lamb cubes and marinate at least 2 hours in refrigerator.
2. Parboil zucchini and onions 3 minutes in a medium-size saucepan; drain.
3. Drain lamb; reserve marinade. Thread lamb, zucchini and onions alternately on 6 long skewers; brush with reserved coffee marinade.
4. Broil or grill, 4 inches from heat, 20 minutes, turning and basting often, or until lamb is tender and done as you like it. Serve with lemon wedges, if you wish.
*Suggested Variation:* Cubed veal can be substituted for the lamb and yellow squash used for the zucchini.

## GREEK CHICKEN LIVERS

*Quick dishes are great for calorie counters. No need to nibble while waiting for a slow kettle to boil.*

Makes 6 servings/**230 calories each.**

- 1 eggplant, sliced ½-inch thick (about 1 pound)
- 1 teaspoon salt
- ¼ cup water
- 1½ pounds chicken livers, cut in half
- 1 medium-size onion, sliced
- 2 tablespoons butter or margarine
- 2 tablespoons all purpose flour
- 1 teaspoon leaf basil, crumbled
- 1 can condensed chicken broth
- 2 tomatoes, peeled and cut into eighths
- 2 tablespoons chopped parsley

1. Season eggplant slices with salt. Overlap slices in a large skillet; pour ¼ cup water over; cover. Bring to boiling; lower heat; steam 5 minutes.
2. Arrange eggplant, overlapping, as a border around edge of heated serving dish; keep warm.
3. Sauté chicken livers and onion in butter or margarine in skillet 6 minutes, or until browned. Stir in flour and basil. Gradually stir in broth.
4. Heat, stirring constantly, until mixture thickens and bubbles 3 minutes. Add tomatoes; cover; reduce heat; simmer 5 minutes. Spoon into center of serving dish with eggplant border. Sprinkle with parsley.

## LAMB CHOPS EN BROCHETTE

*Kabob cooking adds glamour to dinner.*

Makes 6 servings/**328 calories each.**

- 6 lamb shoulder arm or blade chops, 1-inch thick
- ½ cup bottled low calorie Italian salad dressing
- 12 water chestnuts
- 6 slices bacon, halved
- 2 large tomatoes, cut into wedges
- 12 large mushrooms

1. Trim all fat from chops; arrange chops in a shallow glass or ceramic dish; pour Italian dressing over chops; cover dish with plastic wrap. Refrigerate for several hours or overnight, turning lamb occasionally.
2. Place lamb chops on 1 long skewer. Wrap water chestnuts in bacon; then alternate bacon-wrapped water chestnuts, tomato wedges and mushrooms on 2 long skewers.
3. Grill chops, 4 inches from heat, 16 to 20 minutes, or until done as you like them, turning and brushing frequently with marinade. Grill vegetables 7 minutes, or until crisply tender, turning frequently and brushing with remaining marinade.

## SAMOA CHICKEN

*Sweet and spicy, this modern-day version of a South Seas classic is extra easy when made in a microwave oven.*

Microwave for 23 minutes.
Makes 4 servings/**257 calories each.**

 1 broiler-fryer, cut up (2½ pounds)
 ¼ cup soy sauce
 ¼ cup dry white wine
 1 tablespoon Worcestershire sauce
 1 clove garlic, minced
 ¼ teaspoon ground ginger
   Dash liquid red pepper seasoning

1. Place chicken pieces in a deep glass bowl. Combine soy sauce, wine, Worcestershire sauce, garlic, ginger and red pepper seasoning in a small bowl; pour over chicken. Cover bowl with plastic wrap; marinate at least 2 hours in refrigerator.
2. Arrange chicken pieces in a 12-cup shallow glass baking dish. (Place large pieces in corners and smaller ones in the center.)
3. Microwave 23 minutes, rotating the dish several times, or until chicken is tender. Allow to stand 5 minutes before serving. Garnish with orange slices, if you wish.

## BURGUNDY BURGERS

*Don't worry about the wine calories; most of them evaporate during the cooking.*

Makes 8 servings/**203 calories each.**

 2 pounds ground round
 ½ cup cracked ice
 1 tablespoon instant minced onion
 2 teaspoons garlic salt
 ¼ teaspoon seasoned pepper
 1 tablespoon vegetable oil
 1 can (8 ounces) sliced mushrooms
 ¼ cup cold water
 2 tablespoons all purpose flour
 ¾ cup dry red Burgundy
 2 tablespoons parsley
 ½ teaspoon leaf thyme, crumbled

1. Combine ground beef, ice, onion, garlic salt and pepper in a large bowl. Shape into 8 oval steaks.
2. Heat oil in a large nonstick skillet; brown the beefburgers quickly on both sides. Lower heat; continue cooking about 5 minutes longer, or until burgers are medium rare. Remove to serving platter; keep warm.
3. Drain mushrooms, reserving liquid. Combine mushroom liquid with water, flour, wine, parsley and thyme in a 2-cup measure. Pour into skillet; stir until well blended.
4. Cook over medium heat, stirring constantly, until sauce thickens and bubbles 1 minute; add mushrooms and cook until mushrooms are hot, about 5 minutes longer. Serve sauce over beefburgers.

## ROCK LOBSTER HONG KONG

*Chinese vegetables and soy sauce team with succulent lobster tails for a main dish salad.*

Makes 6 servings/**112 calories each.**

 3 packages (4 ounces each) frozen Rock lobster tails
 2 cups sliced celery
 1 can (16 ounces) mixed Chinese vegetables, drained
 1 can (8½ ounces) water chestnuts, drained and sliced
 1 can (16 ounces) bean sprouts, drained
 1½ teaspoons salt
 ¼ teaspoon pepper
 1 tablespoon lemon juice
 1½ teaspoons soy sauce
 ¼ cup bottled low calorie coleslaw dressing
 4 cups broken lettuce

1. Drop frozen lobster tails into boiling salted water in a large saucepan. Return to boiling; cook 3 minutes. Drain and drench with cold water.
2. Remove underside membrane with scissors and pull out meat in one piece. Slice meat into ½-inch pieces.
3. Combine lobster, celery, Chinese vegetables, sliced water chestnuts, bean sprouts, salt, pepper, lemon juice, soy sauce and coleslaw dressing in a large bowl; toss to coat well; cover with plastic wrap; chill to blend flavors.
4. Line a large salad bowl with lettuce; spoon lobster mixture over.

## PORK CHOPS SEVILLE

*Orange juice and marjoram are perfect in this quick-cooking pork dish.*

Makes 6 servings/**283 calories each.**

 6 thin lean pork chops (1½ pounds)
 1 medium-size onion, chopped (½ cup)
 ½ cup orange juice
 1 envelope or teaspoon instant chicken broth
 1 teaspoon leaf marjoram, crumbled
 ¼ teaspoon lemon pepper

1. Trim any remaining fat from chops. Sprinkle salt in bottom of a large heavy skillet; heat skillet. Add chops, 3 at a time; brown 5 minutes on each side; remove and reserve; pour off all but 1 tablespoon pan drippings.
2. Sauté onion until soft in same pan; add orange juice, instant chicken broth, marjoram and lemon pepper and stir until smooth. Return chops to pan; cover skillet.
3. Simmer 30 minutes, or until chops are tender when pierced with a two-tined fork. Serve with orange slices, if you wish. Garnish serving platter with fresh watercress, if you wish.

## FLORIDA BAKED FILLETS

*Tangy citrus and delicate fish make a delicious flavor combination.*

Bake at 350° for 15 minutes.
Makes 4 servings/**111 calories each.**

 4 small fresh fillets of sole (about 1 pound)
   OR: 1 package (1 pound) frozen fillets of sole, haddock or turbot
 1 teaspoon grated orange rind
 ½ teaspoon salt
 ¼ teaspoon seasoned pepper
 ⅓ cup orange juice
 1 tablespoon butter or margarine

1. Place fresh fillets in a single layer or block of frozen fish in a shallow baking dish. Sprinkle with orange rind, salt and seasoned pepper; pour orange juice into dish; dot with butter or margarine; cover baking dish with aluminum foil.
2. Bake in moderate oven (350°), basting once or twice with juices in dish, 15 minutes for fresh fish and 30 minutes for frozen, or until fish flakes easily when pierced with a fork.
3. Place on a heated serving platter; garnish with orange slices and parsley, if you wish.

## LAMB ITALIANO

*Tomato and onion, garlic and herbs bubble away with chunks of lamb for a special dish —meraviglioso!*

Makes 8 servings/**204 calories each.**

 2 pounds lean lamb shoulder
 1 teapoon salt
 1 large onion, chopped (1 cup)
 2 cloves garlic, minced
 1 can (1 pound, 12 ounces) Italian tomatoes
 1 bay leaf
 ½ teaspoon leaf rosemary, crumbled
 ¼ teaspoon freshly ground pepper

1. Trim any remaining fat from lamb; cut into cubes. Sprinkle salt in bottom of a large heavy skillet; heat skillet. Add lamb, part at a time; brown 5 minutes on each side; remove and reserve; pour off all but 1 tablespoon pan drippings.
2. Sauté onion and garlic in pan until soft; drain liquid from tomatoes into skillet; stir up all cooked-on bits from pan; bring to boiling; let bubble 5 minutes.
3. Add tomatoes, bay leaf, rosemary and pepper; stir to blend; return meat to skillet; cover.
4. Simmer 1 hour, or until meat is tender when pierced with a two-tined fork. Sprinkle with chopped parsley, if you wish.
COOK'S TIP: This dish is even more delicious if made the day before and refrigerated overnight.

## CHICKEN WITH WATERCRESS

*No one will miss the caloric stuffing with tangy watercress filling the bird.*

Microwave 24 minutes.
Makes 4 servings/**309 calories each.**

- 1 large bunch watercress
- 1 broiler-fryer (about 3 pounds)
- ¼ cup bottled low calorie French dressing
- 2 tablespoons diet margarine, melted
- 1 teaspoon salt
- ¼ teaspoon pepper

1. Wash and trim watercress; place stems and a few of the leaves in cavity of broiler-fryer as stuffing; truss chicken. Place chicken in a 10-cup shallow glass baking dish.
2. Combine French dressing, melted margarine, salt and pepper in a cup; brush over chicken to coat well.
3. Microwave 9 minutes; baste bird with pan drippings; rotate pan; cook 9 minutes longer; tip chicken so that juices inside bird run into baking dish; spoon juices over bird.
4. Microwave 6 minutes longer. Cover bird with aluminum foil and allow to stand 10 minutes. Pour juices in baking pan into a small saucepan.
5. Bring pan juices to a quick boil in saucepan. Cut chicken into 4 pieces with poultry shears; line serving platter with remaining watercress; arrange chicken quarters over; pour hot sauce over and serve.

## QUICK MOUSSAKA

*Classic Greek cooking goes diet-style.*

Makes 6 servings/**205 calories each.**

- 1½ pounds lean ground lamb
- 1 eggplant (1 pound), pared and cut into small cubes
- 1 medium-size onion, chopped (½ cup)
- 3 tablespoons chopped parsley
- 1½ teaspoons salt
- 1½ teaspoons leaf oregano, crumbled
- 1 cup canned tomatoes
- 2 tablespoons grated Romano cheese

1. Shape lamb into a large patty; brown in skillet 5 minutes on each side; pour off all fat; break up into chunks with a metal spoon.
2. Add eggplant, onion, parsley, salt and oregano; cook 3 minutes, stirring several times. Add tomatoes, breaking up with a spoon. Mix well. Bring to boiling.
3. Lower heat; cover; simmer 30 minutes, or until eggplant is tender. Uncover; sprinkle with cheese and a little more chopped parsley.

## MEATBALLS IN YOGURT SAUCE

*Ground lamb blends with tomato and yogurt for meatballs, Iranian-style.*

Makes 8 servings/**228 calories each.**

- 2 pounds lean ground lamb
- 1½ teaspoons garlic salt
- 1 egg
- 4 tablespoons tomato paste (from a 6-ounce can)
- 1 cup chopped parsley
- 1 teaspoon pumpkin pie spice
- 2 slices protein bread
- 2 containers (8 ounces each) plain yogurt

1. Combine lamb, garlic salt, egg, tomato paste, parsley and pumpkin pie spice in a large bowl. Dip bread in water; squeeze out excess. Add to meat mixture; mix well. Use a teaspoon to shape into small meatballs. Place on rack in broiler pan.
2. Broil, 3 inches from heat; 10 minutes, turning frequently to brown evenly on all sides.
3. Heat yogurt in a large skillet over low heat; do not allow to boil. Stir in meatballs. Garnish with some additional chopped parsley, if you wish.
COOK'S TIP: These meat balls are also perfect for a party appetizer.

## BEEF STUFFED PEPPERS

*Here's a recipe for the first green peppers from the garden.*

Bake at 350° for 30 minutes.
Makes 4 servings/**230 calories each.**

- 4 large green peppers
- 1 pound ground round
- ¼ cup precooked rice
- ⅓ cup water
- 1 medium-size onion, chopped (½ cup)
- 2 cans (8 ounces each) tomato sauce
- ½ cup water
- 1 teaspoon leaf basil, crumbled
- ½ teaspoon garlic salt
- ⅛ teaspoon seasoned pepper

1. Slice tops from green peppers; remove seeds, leaving shells intact. Cook 3 minutes in boiling water; drain.
2. Sprinkle salt on a large skillet. Heat pan; press beef into pan to cover surface; brown 5 minutes; cut into wedges; turn; brown 5 minutes; drain off all fat; break meat into tiny pieces.
3. Stir in rice, the ⅓ cup water, onion and ½ cup of the tomato sauce. Stuff mixture into pepper shells. Place peppers in 6-cup shallow casserole.
4. Combine remaining tomato sauce, the ½ cup water, basil, garlic salt and pepper in a bowl. Pour over peppers.
5. Bake in moderate oven (350°) 30 minutes, or until peppers are tender.

## OVEN FRIED CHICKEN

*Crisp and crunchy chicken every time, thanks to a mix you make yourself.*

Bake at 375° for 45 minutes.
Makes 8 servings/**183 calories each.**

- ½ cup dry bread crumbs
- 1 teaspoon onion powder
- 1 teaspoon seasoned salt
- ¼ teaspoon lemon pepper
- 2 tablespoons vegetable oil
- 2 broiler-fryers, cut up (about 2½ pounds each)

1. Combine bread crumbs, onion powder, seasoned salt and lemon pepper in a small bowl; stir in vegetable oil with a fork until well blended. Place mixture in a plastic bag.
2. Moisten chicken pieces with water and shake in the bag, a few pieces at a time.
3. Arrange coated chicken pieces, skin-side up, in a single layer on a nonstick cookie sheet.
4. Bake in moderate oven (375°) 45 minutes, or until chicken is golden, adding absolutely no other fats or oils. (Don't be alarmed if the chicken seems dry for the first 20 minutes; then the coating starts to work, and at the end of the baking period, it will be crisp and perfect.
COOK'S TIP: A teaspoon leaf oregano, ¼ teaspoon garlic powder or 1 tablespoon sesame seeds can be added to the coating mix for a variety of fried chicken dishes.

## CURRIED FISH BAKE

*No need to thaw frozen fish; just place the frozen block on a wooden board and cut into pieces with a large sharp knife.*

Bake at 350° for 1 hour, 15 minutes.
Makes 6 servings/**235 calories each.**

- 2 packages (1 pound each) frozen cod, haddock or turbot
- 2 large onions, chopped (2 cups)
- 1 clove garlic, minced
- 2 tablespoons butter or margarine
- 1 teaspoon curry powder
- 3 medium-size apples, pared, quartered, cored and sliced
- ¾ cup water
- 2 teaspoons salt
- ⅛ teaspoon pepper

1. Cut cod evenly into 6 pieces; place in a 6-cup shallow baking dish.
2. Sauté onions and garlic in butter or margarine until soft in a medium-size skillet; stir in curry powder; cook 2 minutes; stir in apples, water, salt and pepper. Heat, stirring constantly, to boiling; spoon over fish; cover.
3. Bake in moderate oven (350°) 1 hour and 15 minutes, or until fish flakes easily.

106

## GRILLED LEMON CHICKEN

*Great on the backyard grill. Even non-dieters will love the fresh taste this baste gives chicken.*

Makes 8 servings/**293 calories each.**

- ½ cup lemon juice
- 2 tablespoons butter or margarine, melted
- 1 teaspoon leaf thyme, crumbled
  OR: 1 tablespoon minced fresh thyme
- ¼ teaspoon liquid red pepper seasoning
- 2 broiler-fryers, quartered (about 2½ pounds each)
  Salt
  Freshly ground pepper

1. Combine lemon juice, butter or margarine, thyme and red pepper seasoning in a small bowl.
2. Sprinkle the chickens with salt and pepper. Place chickens, bone-side down, on the grill 6-inches from hot coals. Brush with the basting sauce.
3. Grill for 40 minutes, turning often. Baste frequently with the sauce. Serve with the remaining basting sauce poured over the chickens.
**Note:** Adjust the heat if chicken is cooking too fast.

## FRITTATA DI VEGETALI

*A luncheon omelet chock full of nutritious mustard greens.*

Makes 4 servings/**202 calories each.**

- 1 package (10 ounces) frozen chopped mustard greens or kale
- 1 medium-size onion, chopped (½ cup)
- 1 clove garlic, minced
- 2 tablespoons grated Parmesan cheese
  Salt and pepper
- 8 eggs
- ¼ cup skim milk
  Vegetable spray on (see Cook's Guide, page 127)

1. Cook mustard greens, following label directions; drain well. Combine with onion, garlic, Parmesan cheese, salt and pepper in a medium-size bowl until well blended.
2. Beat eggs and milk until light and fluffy with a wire whip in a medium-size bowl; stir into mustard greens.
3. Spray a large skillet with vegetable spray on, following label directions. Heat pan until hot over medium heat. Pour in egg mixture; cook until brown on underside and dry on top; loosen around edge with a spatula; invert onto cookie sheet; slide back into skillet.
4. Cook 3 minutes, or until brown. Cut into wedges to serve.

## SPANISH SNAPPER

*Flounder, haddock or cod can be used in place of the red snapper in this pungent microwave oven recipe.*

Microwave 12 minutes.
Makes 6 servings/**162 calories each.**

- 2 pounds fresh or frozen red snapper fillets
- 1 small tomato, chopped
- 1 medium-size onion, chopped (½ cup)
- 1 small green pepper, halved, seeded and chopped
- 1 can (3 or 4 ounces) mushroom pieces, drained
- 1 clove garlic, minced
- ½ teaspoon leaf oregano, crumbled
  Dash liquid red pepper seasoning
- ½ cup bottled low calorie Italian salad dressing
- ¼ cup dietetic chili sauce
  Salt and pepper

1. Defrost fish, if frozen, in a 12x7x2-inch glass baking dish; remove fish from dish.
2. Combine tomato, onion, green pepper, mushrooms, garlic, oregano and red pepper seasoning in same baking dish; stir in salad dressing to blend well; cover with plastic wrap.
3. Microwave 6 minutes. Place fish over vegetables, spooning part of mixture over; spread chili sauce on top of fish and vegetables; cover.
4. Microwave 6 minutes; taste sauce and season with salt and pepper. Let stand 4 minutes before serving.

## ALOHA LAMBURGERS

*Ground lamb contains fewer calories than ground beef, even when topped with pineapple rings.*

Makes 6 servings/**223 calories each.**

- 1½ pounds ground lamb
- 1 egg
- 1 green pepper, finely chopped
- 1 medium-size onion, chopped (½ cup)
- 1 tablespoon soy sauce
- 1 teaspoon salt
  Pinch pepper
- 6 slices pineapple in pineapple juice (from a 1-pound, 4-ounce can)

1. Combine ground lamb, egg, green pepper, onion, soy sauce, salt, pepper and 2 tablespoons of juice from pineapple in a large bowl. Mix well. Shape into 6 patties; place on rack of broiler pan.
2. Broil, 3 inches from heat, about 5 minutes on each side. Top each patty with a drained pineapple slice; brush lightly with additional soy sauce; broil about 1 minute longer to lightly brown pineapple.

## HALIBUT IN YOGURT

*Try this with salmon, too, or any favorite fish steak.*

Bake at 350° for 25 minutes.
Makes 4 servings/**172 calories each.**

- 1 package (1 pound) frozen halibut
- ½ cup dry white wine
- 1 envelope or teaspoon instant chicken broth
- ½ cup boiling water
- ½ teaspoon dillweed
- ¼ teaspoon salt
- ⅛ teaspoon pepper
- 2 tablespoons chopped parsley
- 1 container (8 ounces) plain yogurt

1. Place frozen halibut in a shallow 6-cup baking dish. Pour wine over. Dissolve instant chicken broth in boiling water in a 1-cup measure; pour over fish. Sprinkle with dillweed, salt, pepper and parsley.
2. Bake in moderate oven (350°) 25 minutes, or until fish flakes easily with a fork. Baste several times with liquid. Drain liquid from baking dish; measure ⅔ cup into a saucepan. Bubble over high heat until reduced to ⅓ cup. Stir into yogurt in a small bowl; return to saucepan; heat just until hot. Spoon sauce over fish and serve.

## COUNTRY FARM CHICKEN

*Rosy tomatoes and bright green pepper makes a colorful sauce for this easy-on-the-calories microwave recipe.*

Microwave 21 minutes.
Makes 4 servings/**279 calories each.**

- 1 broiler-fryer, cut up (2½ pounds)
- 1 tablespoon all purpose flour
- 1 teaspoon salt
- 1 teaspoon paprika
- 1 teaspoon leaf thyme, crumbled
- ¼ teaspoon seasoned pepper
- 1 tablespoon vegetable oil
- 2 large tomatoes, chopped
- 1 medium-size green pepper, halved, seeded and coarsely chopped
- ¼ pound mushrooms, chopped
- 1 cup chicken broth

1. Season chicken with a mixture of flour, salt, paprika, thyme and seasoned pepper.
2. Arrange chicken pieces, skin-side up, in a 12-cup shallow glass-ceramic baking dish; drizzle with oil; sprinkle tomatoes, green pepper and mushrooms over; pour broth in; cover with plastic wrap.
3. Microwave 8 minutes; rotate dish; microwave 8 minutes; uncover; cook 5 minutes longer.
**COOK'S TIP:** For a crisply coated chicken, place dish in broiler of conventional oven, 4 inches from heat, for 5 minutes.

## ROSY PINEAPPLE CHICKEN

*Paprika and pineapple are a distinctive flavor team for tender chicken.*

Microwave for 20 minutes.
Makes 4 servings/**281 calories each.**

1 broiler-fryer, cut up (3 pounds)
1 teaspoon salt
¾ teaspoon leaf rosemary, crumbled
¼ teaspoon seasoned pepper
2 tablespoons chopped shallots
1 can (8¼ ounces) crushed
    pineapple in pineapple juice
1 teaspoon paprika
½ teaspoon ground ginger

1. Rub chicken pieces with salt, rosemary and pepper; arrange chicken pieces in a 12-cup shallow glass baking dish. (Place large pieces in corners and smaller ones in the center.) Sprinkle shallots over chicken.
2. Combine crushed pineapple and juice, paprika and ginger in a small bowl; spoon over chicken.
3. Microwave 20 to 22 minutes, rotating the dish several times, or until chicken is tender. Allow to stand 4 minutes before serving.

## DOUBLE BOILER SOUFFLÉ

*It puffs beautifully and holds up well, even if dinnertime is delayed.*

Makes 4 servings/**187 calories each.**

1 can (about 6¼ ounces) crab meat
1 teaspoon grated onion
⅛ teaspoon curry powder
2 tablespoons diet margarine
2 tablespoons all purpose flour
½ teaspoon salt
⅔ cup skim milk
1 tablespoon chopped parsley
4 eggs, separated

1. Drain crab meat and flake, removing bony tissue, if any.
2. Sauté onion with curry powder in margarine 1 minute in a small saucepan; stir in flour and salt; cook, stirring constantly, just until bubbly. Stir in milk; continue cooking and stirring until sauce thickens and bubbles 3 minutes; remove from heat. Stir in flaked crab meat and parsley; let cool a few minutes.
3. Beat egg whites until they form soft peaks in a medium-size bowl with electric mixer at high speed.
4. Beat egg yolks until creamy thick in a second medium-size bowl; blend in cooled crab sauce; fold in beaten egg whites with wire whip until no streaks of white remain. Pour into the top of an 8-cup ungreased double-boiler; place over simmering water; cover double-boiler.
5. Cook, keeping water simmering all the time, 1 hour, or until soufflé is firm on top. Serve at once. (If soufflé must stand, cover and keep hot over simmering water.)
COOK'S TIP: If you don't have a double-boiler, pour soufflé mixture into an 8-cup saucepan; cover. Place in a large skillet; carefully pour in boiling water to a depth of about one inch. Keep water simmering all the time, adding more boiling water, as needed.

## CLAM SOUFFLÉ

*This delicate seafood soufflé even has a rich leek sauce counted into the calories.*

Bake at 350° for 50 minutes.
Makes 4 servings/**251 calories each.**

1 can (about 8 ounces) minced
    clams
    Skim milk
¼ cup all purpose flour
1 teaspoon salt
    Dash liquid red pepper seasoning
4 eggs, separated
    Leek Sauce (recipe follows)

1. Grease a 4-cup soufflé or straight-sided baking dish well.
2. Drain liquid from clams into a 1-cup measure; add skim milk to make 1 cup. Set clams aside. Combine liquid with flour, salt and red pepper seasoning in a small saucepan; cook, stirring constantly, until mixture thickens and boils 1 minute; remove from heat. Let cool.
3. Beat egg whites just until they form soft peaks in a medium-size bowl.
4. Beat egg yolks until creamy thick in a large bowl; beat in cooled sauce very slowly; stir in minced clams, then fold in beaten egg whites with wire whip until no streaks of white remain. Pour into prepared dish.
5. Set dish in a larger baking pan; place on oven shelf; carefully pour boiling water into baking pan to a depth of about an inch.
6. Bake in moderate oven (350°) 50 minutes, or until puffy and firm and golden on top. Remove from pan of water. Serve at once with LEEK SAUCE.

LEEK SAUCE: Makes 1½ cups/**15 calories per tablespoon.** Trim root and tip from 1 medium-size leek, then thinly slice leek. (It should measure about 1 cup.) If leeks are not available in your area, use 1 medium-size onion, peeled and coarsely chopped. Parboil leek or onion in water to cover in a small saucepan 5 minutes; drain well. Combine 1 cup skim milk, 2 tablespoons butter or margarine, 2 tablespoons all purpose flour and ¼ teaspoon salt in a small saucepan. Cook, stirring constantly, until sauce thickens and bubbles 3 minutes. Stir in drained leek or onion; simmer 10 minutes to blend flavors.

## CANTONESE CHICKEN

*Tender chicken breasts are marinated in soy and ginger, then grilled to a crisp perfection.*

Makes 8 servings/**170 calories each.**

4 whole chicken breasts, split
    (about 10 ounces each)
1 cup dry Sherry
2 tablespoons vegetable oil
1 tablespoon soy sauce
½ teaspoon salt
⅛ teaspoon pepper
¼ teaspoon sugar
4 slices fresh ginger root

1. Skin chicken breasts, if you wish.
2. Combine Sherry, oil, soy sauce, salt, pepper, sugar and ginger root in a large bowl; add chicken breasts. Marinate for 4 hours in refrigerator.
3. Drain chicken; reserve marinade.
4. Broil or grill, 4-inches from heat, turning and basting once, 15 minutes, or until chicken is golden.
5. Bring remaining marinade to boiling in a small saucepan; spoon over chicken breasts, just before serving. Serve over shredded lettuce.

## SKILLET GINGERED LAMB

*Look for fresh ginger root in your supermarket's produce department.*

Makes 8 servings/**266 calories each.**

2 pounds lean lamb, trimmed of fat
    and cut into thin strips
1 tablespoon vegetable oil
1 bunch green onions, sliced
    lengthwise
3 cans (4 ounces each) whole
    mushrooms
1 can (8 ounces) water chestnuts,
    drained and sliced
1 can (5 ounces) bamboo shoots,
    drained
½ cup soy sauce
3 tablespoons shredded whole
    ginger root
    OR: 2 teaspoons ground ginger
2 tablespoons cornstarch
    Water

1. Brown lamb quickly in hot oil in a large skillet or wok, stirring constantly. Remove lamb and reserve.
2. Brown onions in skillet. Drain mushrooms, reserving liquid. Add lamb, mushrooms, water chestnuts, bamboo shoots, soy sauce and ginger to onions in skillet. Heat, stirring constantly, until bubbly hot.
3. Dissolve cornstarch in ¼ cup cold water in a 2-cup measure; add mushroom liquid and enough water to measure two cups. Blend into lamb mixture; cook, stirring constantly, until sauce thickens and bubbles 1 minute. Serve over shredded lettuce, rather than rice, to save calories and add extra crunch.

## SPRING VEAL RAGOÛT

*Bright spring vegetables add the perfect touch to delicate veal.*

Makes 4 servings/**387 calories each.**

    1 pound lean veal shoulder
    1 large onion, thinly sliced
    2 cups shredded lettuce
    1 teaspoon salt
      Dash of pepper
    ½ teaspoon leaf rosemary, crumbled
    1 envelope or teaspoon instant
      chicken broth
    1 cup water
    8 small new potatoes
    2 medium-size yellow squash
    ½ pound green beans
    2 tablespoons cornstarch
    ¼ cup water

1. Trim all fat from veal, then cut veal into ½-inch cubes.
2. Combine veal with onion, lettuce, salt, pepper, rosemary, instant chicken broth and the 1 cup water in a kettle or Dutch oven. Bring to boiling, cover. Simmer 1 hour, or until veal is tender.
3. While veal cooks, scrub potatoes well; cut off a band of skin around middle of each. Trim squash and thinly slice. Tip beans and cut diagonally into ½-inch-long pieces.
4. Place potatoes on top of meat mixture; cook 30 minutes, or until tender. Cook squash and green beans in slightly salted boiling water in separate medium-size saucepans 10 minutes, or until crisply tender; drain; keep hot.
5. Smooth cornstarch and the ¼ cup water to a paste in a cup; stir into hot meat mixture. Cook, stirring constantly, until broth thickens and bubbles 3 minutes.
6. Spoon meat mixture and potatoes, dividing evenly, on each of 4 heated serving plates; spoon green beans and yellow squash around edges.

## EGG SALAD CUPS

*Egg salad with a difference. It's made with chopped radishes and celery and piled high into tomato cups.*

Makes 4 servings/**156 calories each.**

    4 hard cooked eggs, coarsely
      chopped
    ½ cup chopped radishes
    ½ cup chopped celery
    3 tablespoons imitation
      mayonnaise
    1 teaspoon salt
    1 teaspoon prepared mustard
    ⅛ teaspoon lemon pepper
    ½ teaspoon Worcestershire sauce
    4 large ripe firm tomatoes
      Leaf lettuce

1. Combine eggs, radishes, celery, im-itation mayonnaise, salt, mustard, pepper and Worcestershire sauce in small bowl.
2. Cut thin slice from stem end of tomatoes; scoop out centers, leaving shells about ¼-inch thick; sprinkle shells lightly with salt.
3. Fill with egg salad mixture; serve on lettuce on chilled salad plates.

## ORIENTAL PORK PLATTER

*Not the usual way to use up the Sunday roast, but so good.*

Makes 6 servings/**260 calories each.**

    12 thin slices cooked pork
    ½ cup dry Sherry
    ¼ cup soy sauce
    1 tablespoon peanut or vegetable
      oil
    2 medium-size onions, sliced
    2 medium-size green peppers,
      halved, seeded and cut into
      cubes
    2 yellow squash, sliced
    ½ pound mushrooms, sliced
      OR: 1 can (6 ounces) sliced
      mushrooms
    1½ cups water
    1 envelope or teaspoon instant
      chicken broth
    2 teaspoons salt
    1 can (5 ounces) water chestnuts,
      drained and sliced
    1 can (4 ounces) pimiento, drained
      and chopped
    2 tablespoons cornstarch
    ¼ cup cold water
    1 head romaine, shredded

1. Place pork slices in a shallow pan; combine Sherry and soy sauce and pour over meat. Marinate 30 minutes.
2. Heat oil in a large nonstick skillet; brown pork quickly in oil; remove from skillet and keep warm.
3. Sauté onions in same skillet just until soft; add green peppers and yellow squash; sauté 2 minutes; add mushrooms and sauté 2 minutes. Add marinade from pork, 1½ cups water, instant chicken broth and salt.
4. Bring to boiling; cover skillet; lower heat; simmer 5 minutes, or just until vegetables are crisply tender. Add water chestnuts and pimiento.
5. Combine cornstarch and cold water to make a smooth paste. Stir into bubbling liquid in skillet. Cook, stirring constantly, 1 minute. Return pork slices; heat 1 minute, or just until thoroughly hot.
6. Line a heated serving platter with shredded romaine and spoon vegetable mixture over, reserving some of the sauce; arrange pork slices over vegetables and spoon sauce over.
COOK'S TIP: Slices of cooked chicken, turkey, veal or lamb can be used in place of the pork for delicious variations of this recipe.

## SUN GOLD EGG MOLD

*Hard cooked eggs crown a tangy molded egg and pimiento salad.*

Makes 6 servings/**134 calories each.**

    1 envelope unflavored gelatin
    ¼ cup water
    1 can (about 14 ounces) chicken
      broth
    1 teaspoon Worcestershire sauce
    2 pimientos (from a 4-ounce can)
    5 hard cooked eggs, shelled
    ½ cup diced celery
    1 teaspoon grated onion
    ¼ cup imitation mayonnaise or salad
      dressing
    1 tablespoon prepared mustard
    2 tablespoons lemon juice
    1 teaspoon salt

1. Soften gelatin in water in a small saucepan; heat over low heat, stirring constantly, just until gelatin dissolves. Stir in chicken broth and Worcestershire sauce. Chill 30 minutes.
2. Cut 6 one-inch-long strips of pimiento; arrange, petal fashion, in the bottom of a 4-cup mold. Chop remaining pimiento; reserve.
3. Spoon 1 cup of the thickened gelatin over pimiento in mold. Slice 2 of the hard-cooked eggs lengthwise; press 6 of the largest slices into gelatin around side of mold. Chill again until sticky and firm.
4. While gelatin chills, chop remaining whole eggs and slices; place in a medium-size bowl with reserved chopped pimiento, celery, onion, mayonnaise, mustard, lemon juice and salt. Mix well, then fold in remaining thickened gelatin.
5. Spoon over sticky and firm layer in mold. Chill until firm.
6. Unmold by running a sharp tipped knife around edge, then dipping *quickly* in and out of a pan of hot water; invert onto a serving plate.

## DIET DO'S

### HOW MANY CALORIES DO YOU NEED?

To determine the approximate number of calories needed daily to maintain your weight, follow the chart below. Find your age and sex; multiply your weight by the corresponding number.

| Age | Calorie multiplier |
| --- | --- |
| Males, 15-18 | 22 |
| Females, 15-18 | 18 |
| Males, 19-22 | 20 |
| Females, 19-22 | 16 |
| Males, 23-50 | 18 |
| Females, 23-50 | 16 |
| Males, over 51 | 16 |
| Females, over 51 | 14 |

*Source: *The Food Counter's Guide,* by Ronald M. Deutsch

## PUFFY ITALIAN OMELET

*It's subtly flavored with tender green onions and Parmesan cheese.*

Bake at 350° for 10 minutes.
Makes 6 servings/**194 calories each.**

- 2 slices slightly dry bread
- ½ cup skim milk
- 1 bunch green onions, washed, trimmed and finely chopped
- 2 tablespoons olive or vegetable oil
- 6 eggs
- 2 egg whites
- ½ teaspoon salt
- ¼ teaspoon pepper
- ¼ cup grated Parmesan cheese
- 2 tablespoons finely chopped parsley

1. Place bread in shallow pan; pour milk over; let soak, then pull apart into coarse crumbs.
2. Sauté onions in oil in a 10-inch nonstick skillet with ovenproof or removable handle 5 minutes; remove from heat.
3. Separate eggs, putting whites into large bowl of electric mixer; place yolks into a medium-size bowl. Add extra egg whites to large bowl.
4. Beat egg whites with salt and pepper with electric mixer at high speed, until they stand in firm peaks.
5. Beat egg yolks until light with mixer at medium speed; stir in sautéed onions, bread crumb mixture, cheese and parsley. Fold mixture into egg whites with wire whip until no streaks of white or yellow remain.
6. Pour into skillet; cook over low heat 10 minutes; or until mixture is set on bottom.
7. Bake in moderate oven (350°) 10 minutes, or until puffy and golden on top. Cut into wedges with sharp knife; serve immediately.

## BROILED CORNISH HENS

*Cornish hens don't dry out, when you lavishly baste them with soy sauce.*

Makes 6 servings/**313 calories each.**

- 3 frozen Rock Cornish game hens (about 1½ pounds each), thawed
- ½ cup soy sauce
- 1½ cups water
- 2 green onions, trimmed and chopped
- ¼ teaspoon crushed red pepper
- 1 small head romaine, shredded (about 4 cups)
- 2 tablespoons dry sherry

1. Cut hens in half with poultry shears or kitchen scissors. Place in a shallow broiling pan, without rack.
2. Combine soy sauce, ½ cup of the water, green onions and red pepper; pour over hens. Marinate 1 hour.
3. Broil hens, 4 inches from heat, turning often and basting with marinade, 40 minutes, or until hens are a rich brown.
4. Line a heated serving platter with shredded romaine. Arrange hens on romaine; keep warm.
5. Stir remaining 1 cup water and sherry into broiling pan.
6. Cook, stirring and scraping cooked-on bits from sides of pan, until liquid comes to boiling. Spoon over hens.

## DIET DO'S

### EYE CATCHERS

Try one of the following low calorie garnishes to spruce up your food:
- Carrot curls: Pare carrot; cut long, thin shavings with vegetable parer; roll up and fasten with wooden picks. Chill in ice water; remove picks.
- Cucumber cartwheels: Wash cucumber and thinly slice, but do not pare. Serrate edge with paring knife.
- Green onion ruffles: Wash green onions; trim off root ends and all but 2 to 3 inches of tops. Beginning at root end, make crisscross cuts deep into stalk up to where green begins to show. Quick-chill in ice water. Drain.
- Lemon, lime or orange cartwheels: Thinly slice; serrate edges with knife.
- Lemon, lime, orange rind roses: With vegetable parer, pare round and round fruit into a long spiral. Roll rind up; not too tightly, shaping into a full-blown "rose."
- Pickle fans: Choose small to medium-size pickles. Make several thin, lengthwise cuts from top to about ¼" from bottom. Spread slices to form a fan.
- Stuffed mushrooms: Wipe mushrooms clean with damp cloth. Twist out stems, scoop out cap with a spoon; peel cap. Fill with grated carrots tossed with bottled low calorie Italian or French dressing.
- Prepare ice cubes, placing mint sprigs or lemon rind in each section.

## WINE POACHED FISH

*Served plain, this fish is super slimming; topped with sauce, it's still low calorie fare.*

Makes 4 servings/**217 calories each.**

- 4 small flounder fillets
  OR: 1 package (1 pound) frozen flounder fillets
  Water
  Salt
  Onion
  Lemon slices
  Bay leaf
  Peppercorns
- 1 cup dry white wine
  Creamy Egg Sauce (recipe follows)

1. Half-fill a large skillet with water; season with salt, a few onion and lemon slices, bay leaf and peppercorns. Add white wine. Bring to boiling; lower heat to keep water just at simmering.
2. Place fish on a large piece of foil for easy handling; lower into simmering water; cover pan. Simmer 5 minutes for ½-inch thick fillets or 15 minutes for frozen fish. (Watch carefully, as overcooking toughens delicate fish.)
3. Test for doneness: Stick a fork into thickest part of fish; it should separate easily into flakes. Lift up foil and remove from pan to drain; reserve poaching liquid; keep fish warm.
4. When ready to serve, spoon CREAMY EGG SAUCE over fish.

**CREAMY EGG SAUCE:** Makes about 2 cups/**15 calories per tablespoon.** Hard-cook 2 eggs; shell and chop; set aside. Melt 2 tablespoons butter or margarine in a small saucepan; blend in 2 tablespoons all purpose flour and ¾ teaspoon salt. Cook, stirring constantly, until mixture bubbles. Stir in 1½ cups poaching liquid, ½ cup evaporated skim milk and 1 teaspoon Worcestershire sauce; cook, stirring constantly, until sauce thickens and bubbles 3 minutes. Stir in chopped eggs.

## CRUNCHY CHEF'S SALAD

*Sauerkraut adds a German touch to the classic chef's salad.*

Makes 6 servings/**264 calories each.**

- 1 cup plain yogurt
- ¼ cup imitation mayonnaise
- 3 tablespoons catsup
- 1 teaspoon salt
- ¼ teaspoon pepper
- 1 can (1 pound, 12 ounces) sauerkraut, well drained
- 3 cups broken lettuce
- 2 cups cooked turkey or chicken, cubed
- 1 package (8 ounces) Muenster cheese slices, cut into strips
- 2 hard cooked eggs, shelled and sliced
- 1 tomato, cut into wedges

1. Combine yogurt, imitation mayonnaise, catsup, salt and pepper in a small bowl. Chill to blend flavors.
2. Combine sauerkraut and ¾ cup dressing in a small bowl; toss well.
3. Place lettuce in a large bowl. Top with some of the sauerkraut mixture. Arrange turkey or chicken, cheese, eggs and tomato, in spoke-fashion, on top of lettuce. Place remaining kraut in the center; cover with plastic wrap. Chill until serving time.
4. Toss salad until well mixed. Serve with remaining dressing.

## BARBECUED FRANKS

*Chili powder and mustard blend with tomato sauce to make a tangy sauce.*

Makes 6 servings/**261 calories each.**

- 1 package (1 pound) frankfurters, cut in 1-inch pieces
- 1 small onion, chopped (¼ cup)
- ½ teaspoon salt
  Pinch pepper
- 1 teaspoon chili powder
- 1 teaspoon dry mustard
- 1 can (8 ounces) tomato sauce

1. Brown frankfurters and onions slowly in a large nonstick skillet. Drain off excess fat.
2. Add salt, pepper, chili powder and dry mustard; cook 2 minutes, stirring constantly; pour tomato sauce into skillet. Mix well. Simmer 10 minutes to blend flavors.

## OVEN-FRIED FISH

*Here's a low calorie version of everyone's favorite fish dish.*

Bake at 450° for 12 minutes.
Makes 8 servings/**146 calories each.**

- 2 packages (1 pound each) frozen flounder, sole or perch fillets, thawed
- ½ cup fine dry bread crumbs
- 1 teaspoon seasoned salt
- ⅛ teaspoon seasoned pepper
- 1 tablespoon parsley flakes
- 1 teaspoon paprika
- 2 tablespoons vegetable oil

1. Carefully separate fish into fillets.
2. Combine bread crumbs, salt, pepper, parsley flakes and paprika in a small bowl; add oil. Blend with a fork until thoroughly combined. Spread on wax paper.
3. Press the fish fillets into crumb mixture to coat both sides. Place on a large cookie sheet.
4. Bake in a very hot oven (450°) 12 minutes, or until golden brown.

## MEAT LOAF ITALIANO

*Puréed vegetables add moistness with little calories to this pungent meat loaf. You can oven bake eggplant to serve with it.*

Bake at 375° for 50 minutes.
Makes 6 servings/**260 calories each.**

- 1½ pounds lean ground round
- 1 jar (about 5 ounces) baby-pack strained carrots
- ½ cup tomato juice
- ¼ cup chopped parsley
- 1 small onion, chopped (¼ cup)
- 1½ teaspoons salt
- 1 teaspoon mixed Italian herbs, crumbled

1. Mix beef, carrots, tomato juice,

parsley, onion, salt and mixed Italian herbs just until blended in a large bowl. Form into a thick round patty about 8-inches in diameter; place on rack in broiler pan or set on a wire rack in a shallow baking pan.
2. Bake in moderate oven (375°) 50 minutes, or until brown. Slice patty into 6 wedges.

# MORE WITH SALADS AND VEGETABLES

## LEMON DRESSING

*Serve with Boston lettuce and melon balls for a cooling summer salad.*

Makes 1 cup/**9 calories per tablespoon.**

- 1 teaspoon unflavored gelatin (from 1 envelope)
- 1 tablespoon cold water
- ¼ cup boiling water
- 2 tablespoons sugar
- ½ teaspoon salt
- 1 teaspoon grated lemon rind
- ½ cup lemon juice
- 1 teaspoon dry mustard
- ¼ teaspoon garlic salt
  Pinch white pepper
- ¼ teaspoon Worcestershire sauce

1. Sprinkle gelatin over cold water in small bowl to soften. Add boiling water; stir until gelatin is dissolved.
2. Add sugar and salt; stir.
3. Combine gelatin mixture with lemon rind and juice, dry mustard, garlic salt, white pepper and Worcestershire sauce in a 2-cup jar with a screw top. Shake well; serve at room temperature.

## THOUSAND ISLAND DRESSING

*Zesty bits of olives and pickle spark this creamy dressing. Serve with wedges of iceberg lettuce.*

Makes ¾ cup/**12 calories per tablespoon.**

- 1 egg
- ¼ cup skim milk
- 2 tablespoons cider vinegar
- ½ teaspoon paprika
- ½ teaspoon salt
- ¼ teaspoon dry mustard
- ½ teaspoon chili powder
- 2 tablespoons tomato paste
- 2 tablespoons chopped stuffed olives
- 2 tablespoons chopped dill pickle

1. Combine egg, skim milk, vinegar, paprika, salt, dry mustard, chili powder and tomato paste in container of electric blender; cover. Process at high speed until well mixed.
2. Transfer dressing to small saucepan. Cook over very low heat, stirring constantly, until dressing thickens. Stir in olives and pickle. Chill to blend flavors before serving.

## SQUASH BAKE

*Long, slender slices of yellow squash bake with herbs and a cheese topping.*

Bake at 350° for 15 minutes.
Makes 4 servings/**76 calories each.**

- 2 medium-size yellow squash
- 1 tablespoon butter or margarine
- 1 teaspoon leaf oregano, crumbled
- ½ teaspoon salt
  Dash pepper
- ¼ cup bottled low calorie Italian salad dressing
- 2 tablespoons grated Parmesan cheese

1. Tip squash; cut into thin slices, lengthwise, with a sharp French knife.
2. Brush a 6-cup shallow glass-ceramic or metal baking dish with melted butter or margarine. Lay squash slices in dish; season with oregano, salt and pepper; drizzle with Italian dressing.
3. Bake in moderate oven (350°) 15 minutes, or until squash is tender; sprinkle with Parmesan cheese.
4. Broil, 4 inches from heat, 2 minutes or until golden brown.
COOK'S TIP: Zucchini can be substituted for the yellow squash.

## EGGS EN GELÉE

*Deviled eggs served in shimmering jellied beef broth make a low calorie salad.*

Makes 4 servings/**124 calories each.**

- 1 envelope unflavored gelatin
- 1 can (13¾ ounces) beef broth
- 4 hard-cooked eggs, shelled
- 2 tablespoons imitation mayonnaise
- 1 teaspoon prepared mustard
  Dash salt
  Lettuce

1. Soften gelatin in beef broth in a small saucepan. Heat slowly, stirring constantly, until gelatin dissolves; pour into a shallow pan. Chill 30 minutes, or until syrupy.
2. Cut eggs in half, crosswise; carefully remove yolks and place in a small bowl. Mash well with a fork. Blend in mayonnaise, mustard and salt to make a smooth mixture.
3. Fill egg whites with egg mixture. (Pipe through a pastry bag with a star tip, if you wish.) Place 2 stuffed eggs into each of 4 custard cups.
4. Spoon gelatin syrup over eggs, dividing evenly. Chill at least 4 hours, or until firm.
5. Unmold by running a thin blade knife around edge of each cup; dip cups *quickly* in and out of a pan of hot water. Invert onto lettuce lined salad plates. Serve with a colorful assortment of crisp vegetables, such as carrots, radishes and celery.

## SKILLET OKRA & TOMATOES

*A skillet vegetable dish—from freezer to table in less than half an hour.*

Makes 6 servings/**76 calories each.**

- 2 tablespoons diet margarine
- 1 medium-size onion, chopped (½ cup)
- 1 can (1 pound) tomato wedges
- 1 bag (1 pound) frozen whole okra pods
- ½ teaspoon salt
- ¼ teaspoon pepper

1. Melt diet margarine in a large heavy skillet. Sauté chopped onion until soft.
2. Add tomatoes, okra, salt and pepper; cover. Cook, stirring several times, 20 to 25 minutes, or until okra is tender.

## RED CABBAGE SLAW

*Colorful and vitamin-rich red cabbage makes a perfect salad choice.*

Makes 6 servings/**45 calories each.**

- 1 medium-size head red cabbage, shredded
- 1 medium-size onion, minced (½ cup)
- 1 medium-size green pepper, halved seeded and chopped (½ cup)
- 1 medium-size carrot, pared and shredded
- ½ cup plain yogurt (from an 8-ounce container)
- 3 tablespoons lemon juice
- 1½ teaspoons salt
- ¼ teaspoon garlic powder
- ¼ teaspoon lemon pepper

1. Toss cabbage, onion, green pepper and carrot together in a large bowl.
2. Combine yogurt, lemon juice, salt, garlic powder and pepper in a small bowl; fold into the vegetables. Chill.

## MARINATED ARTICHOKES

*Artichokes should be high on a dieter's list of vegetables because they're high in nutrition, yet low in calories.*

Makes 4 servings/**40 calories each.**

- 4 medium-size artichokes
- 6 whole allspice
- 1 bay leaf
- 1 teaspoon salt
- 1 tablespoon olive or vegetable oil

1. Wash artichokes; cut stems and snip about 1 inch from tips of leaves with scissors. Stand artichokes upright in a large saucepan; add allspice, bay leaf, salt, oil and enough water to half fill pan; cover.
2. Bring to boiling; lower heat; cook 40 minutes, or until tender when pierced with a fork. Allow artichokes

to cool in liquid. Lift out and set on paper towels to drain.
3. Open each artichoke and remove choke from bottom with a teaspoon. Chill until serving time.
4. Place each artichoke on a large plate. Serve plain, since cooking water marinates the artichokes. Garnish with lemon wedge, if you wish.

## MOLDED TURKEY CROWN

*Molded in two layers, it turns out with a shimmery avocado topping over a crunchy and creamy turkey salad.*

Makes 6 servings/**265 calories each.**

**Avocado Layer**
- 1 envelope unflavored gelatin
- 1 cup water
- ¾ cup cold water
- 3 tablespoons lemon juice
- 2 drops liquid red pepper seasoning
- 1 avocado, halved, pitted, peeled and diced

**Turkey Layer**
- 1 envelope unflavored gelatin
- 1 envelope or teaspoon instant chicken broth
- ½ teaspoon salt
- ½ teaspoon dillweed
- 5 drops liquid red pepper seasoning
- 1½ cups water
- ½ cup imitation mayonnaise
- 2 cups diced cooked turkey
- ½ cup thinly sliced celery
- ¼ cup chopped water chestnuts

1. Make avocado layer: Soften gelatin in 1 cup water in a small saucepan. Heat, stirring constantly, until gelatin dissolves; stir in the ¾ cup cold water, lemon juice and liquid red pepper seasoning.
2. Chill 30 minutes, or just until as thick as unbeaten egg white; fold in diced avocado; pour into an 8-cup tube mold. Chill 30 minutes, or just until sticky and firm.
3. Make turkey layer: Soften gelatin with instant chicken broth, salt, dillweed and liquid red pepper seasoning in water in a medium-size saucepan; heat, stirring constantly, just until gelatin dissolves. Remove saucepan from heat.
4. Beat in imitation mayonnaise until smooth; fold in turkey, celery and water chestnuts. Cool. Spoon over sticky and firm avocado layer. Chill at least 3 hours, or until firm. (Overnight is best.)
5. To unmold, run a sharp tipped thin bladed knife around top of mold, then dip mold *very quickly* in and out of a pan of hot water. Cover mold with a large serving plate; turn upside down, then carefully lift off mold. Garnish center with a few salad greens, if you wish.

## CURRY TOMATO DRESSING

*Try this dressing over red and green pepper rings on a bed of shredded lettuce; it's also great as a party dip.*

Makes ½ cup/**15 calories per tablespoon.**

- ⅓ cup cream-style cottage cheese
- ¼ cup buttermilk
- 1 tablespoon catsup
- ½ teaspoon curry powder
- ½ teaspoon Worcestershire sauce
- ¼ teaspoon salt

Combine cottage cheese, buttermilk, catsup, curry powder, Worcestershire sauce and salt in container of electric blender; cover container; process at high speed until smooth, scraping sides with rubber spatula, if necessary. Refrigerate in covered container before serving.

## GERMAN SAUERKRAUT

*This is the special Bavarian way of serving zestful sauerkraut.*

Makes 4 servings/**74 calories each.**

- 1 can (1 pound) sauerkraut
- 1 medium-size onion, chopped (½ cup)
- 1 clove garlic, minced
- 1 tablespoon vegetable shortening
  Dash sugar
- 1 teaspoon caraway seeds, crushed
- 1 cup beef broth
- 1 small potato, pared and grated

1. Drain sauerkraut and rinse under running water, if you wish; drain.
2. Sauté onion and garlic in hot shortening in a large saucepan until soft. Stir in drained sauerkraut, sugar, caraway seeds and broth.
3. Bring to boiling; lower heat; cover saucepan; simmer 20 minutes. Stir in grated potato; cook 10 minutes or until flavors blend.

## PARSLEY CUCUMBERS

*Cooked cucumbers? Yes, they're delicious poached in broth.*

Makes 4 servings/**40 calories each.**

- 2 large firm cucumbers
- 1 cup beef broth
- 2 tablespoons diet margarine
- 2 tablespoons chopped parsley

1. Pare cucumbers; quarter, lengthwise; remove seeds; cut quarters into 2-inch pieces.
2. Combine cucumbers and broth in a medium-size saucepan; bring to boiling; cover saucepan; simmer 2 minutes, or until crisply tender.
3. Drain broth into a jar and use to make soup. Toss margarine and parsley with cucumbers in saucepan until margarine melts.

## EGGPLANT AU GRATIN

*Eggplant tastes so hearty, you'd think it was loaded with calories; actually there are only 92 in a 1 pounder.*

Bake at 400° for 25 minutes.
Makes 6 servings/**99 calories each.**

1 small eggplant (about 1 pound)
½ pound mushrooms, sliced
2 tablespoons butter or margarine
2 tablespoons lemon juice
1 tablespoon all purpose flour
½ cup evaporated skim milk
1 egg
2 tablespoons water
1 teaspoon salt
¼ teaspoon pepper
    Dash ground nutmeg
    Dash liquid red pepper seasoning
1 tablespoon fine dry bread crumbs
1 tablespoon grated Parmesan cheese

1. Cut eggplant into 1-inch slices; pare and cube. Cook in boiling salted water 5 minutes; drain.
2. Sauté mushrooms in 1 tablespoon of the butter or margarine and lemon juice until mushrooms wilt. Stir in flour until well blended; stir in milk; cook, stirring constantly, until sauce thickens and bubbles 3 minutes.
3. Beat egg and water in a cup; stir into sauce; cook, stirring constantly, 1 minute; add drained eggplant with salt, pepper, nutmeg and red pepper seasoning; stir to mix well. Spoon mixture into an 8-inch pie plate.
4. Combine remaining butter, bread crumbs and Parmesan cheese in a cup; sprinkle over eggplant mixture.
5. Bake in hot oven (400°) 25 minutes, or until golden brown. Cut into wedges to serve.

## ZUCCHINI PROVENÇAL

*This is a new way to make an omelet.*

Makes 4 servings/**165 calories each.**

2 tablespoons olive or vegetable oil
1 large onion, thinly sliced
6 medium-size zucchini, tipped and sliced
1 clove garlic, minced
1 teaspoon leaf oregano, crumbled
3 eggs
1 teaspoon salt
¼ teaspoon pepper

1. Heat oil in a large skillet; add onions; lower heat; cover skillet; steam 7 minutes. Add zucchini, garlic and oregano; cover; steam 20 minutes, or until very soft; mash zucchini slightly.
2. Beat eggs with salt and pepper in a bowl; pour into skillet; cook 3 minutes, or just until eggs are set. Spoon onto heated serving plates. Garnish with parsley sprigs.

## KATHY'S RATATOUILLE MOLD

*Kathy Hadda created this picnic dish for an outdoor concert last summer in New York City's Central Park.*

Makes 8 servings/**71 calories each.**

2 cups Ratatouille Nicolse (recipe, page 77)
1 medium-size green pepper, halved, seeded and chopped
1 medium-size red pepper, halved, seeded and chopped
2 envelopes unflavored gelatin
¼ cup dry Sherry
2 cups chicken broth (made with 3 envelopes or teaspoons instant chicken broth and 2 cups boiling water)
1 can (6 ounces) tomato paste
1 tablespoon lemon juice
1 tablespoon Worcestershire sauce
1 teaspoon salt
    Few drops liquid red pepper seasoning
2 large stalks celery, finely chopped (1½ cups)
2 large carrots, pared and finely chopped (2 cups)
1 large cucumber, pared and finely chopped (2 cups)

1. Combine RATATOUILLE NIÇOISE and chopped green and red peppers in a medium-size saucepan; bring to boiling; lower heat; simmer 15 minutes.
2. Soften gelatin in Sherry in small saucepan 2 minutes; cook over low heat, stirring constantly, 3 minutes, or until gelatin dissolves.
3. Place half the ratatouille mixture and 1 cup of the chicken broth in the container of an electric blender; cover; process at high speed 30 seconds, or until smooth; repeat with remaining ratatouille mixture and chicken broth.
4. Combine blended vegetables and softened gelatin in medium-size bowl until well blended. Add tomato paste, lemon juice, Worcestershire sauce, salt and liquid red pepper seasoning; stir until well blended; chill 30 minutes, or until just the consistency of unbeaten egg white.
5. Add chopped celery, carrot and cucumber to syrupy gelatin mixture. Spoon into an 8-cup mold or bowl. Chill 4 hours, or until firm.
6. Just before serving, run a thin bladed knife around top of mold; then dip mold *very quickly* in and out of a pan of hot water. Invert onto serving plate; carefully lift off mold. Garnish with cucumber cartwheels and carrot curls, if you wish.
COOK'S TIPS: Gelatin is dissolved when all the granules disappear and liquid is clear. For picnics, carry KATHY'S RATATOUILLE MOLD in mold, covered tightly with aluminum foil; spoon out individual helpings at serving time.

# MORE DESSERTS

## MICHIGAN CHERRY ROLL

*Just to prove that all gorgeous desserts aren't loaded with calories.*

Bake at 400° for 8 minutes.
Makes 10 servings/**135 calories each.**

½ cup cake flour
¾ teaspoon baking powder
¼ teaspoon salt
3 eggs
½ cup granulated sugar
1 teaspoon vanilla
2 tablespoons 10X (confectioners' powdered) sugar
1 cup cherry pie filling (from a 1-pound can)

1. Grease a 15x10x1-inch jelly roll pan; line with wax paper; grease.
2. Measure cake flour, baking powder and salt into sifter.
3. Beat eggs until foamy light and double in volume in small bowl of electric mixer at high speed; beat in sugar, 1 tablespoon at a time, until mixture is thick; stir in vanilla.
4. Sift flour mixture over and fold in with wire whip until no streaks of white remain. Spread evenly in pan.
5. Bake in hot oven (400°) 8 minutes, or until center springs back when lightly pressed with fingertip.
6. Loosen cake around edges with a sharp knife; invert cake onto a clean towel dusted with 1 tablespoon of the 10X sugar; peel off wax paper. Starting at one short end of cake, roll up; wrap in towel; cool completely.
7. Unroll cake carefully; spread evenly with filling; reroll; dust top with remaining 1 tablespoon 10X sugar.
8. Cut crosswise into 10 slices.

## PERSIAN FRUIT DESSERT

*Just a few nuts add the perfect touch to this colorful fruit medley.*

Makes 8 servings/**104 calories each.**

1 small ripe honeydew
1 small ripe cantaloupe
1 pint strawberries
1 cup seedless green grapes
3 tablespoons finely chopped pistachio nuts
1 cup orange juice
2 tablespoons brandy
1 tablespoon rose water (optional)

1. Slice, pare and seed melons; cut into 1-inch cubes. Wash and hull strawberries.
2. Combine melon cubes, whole strawberries, grapes and nuts in a large glass bowl.
3. Pour orange juice over fruits with brandy and rose water; mix well. Cover bowl with plastic wrap. Chill several hours to blend flavors.

## MEAT GROUP

| | Measure or Weight | Calories | Protein grams | Fat grams | Saturated Fatty Acids grams | Polyunsaturated Fatty Acids grams | Cholesterol mg. | Carbohydrates grams | Calcium mg. | Iron mg. | Vitamin A I.U. | Vitamin B/Thiamin mg. | Vitamin B/Riboflavin mg. | Vitamin B/Niacin mg. | Vitamin C/Ascorbic Acid mg. |
|---|---|---|---|---|---|---|---|---|---|---|---|---|---|---|---|
| Chicken, broiled, no skin | 3 oz. | 115 | 20 | 3 | 1 | 1 | 50 | 0 | 8 | 1.4 | 80 | 0.05 | 0.16 | 7.4 | — |
| Cod fillet, poached | 3 oz. | 89 | 20 | # | # | # | — | 0 | 11 | 0.45 | 0 | 0.07 | 0.08 | 2.5 | 2 |
| Tuna, in oil, drained | 3 oz. | 170 | 24 | 7 | 2 | 1 | 60 | 0 | 7 | 1.6 | 70 | 0.04 | 0.10 | 10.1 | — |
| Shrimp, canned | 3 oz. | 100 | 21 | 1 | — | — | 106 | 1 | 98 | 2.6 | 50 | 0.01 | 0.03 | 1.5 | — |
| Ground beef, lean | 3 oz. | 185 | 23 | 10 | 5 | trace | 60 | 0 | 10 | 3.0 | 20 | 0.08 | 0.20 | 5.1 | — |
| Lamb, roast, lean | 3 oz. | 165 | 24 | 6 | 4 | trace | 60 | 0 | 11 | 1.7 | — | 0.14 | 0.25 | 5.3 | — |
| Veal, roast, med. fat | 3 oz. | 186 | 23 | 14 | 7 | trace | 77 | 0 | 10 | 2.9 | — | 0.11 | 0.26 | 6.6 | — |
| Pork, roast, lean | 3 oz. | 219 | 25 | 13 | 4 | 1 | 60 | 0 | 11 | 3.2 | 0 | 0.91 | 0.26 | 5.5 | — |
| Ham, boiled | 3 oz. | 203 | 17 | 15 | 6 | 2 | 60 | 0 | 9 | 2.4 | 0 | 0.38 | 0.14 | 2.3 | — |
| Bacon, crisp | 2 slices | 100 | 5 | 8 | 3 | 1 | ★ | 1 | 2 | 0.5 | 0 | 0.08 | 0.05 | 0.8 | — |
| Beef liver, cooked | 3 oz. | 158 | 23 | 9 | — | — | 257 | 5 | 9 | 7.5 | 45,420 | 0.23 | 3.56 | 14.1 | 23 |
| Bologna | 1 slice | 100 | 3 | 7 | ★ | # | ★ | trace | 2 | 0.5 | — | 0.04 | 0.06 | 0.7 | — |
| Frankfurter, 8 per pound | 1 | 179 | 7 | 15 | ★ | # | ★ | 1 | 3 | 0.8 | — | 0.08 | 0.11 | 1.4 | — |
| Egg | 1 large | 80 | 6 | 6 | 2 | trace | 275 | trace | 27 | 1.1 | 590 | 0.05 | 0.15 | trace | 0 |
| Red kidney beans, cooked | 1 cup | 230 | 15 | 1 | — | — | 0 | 42 | 74 | 4.6 | 10 | 0.13 | 0.10 | 1.5 | — |
| Split green peas, cooked | 1 cup | 290 | 20 | 1 | — | — | 0 | 52 | 28 | 4.2 | 100 | 0.37 | 0.22 | 2.2 | — |
| Peanut butter | 1 tbsp. | 95 | 4 | 8 | 2 | 2 | 0 | 3 | 9 | 0.3 | — | 0.02 | 0.02 | 2.4 | 0 |
| Peanuts | ¼ cup | 170 | 9 | 18 | 4 | 5 | 0 | 7 | 27 | 0.8 | — | 0.11 | 0.05 | 6.1 | 0 |
| Walnuts | ¼ cup | 198 | 6 | 19 | 1 | 9 | 0 | 5 | trace | 1.9 | 95 | 0.07 | 0.04 | 0.2 | — |
| Coconut | ¼ cup | 124 | 1 | 11 | 10 | trace | 0 | 3 | 4 | 0.5 | — | 0.02 | 0.01 | 0.2 | 1 |

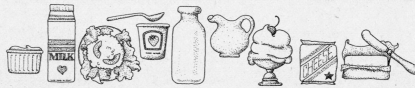

## DAIRY FOODS GROUP

| | Measure or Weight | Calories | Protein grams | Fat grams | Saturated Fatty Acids grams | Polyunsaturated Fatty Acids grams | Cholesterol mg. | Carbohydrates grams | Calcium mg. | Iron mg. | Vitamin A I.U. | Vitamin B/Thiamin mg. | Vitamin B/Riboflavin mg. | Vitamin B/Niacin mg. | Vitamin C/Ascorbic Acid mg. |
|---|---|---|---|---|---|---|---|---|---|---|---|---|---|---|---|
| Skim milk, non-fat | 1 cup | 90 | 9 | trace | — | — | 7 | 12 | 296 | 0.1 | 10 | 0.09 | 0.44 | 0.2 | 2 |
| Whole milk | 1 cup | 160 | 9 | 9 | 5 | trace | 27 | 12 | 288 | 0.1 | 350 | 0.07 | 0.41 | 0.2 | 2 |
| Buttermilk | 1 cup | 90 | 9 | trace | — | — | 7 | 12 | 296 | 0.1 | 10 | 0.10 | 0.44 | 0.2 | 2 |
| Chocolate drink | 1 cup | 190 | 8 | 6 | 3 | trace | ★ | 27 | 270 | 0.5 | 210 | 0.10 | 0.40 | 0.3 | 3 |
| Evaporated milk | 1 tbsp. | 22 | 1 | 1 | 1 | trace | ★ | 1 | 40 | trace | 50 | trace | 0.05 | trace | trace |
| Light cream | 1 tbsp. | 30 | 1 | 3 | 2 | trace | ★ | 1 | 15 | trace | 130 | trace | 0.02 | trace | trace |
| Heavy cream | 1 tbsp. | 55 | trace | 6 | 3 | trace | ★ | 1 | 11 | trace | 230 | trace | 0.02 | trace | trace |
| Powdered imit. cream | 1 tbsp. | 30 | trace | 3 | 2 | 0 | # | 3 | 3 | trace | trace | — | — | — | — |
| Pressurized imit. cream | ¼ cup | 48 | trace | 4 | 4 | 0 | # | 2 | 1 | — | 85 | — | 0 | — | — |
| Pressurized wh. cream | ¼ cup | 39 | trace | 4 | 2 | trace | ★ | 2 | 17 | — | 142 | — | 0.01 | — | — |
| Dairy sour cream | 1 tbsp. | 25 | trace | 2 | 1 | trace | ★ | 1 | 12 | trace | 100 | trace | 0.02 | trace | trace |
| Yogurt, part skim milk | 1 cup | 120 | 8 | 4 | 2 | trace | ★ | 13 | 294 | 0.1 | 170 | 0.10 | 0.44 | 0.2 | 2 |
| Ice milk | ½ cup | 130 | 3 | 4 | 2 | trace | ★ | 15 | 102 | 0.05 | 140 | 0.04 | 0.15 | 0.05 | trace |
| Ice cream, regular | ½ cup | 148 | 3 | 7 | 4 | trace | 30 | 14 | 97 | 0.05 | 295 | 0.03 | 0.14 | 0.05 | trace |
| Baked custard | ½ cup | 142 | 7 | 8 | 4 | 1 | 150a | 15 | 150 | 0.6 | 465 | 0.06 | 0.25 | 0.2 | trace |
| Cottage cheese, dry | ½ cup | 97 | 17 | 1 | trace | trace | # | 3 | 90 | 0.4 | 10 | 0.03 | 0.28 | 0.1 | 0 |
| Cottage cheese, creamed | ½ cup | 120 | 17 | 5 | 3 | trace | 19 | 4 | 115 | 0.35 | 210 | 0.04 | 0.32 | 0.1 | 0 |
| Process. Amer. cheese | 1 oz. | 105 | 7 | 9 | 5 | trace | 24 | 1 | 198 | 0.3 | 350 | 0.01 | 0.12 | trace | 0 |
| Cheddar cheese | 1 oz. | 115 | 7 | 9 | 5 | trace | 28 | 1 | 17 | 0.06 | 437 | 0.01 | 0.13 | trace | 0 |
| Cream cheese | 1 oz. | 107 | 2 | 11 | 6 | trace | 34 | 1 | 17 | 0.06 | 437 | 0.01 | 0.06 | 0.03 | 0 |

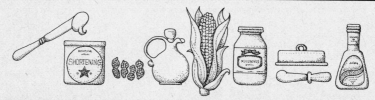

## FATS and OILS

| | Measure or Weight | Calories | Protein grams | Fat grams | Saturated Fatty Acids grams | Polyunsaturated Fatty Acids grams | Cholesterol mg. | Carbohydrates grams | Calcium mg. | Iron mg. | Vitamin A I.U. | Vitamin B/Thiamin mg. | Vitamin B/Riboflavin mg. | Vitamin B/Niacin mg. | Vitamin C/Ascorbic Acid mg. |
|---|---|---|---|---|---|---|---|---|---|---|---|---|---|---|---|
| Butter | 1 tbsp. | 100 | trace | 12 | 6 | trace | 36 | trace | 3 | 0 | 470 | — | — | — | 0 |
| Margarine, regular | 1 tbsp. | 100 | trace | 12 | 2 | 3 | 0 | trace | 3 | 0 | 470 | — | — | — | 0 |
| Margarine, liq. oil, 1st ing. | 1 tbsp. | 100 | trace | 11 | 2 | 4 | 0 | trace | 3 | 0 | 470 | — | — | — | 0 |
| Hydro. veg. shortening | 1 tbsp. | 125 | 0 | 13 | 3 | 3 | 0 | 0 | 0 | 0 | — | 0 | 0 | 0 | — |
| Lard | 1 tbsp. | 125 | 0 | 13 | 5 | 1 | 12 | 0 | 0 | 0 | 0 | 0 | 0 | 0 | — |
| Corn oil | 1 tbsp. | 125 | 0 | 14 | 1 | 7 | 0 | 0 | 0 | 0 | — | 0 | 0 | 0 | — |
| Cottonseed oil | 1 tbsp. | 125 | 0 | 14 | 4 | 7 | 0 | 0 | 0 | 0 | — | 0 | 0 | 0 | — |
| Peanut oil | 1 tbsp. | 125 | 0 | 14 | 3 | 4 | 0 | 0 | 0 | 0 | — | 0 | 0 | 0 | — |
| Mayonnaise | 1 tbsp. | 100 | trace | 11 | 2 | 6 | # | trace | 3 | 0.1 | 40 | trace | 0.01 | trace | — |
| French dressing | 1 tbsp. | 65 | trace | 6 | 1 | 3 | 0 | 3 | 2 | 0.1 | — | — | — | — | — |

Symbols: — indicates value unknown, but probably a measurable amount
★ indicates value unknown, but probably a considerable amount
# indicates value unknown, but probably very little

a—if 2-cup whole-milk, 2-egg recipe, making 4
b—if 1-egg recipe making 12
c—if 2-egg recipe
d—if 3-egg recipe

## FRUIT and VEGETABLE GROUP

| | Measure or Weight | Calories | Protein grams | Fat grams | Saturated Fatty Acids grams | Polyunsaturated Fatty Acids grams | Cholesterol mg. | Carbohydrates grams | Calcium mg. | Iron mg. | Vitamin A I.U. | Vitamin B/Thiamin mg. | Vitamin B/Riboflavin mg. | Vitamin B/Niacin mg. | Vitamin C/Ascorbic Acid mg. |
|---|---|---|---|---|---|---|---|---|---|---|---|---|---|---|---|
| Orange juice | ½ cup | 60 | 1 | trace | — | — | 0 | 15 | 13 | 0.1 | 275 | 0.11 | 0.01 | 0.5 | 60 |
| Grapefruit | ½ med. | 45 | 1 | trace | — | — | 0 | 12 | 19 | 0.5 | 10 | 0.05 | 0.02 | 0.2 | 44 |
| Strawberries | 1 cup | 55 | 1 | 1 | — | — | 0 | 13 | 31 | 1.5 | 90 | 0.04 | 0.10 | 1.0 | 88 |
| Apple | 1 med. | 70 | trace | trace | — | — | 0 | 18 | 8 | 0.4 | 50 | 0.04 | 0.02 | 0.1 | 3 |
| Banana | 1 med. | 85 | 1 | trace | — | — | 0 | 26 | 10 | 0.8 | 230 | 0.06 | 0.07 | 0.8 | 12 |
| Avocado | ½ med. | 167 | 2 | 13 | 1.4 | 1 | 0 | 4 | 9 | 1.4 | 460 | 0.09 | 0.09 | 1.4 | 6 |
| Applesauce, no sugar | ½ cup | 50 | trace | trace | — | — | 0 | 13 | 5 | 0.6 | 50 | 0.03 | 0.01 | 1.0 | 1 |
| Peaches, canned | ½ cup | 90 | trace | trace | — | — | 0 | 26 | 5 | 0.4 | 550 | 0.01 | 0.03 | 0.7 | 3 |
| Pineapple, crushed | ½ cup | 97 | trace | trace | — | — | 0 | 25 | 15 | 0.4 | 60 | 0.10 | 0.03 | 0.3 | 9 |
| Raisins | ¼ cup | 115 | 1 | trace | — | — | 0 | 32 | 26 | 1.5 | 8 | 0.04 | 0.03 | 0.2 | 1 |
| Cabbage, shredded raw | ½ cup | 8 | trace | trace | — | — | 0 | 2 | 17 | 0.1 | 45 | 0.02 | 0.02 | 0.1 | 17 |
| Carrot, raw | 1 med. | 20 | 1 | trace | — | — | 0 | 5 | 18 | 0.4 | 5,500 | 0.03 | 0.03 | 0.3 | 4 |
| Tomato, raw | 1 med. | 35 | 2 | trace | — | — | 0 | 9 | 24 | 0.9 | 1,640 | 0.11 | 0.07 | 1.3 | 42 |
| Green beans, cooked | ½ cup | 15 | 1 | trace | — | — | 0 | 4 | 32 | 0.4 | 340 | 0.04 | 0.06 | 0.3 | 8 |
| Spinach, cooked | ½ cup | 20 | 3 | trace | — | — | 0 | 3 | 83 | 2.0 | 7,290 | 0.07 | 0.12 | 0.5 | 25 |
| Summer squash, cooked | ½ cup | 15 | 1 | trace | — | — | 0 | 4 | 26 | 0.4 | 410 | 0.05 | 0.08 | 0.8 | 10 |
| White potato, boiled | 1 med. | 80 | 3 | trace | — | — | 0 | 21 | 9 | 0.7 | trace | 0.10 | 0.04 | 1.7 | 20 |
| Sweet potato, baked | 1 med. | 155 | 2 | 1 | — | — | 0 | 36 | 44 | 1.0 | 8,910 | 0.10 | 0.07 | 0.7 | 24 |
| Peas, canned | ½ cup | 75 | 5 | trace | — | — | 0 | 16 | 25 | 2.1 | 560 | 0.11 | 0.07 | 1.1 | 11 |
| Corn, canned | ½ cup | 75 | 3 | 1 | — | — | 0 | 20 | 5 | 0.5 | 345 | 0.03 | 0.06 | 1.1 | 6 |

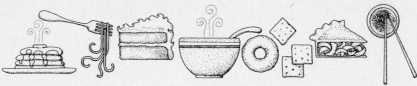

## BREAD and CEREAL GROUP

| | Measure or Weight | Calories | Protein grams | Fat grams | Saturated Fatty Acids grams | Polyunsaturated Fatty Acids grams | Cholesterol mg. | Carbohydrates grams | Calcium mg. | Iron mg. | Vitamin A I.U. | Vitamin B/Thiamin mg. | Vitamin B/Riboflavin mg. | Vitamin B/Niacin mg. | Vitamin C/Ascorbic Acid mg. |
|---|---|---|---|---|---|---|---|---|---|---|---|---|---|---|---|
| White bread, enriched | 1 slice | 70 | 2 | 1 | — | — | # | 13 | 21 | 0.6 | trace | 0.06 | 0.05 | 0.6 | trace |
| Whole wheat bread | 1 slice | 65 | 3 | 1 | — | — | # | 14 | 24 | 0.8 | trace | 0.09 | 0.03 | 0.8 | trace |
| Oatmeal, cooked | ½ cup | 65 | 3 | 1 | — | 1 | 0 | 12 | 11 | 0.7 | 0 | 0.09 | 0.03 | 0.1 | 0 |
| Shredded wheat | 1 | 90 | 2 | 1 | — | — | 0 | 20 | 11 | 0.9 | 0 | 0.06 | 0.03 | 1.1 | 0 |
| Corn flakes | 1 cup | 100 | 2 | trace | — | — | 0 | 21 | 4 | 0.4 | 0 | 0.11 | 0.02 | 0.5 | 0 |
| Sugared corn flakes | 1 cup | 110 | 2 | trace | — | — | 0 | 36 | 5 | 0.4 | 0 | 0.16 | 0.02 | 0.8 | 0 |
| Puffed rice | 1 cup | 55 | 1 | trace | — | — | 0 | 13 | 3 | 0.3 | 0 | 0.07 | 0.01 | 0.7 | 0 |
| Rice, enriched, cooked | ½ cup | 106 | 2 | trace | — | — | 0 | 25 | 10 | 0.9 | 0 | 0.12 | 0.01 | 1.1 | 0 |
| Macaroni, enr., cooked | 1 cup | 155 | 5 | 1 | — | — | 0 | 32 | 8 | 1.3 | 0 | 0.20 | 0.11 | 1.5 | 0 |
| Egg noodles, enriched | ½ cup | 100 | 4 | 1 | trace | trace | ★ | 18 | 8 | 0.5 | 55 | 0.03 | 0.01 | 0.3 | 0 |
| All purpose flour | 1 tbsp. | 25 | 1 | trace | — | — | 0 | 6 | 1 | 0.2 | 0 | 0.03 | 0.02 | 0.2 | 0 |
| Pancake, 4-inch | 1 | 60 | 2 | 2 | trace | trace | 26b | 9 | 27 | 0.4 | 30 | 0.05 | 0.06 | 0.4 | trace |
| Saltines | 4 | 50 | 1 | 1 | — | — | 0 | 8 | 2 | 0.1 | 0 | trace | trace | 0.1 | 0 |
| Graham crackers | 4 | 120 | 2 | 3 | — | — | 0 | 21 | 11 | 0.4 | 0 | 0.01 | 0.06 | 0.4 | 0 |
| Brownie | 1 med. | 120 | 1 | 6 | 1 | 1 | 36c | 10 | 8 | 0.4 | 40 | 0.04 | 0.02 | 0.1 | trace |
| Doughnut | 1 med. | 125 | 3 | 5 | — | # | 15 | 22 | 147 | 0.7 | 0 | 0.12 | 0.07 | 1.0 | trace |
| Angelfood cake | 1/12 | 110 | 3 | trace | — | — | 0 | 32 | 50 | 0.2 | 0 | trace | 0.06 | 0.1 | 0 |
| Yellow cake, choc. icing | 1/12 | 366 | 4 | 13 | 4 | 2 | 69d | 60 | 68 | 0.6 | 160 | 0.02 | 0.08 | 0.2 | trace |
| Apple pie | ⅛ | 306 | 3 | 13 | 4 | 3 | # | 45 | 9 | 0.4 | 35 | 0.03 | 0.03 | 0.4 | 1 |
| Lemon meringue pie | ⅛ | 269 | 4 | 10 | 4 | 2 | 103d | 40 | 15 | 0.5 | 175 | 0.04 | 0.09 | 0.2 | 4 |

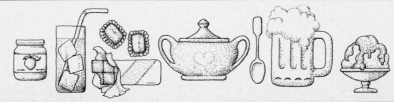

## SUGARS, SWEETS and BEVERAGES

| | Measure or Weight | Calories | Protein grams | Fat grams | Saturated Fatty Acids grams | Polyunsaturated Fatty Acids grams | Cholesterol mg. | Carbohydrates grams | Calcium mg. | Iron mg. | Vitamin A I.U. | Vitamin B/Thiamin mg. | Vitamin B/Riboflavin mg. | Vitamin B/Niacin mg. | Vitamin C/Ascorbic Acid mg. |
|---|---|---|---|---|---|---|---|---|---|---|---|---|---|---|---|
| Granulated sugar | 1 tbsp. | 45 | 0 | 0 | — | — | 0 | 11 | 0 | trace | 0 | 0 | 0 | 0 | 0 |
| Brown sugar | 1 tbsp. | 51 | 0 | 0 | — | — | 0 | 13 | 12 | 0.5 | 0 | trace | trace | trace | 0 |
| Jelly | 1 tbsp. | 55 | trace | trace | — | — | 0 | 13 | 4 | 0.3 | trace | trace | 0.01 | trace | 1 |
| Syrup, corn, blend | 1 tbsp. | 60 | 0 | 0 | — | — | 0 | 15 | 9 | 0.8 | 0 | 0 | 0 | 0 | 0 |
| Molasses, light | 1 tbsp. | 50 | — | — | — | — | 0 | 13 | 33 | 0.9 | — | 0.01 | 0.01 | trace | — |
| Choc. fudge topping | 2 tbsp. | 125 | 2 | 5 | 3 | trace | # | 20 | 48 | 0.5 | 60 | 0.02 | 0.08 | 0.2 | trace |
| Milk choc. candy | 1 oz. | 150 | 2 | 9 | 5 | trace | # | 16 | 65 | 0.3 | 80 | 0.02 | 0.10 | 0.1 | trace |
| Cola beverage | 12 oz. | 145 | 0 | 0 | — | — | 0 | 37 | | | | 0 | 0 | 0 | 0 |
| Beer | 12 oz. | 150 | 1 | 0 | — | — | 0 | 14 | 18 | trace | — | 0.01 | 0.11 | 2.2 | — |
| Scotch/80 proof | 1½ oz. | 120 | | | | | 0 | trace | — | — | — | — | — | — | — |

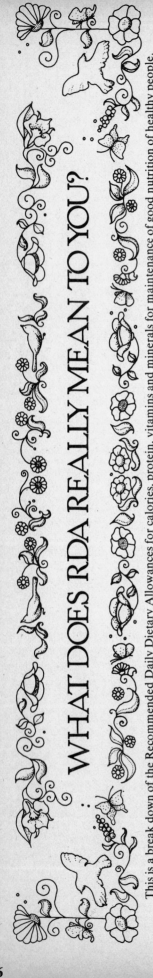

# WHAT DOES RDA REALLY MEAN TO YOU?

This is a break down of the Recommended Daily Dietary Allowances for calories, protein, vitamins and minerals for maintenance of good nutrition of healthy people.

| Group | Age (years) | Weight (kg) | Weight (lbs) | Height (cm) | Height (in) | Energy (kcal)[b] | Protein (g) | Vit. A Activity (RE)[c] | Vit. A Activity (IU) | Vit. D (IU) | Vit. E Activity[e] (IU) | Ascorbic Acid (mg) | Folacin[f] (μg) | Niacin (mg) | Riboflavin (mg) | Thiamin (mg) | Vit. B6 (mg) | Vit. B12 (μg) | Calcium (mg) | Phosphorus (mg) | Iodine (μg) | Iron (mg) | Magnesium (mg) | Zinc (mg) |
|---|---|---|---|---|---|---|---|---|---|---|---|---|---|---|---|---|---|---|---|---|---|---|---|---|
| Infants | 0.0-0.5 | 6 | 14 | 60 | 24 | kg × 117 | kg × 2.2 | 420[d] | 1,400 | 400 | 4 | 35 | 50 | 5 | 0.4 | 0.3 | 0.3 | 0.3 | 360 | 240 | 35 | 10 | 60 | 3 |
| | 0.5-1.0 | 9 | 20 | 71 | 28 | kg × 108 | kg × 2.0 | 400 | 2,000 | 400 | 5 | 35 | 50 | 8 | 0.6 | 0.5 | 0.4 | 0.3 | 540 | 400 | 45 | 15 | 70 | 5 |
| Children | 1-3 | 13 | 28 | 86 | 34 | 1,300 | 23 | 400 | 2,000 | 400 | 7 | 40 | 100 | 9 | 0.8 | 0.7 | 0.6 | 1.0 | 800 | 800 | 60 | 15 | 150 | 10 |
| | 4-6 | 20 | 44 | 110 | 44 | 1,800 | 30 | 500 | 2,500 | 400 | 9 | 40 | 200 | 12 | 1.1 | 0.9 | 0.9 | 1.5 | 800 | 800 | 80 | 10 | 200 | 10 |
| | 7-10 | 30 | 66 | 135 | 54 | 2,400 | 36 | 700 | 3,300 | 400 | 10 | 40 | 300 | 16 | 1.2 | 1.2 | 1.2 | 2.0 | 800 | 800 | 110 | 10 | 250 | 10 |
| Males | 11-14 | 44 | 97 | 158 | 63 | 2,800 | 44 | 1,000 | 5,000 | 400 | 12 | 45 | 400 | 18 | 1.5 | 1.4 | 1.6 | 3.0 | 1,200 | 1,200 | 130 | 18 | 350 | 15 |
| | 15-18 | 61 | 134 | 172 | 69 | 3,000 | 54 | 1,000 | 5,000 | 400 | 15 | 45 | 400 | 20 | 1.8 | 1.5 | 2.0 | 3.0 | 1,200 | 1,200 | 150 | 18 | 400 | 15 |
| | 19-22 | 67 | 147 | 172 | 69 | 3,000 | 54 | 1,000 | 5,000 | 400 | 15 | 45 | 400 | 20 | 1.8 | 1.5 | 2.0 | 3.0 | 800 | 800 | 140 | 10 | 350 | 15 |
| | 23-50 | 70 | 154 | 172 | 69 | 2,700 | 56 | 1,000 | 5,000 | | 15 | 45 | 400 | 18 | 1.6 | 1.4 | 2.0 | 3.0 | 800 | 800 | 130 | 10 | 350 | 15 |
| | 51+ | 70 | 154 | 172 | 69 | 2,400 | 56 | 1,000 | 5,000 | | 15 | 45 | 400 | 16 | 1.5 | 1.2 | 2.0 | 3.0 | 800 | 800 | 110 | 10 | 350 | 15 |
| Females | 11-14 | 44 | 97 | 155 | 62 | 2,400 | 44 | 800 | 4,000 | 400 | 12 | 45 | 400 | 16 | 1.3 | 1.2 | 1.6 | 3.0 | 1,200 | 1,200 | 115 | 18 | 300 | 15 |
| | 15-18 | 54 | 119 | 162 | 65 | 2,100 | 48 | 800 | 4,000 | 400 | 12 | 45 | 400 | 14 | 1.4 | 1.1 | 2.0 | 3.0 | 1,200 | 1,200 | 115 | 18 | 300 | 15 |
| | 19-22 | 58 | 128 | 162 | 65 | 2,100 | 46 | 800 | 4,000 | 400 | 12 | 45 | 400 | 14 | 1.4 | 1.1 | 2.0 | 3.0 | 800 | 800 | 100 | 18 | 300 | 15 |
| | 23-50 | 58 | 128 | 162 | 65 | 2,000 | 46 | 800 | 4,000 | | 12 | 45 | 400 | 13 | 1.2 | 1.0 | 2.0 | 3.0 | 800 | 800 | 100 | 18 | 300 | 15 |
| | 51+ | 58 | 128 | 162 | 65 | 1,800 | 46 | 800 | 4,000 | | 12 | 45 | 400 | 12 | 1.1 | 1.0 | 2.0 | 3.0 | 800 | 800 | 80 | 10 | 300 | 15 |
| Pregnant | | | | | | +300 | +30 | 1,000 | 5,000 | 400 | 15 | 60 | 800 | +2 | +0.3 | +0.3 | 2.5 | 4.0 | 1,200 | 1,200 | 125 | 18+[h] | 450 | 20 |
| Lactating | | | | | | +500 | +20 | 1,200 | 6,000 | 400 | 15 | 80 | 600 | +4 | +0.5 | +0.3 | 2.5 | 4.0 | 1,200 | 1,200 | 150 | 18 | 450 | 25 |

Data from RECOMMENDED DAILY DIETARY ALLOWANCES[a], Revised 1974. FOOD AND NUTRITION BOARD, NATIONAL ACADEMY OF SCIENCES–NATIONAL RESEARCH COUNCIL.

[a] The allowances are intended to provide for individual variations among most normal persons as they live in the United States under usual environmental stresses. Diets should be based on a variety of common foods in order to provide other nutrients for which human requirements have been less well defined.

[b] Kilojoules (kJ) = 4.2 × kcal.

[c] Retinol equivalents.

[d] Assumed to be all as retinol in milk during the first six months of life. All subsequent intakes are assumed to be half as retinol and half as β-carotene when calculated from international units. As retinol equivalents, three fourths are as retinol and one fourth as β-carotene.

[e] Total vitamin E activity, estimated to be 80 percent as β-tocopherol and 20 percent other tocopherols. See text for variation in allowances.

[f] The folacin allowances refer to dietary sources as determined by Lactobacillus casei assay. Pure forms of folacin may be effective in doses less than one fourth of the recommended dietary allowance.

[g] Although allowances are expressed as niacin, it is recognized that on the average 1 mg of niacin is derived from each 60 mg of dietary tryptophan.

[h] This increased requirement cannot be met by ordinary diets; therefore, the use of supplemental iron is recommended.

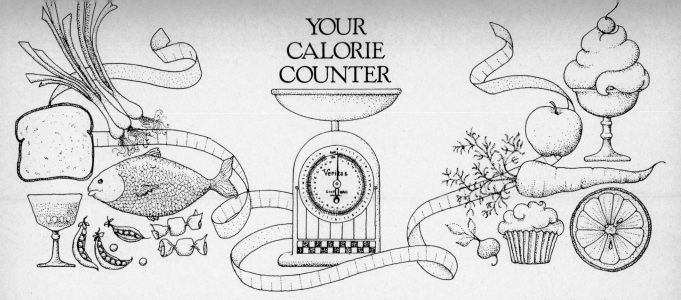

# YOUR CALORIE COUNTER

## FOOD—COUNT—AMOUNT

### A

| Food | Count | Amount |
|---|---|---|
| ALMONDS, shelled, | 850 | 1 cup |
| salted | 83 | 10 nuts |
| ANCHOVIES, fillets | 28 | 4 |
| APPLE | 70 | 1 med. |
| Apple butter | 33 | 1 tbsp. |
| Apple juice | 120 | 1 cup |
| Applesauce, canned, | | |
| sweetened | 230 | 1 cup |
| calories reduced | 100 | 1 cup |
| APRICOTS, | | |
| fresh | 55 | 3 |
| canned in heavy syrup | 110 | ½ cup |
| calories reduced | 56 | ½ cup |
| dried | 90 | 10 |
| Apricot nectar, canned | 140 | 1 cup |
| ARTICHOKES, cooked | 30 | 1 med. |
| frozen, hearts, cooked | 22 | ½ cup |
| Asparagus, fresh, cooked | 20 | 6 spears |
| canned | 20 | 6 spears |
| frozen, spears, cooked | 23 | 5 |
| AVOCADO, | 245 | ½ med. |
| diced | 186 | ½ cup |

### B

| Food | Count | Amount |
|---|---|---|
| BACON, broiled or fried | 100 | 2 slices |
| Canadian, lean, broiled | 50 | 3 slices |
| BAMBOO SHOOTS | 41 | 1 cup |
| BANANA | 85 | 1 |
| BARLEY, pearl, cooked | 142 | 1 cup |
| BEAN SPROUTS, canned | 20 | ½ cup |
| BEANS, baked, with pork | | |
| and molasses | 325 | 1 cup |
| with pork in tomato sauce | 295 | 1 cup |
| BEANS, green or wax | | |
| fresh cut, cooked | 15 | ½ cup |
| canned, cut | 14 | ½ cup |
| frozen, cut, cooked | 18 | ½ cup |
| kidney, canned | 230 | 1 cup |
| lima, fresh, cooked | 180 | 1 cup |
| frozen, cooked | 94 | ½ cup |
| BEEF, brisket, fresh | 266 | 1 slice |
| corned | 266 | 1 slice |
| pot roast, blade | 306 | 1 slice |
| rib roast | 243 | 1 slice |
| rump | 235 | 1 slice |
| sirloin | 186 | 1 slice |
| steak, cubed, raw | 793 | 12 oz. |
| steak, club, raw | 305 | 6 oz. |
| steak, flank | 200 | 3 slices |
| porterhouse | 412 | 1 piece |
| round | 406 | 1 piece |
| ground, round, raw | 271 | 6 oz. |
| sirloin | 353 | 1 piece |
| stew meat, chuck, | | |

| Food | Count | Amount |
|---|---|---|
| boneless, raw | 421 | 4 oz. |
| Beef and vegetable stew | | |
| canned | 210 | 1 cup |
| beef broth, canned, | | |
| condensed | 66 | 1 can |
| envelope instant | 10 | 1 |
| canned corned beef | 185 | 3 oz. |
| canned corned beef hash | 155 | 3 oz. |
| beef potpie, frozen | 436 | 8 oz. |
| Beef TV Dinner | 350 | 1 |
| BEER | 100 | 1 cup |
| BEETS, cooked, diced | 50 | 1 cup |
| BISCUITS, baking powder | 129 | 1 |
| BLACKBERRIES, fresh | 43 | ½ cup |
| frozen, unsweetened | 55 | ½ cup |
| BLUEBERRIES, fresh | 43 | ½ cup |
| frozen, sweetened | 129 | ½ cup |
| frozen, unsweetened | 45 | ½ cup |
| BOLOGNA | 87 | 1 slice |
| BRAN FLAKES, 40% | 95 | ¾ cup |
| BRANDY | 120 | 2 oz. |
| BRAZIL NUTS, shelled | 100 | 4 |
| BREAD | | |
| Boston brown | 100 | 1 slice |
| cracked wheat | 60 | 1 slice |
| French | 108 | 1 piece |
| Italian | 108 | 1 piece |
| pumpernickel | 65 | 1 slice |
| raisin, unfrosted | 80 | 1 slice |
| rye | 65 | 1 slice |
| white, enriched | 70 | 1 slice |
| whole wheat | 65 | 1 slice |
| bread crumbs, dry | 345 | 1 cup |
| soft | 140 | 1 cup |
| BROCCOLI, fresh, spears, | | |
| cooked | 40 | 4 |
| frozen, chopped, cooked | 25 | ½ cup |
| frozen, spears, cooked | 26 | 3 |
| BROWNIES | 120 | 1 |
| BRUSSELS SPROUTS, | | |
| fresh, cooked | 45 | 1 cup |
| frozen, cooked | 29 | ½ cup |
| BUTTER | 100 | 1 tbsp. |

### C

| Food | Count | Amount |
|---|---|---|
| CABBAGE, raw, finely | | |
| shredded | 16 | 1 cup |
| cooked, finely shredded | 35 | 1 cup |
| Chinese, raw, | | |
| chopped | 15 | 1 cup |
| cooked, chopped | 20 | 1 cup |
| CAKES | | |
| angel | 110 | 1 wedge |
| chocolate with icing | 445 | 1 wedge |
| cupcake with icing | 185 | 1 |
| plain cake, no icing | 200 | 1 slice |
| poundcake | 140 | 1 slice |
| spongecake | 120 | 1 wedge |
| CANDY | | |

| Food | Count | Amount |
|---|---|---|
| caramels | 42 | 1 |
| chocolate creams | 47 | 1 |
| chocolate fudge | 66 | 1 |
| chocolate mint patty | 40 | 1 |
| marshmallows | 26 | 1 large |
| peanut brittle | 125 | 1 piece |
| CANTALOUPE | 60 | ½ med. |
| balls | 20 | ½ cup |
| CARBONATED DRINKS | 90 | 8 oz. |
| CARROTS, raw, whole | 20 | 1 |
| raw, grated | 45 | 1 cup |
| cooked, diced | 45 | 1 cup |
| CASHEW NUTS, roasted | 164 | 8 |
| CATSUP | 15 | 1 tbsp. |
| CAULIFLOWER, raw | | |
| or cooked flowerets | 25 | 1 cup |
| frozen, flowerets, cooked | 15 | ½ cup |
| CELERY, raw, diced | 15 | 1 cup |
| raw, stalk | 5 | 1 |
| CHEESE | | |
| blue or Roquefort | 105 | 1 oz. |
| Camembert | 86 | 1 oz. |
| Cheddar or American, | | |
| grated | 445 | 1 cup |
| grated | 30 | 1 tbsp. |
| process | 105 | 1 oz. |
| cottage, skim milk | | |
| cream-style | 240 | 1 cup |
| cottage, dry | 195 | 1 cup |
| cream | 55 | 1 tbsp. |
| Parmesan, grated | 31 | 1 tbsp. |
| Swiss, natural | 120 | 1 oz. |
| Swiss, process | 105 | 1 oz. |
| Cheese food, Cheddar | 90 | 1 oz. |
| Cheese, spreads | 35 | 1 tbsp. |
| CHERRIES, sour, canned | 230 | 1 cup |
| sweet, fresh | 80 | 1 cup |
| canned, sweetened | 112 | ½ cup |
| calories reduced | 57 | ½ cup |
| CHICKEN, broiled | | |
| quartered | 248 | 1 piece |
| roast | 115 | 3 slices |
| roast | 101 | 1 leg |
| roast | 147 | 1 thigh |
| Chicken broth, canned | | |
| condensed | 74 | 10 oz. |
| cubes | 6 | 1 |
| envelope instant | 10 | 1 |
| Chicken livers | 146 | ¼ lb. |
| Chicken potpie, frozen | 482 | 8 oz. |
| Chicken TV Dinner | 489 | 1 |
| CHILI CON CARNE | | |
| canned with beans | 335 | 1 cup |
| without beans | 510 | 1 cup |
| CHILI SAUCE | 17 | 1 tbsp. |
| CHOCOLATE, unsweetened | 145 | 1 oz. |
| semisweet pieces | 906 | 6 oz. |
| Chocolate bar, milk, plain | 150 | 1 oz. |
| Chocolate malted milk | | |

| Food | Calories | Amount |
|---|---|---|
| shake with ice cream | 500 | 1½ cups |
| Chocolate milk | 190 | 1 cup |
| Chocolate syrup, thin | 50 | 1 tbsp. |
| CLAMS, raw | 65 | 6 large |
| canned, clams and liquid | 45 | ½ cup |
| Clam juice | 35 | 1 cup |
| COCOA, with whole milk | 235 | 1 cup |
| Cocoa powder | 21 | 1 tbsp. |
| COCONUT, shredded | 335 | 1 cup |
| COD, fresh, poached | 89 | 3 oz. |
| frozen, fillets, poached | 89 | 3 oz. |
| frozen, sticks, breaded | 276 | 5 |
| COLA | 95 | 8 oz. |
| COOKIES | | |
| chocolate wafers | 36 | 1 |
| creme sandwich, chocolate | 54 | 1 |
| fig bars, small | 55 | 1 |
| gingersnaps | 52 | 1 |
| sugar wafers | 10 | 1 |
| vanilla wafers | 18 | 1 |
| CORN FLAKES, plain | 100 | 1 cup |
| presweetened | 110 | ¾ cup |
| CORN, fresh, cooked | 70 | 1 ear |
| canned, cream-style | 92 | ½ cup |
| canned, whole kernel | 70 | ½ cup |
| frozen, whole kernel | 73 | ½ cup |
| CORN MEAL, dry | 420 | 1 cup |
| CORN MUFFINS | 150 | 1 |
| CORN OIL | 125 | 1 tbsp. |
| CORN SYRUP, light or dark | 60 | 1 tbsp. |
| CORNSTARCH | 30 | 1 tbsp. |
| CORNSTARCH PUDDING | | |
| whole milk, chocolate | 67 | ½ cup |
| vanilla or butterscotch | 72 | ½ cup |
| skim milk, chocolate | 45 | ½ cup |
| vanilla or butterscotch | 50 | ½ cup |
| instant chocolate | 183 | ½ cup |
| vanilla or butterscotch | 170 | ½ cup |
| COTTONSEED OIL | 125 | 1 tbsp. |
| CRAB MEAT | 89 | 3 oz. |
| CRACKER MEAL | 45 | 1 tbsp. |
| CRACKERS | | |
| cheese | 34 | 10 |
| graham, plain | 30 | 1 |
| chocolate graham | 56 | 1 |
| oyster | 60 | 20 |
| peanut butter sandwich | 45 | 1 |
| pretzels | 7 | 5 sticks |
| rye wafers | 21 | 1 |
| saltines | 12 | 1 |
| soda | 23 | 1 |
| CRANBERRY JUICE | 160 | 1 cup |
| Cranberry sauce, sweetened, canned, jellied or whole berry | 26 | 1 tbsp. |
| CREAM, half-and-half | 20 | 1 tbsp. |
| heavy or whipping | 55 | 1 tbsp. |
| light, coffee, or table | 30 | 1 tbsp. |
| sour, dairy | 25 | 1 tbsp. |
| CUCUMBER, raw, whole | 30 | 1 |
| raw, sliced | 5 | 6 slices |
| CUSTARD baked with whole milk | 304 | 1 cup |

**D**

| Food | Calories | Amount |
|---|---|---|
| DATES, dry, whole | 100 | 5 |
| DOUGHNUTS, cake type | 125 | 1 |
| DUCK, roast | 165 | 3 slices |

**E**

| Food | Calories | Amount |
|---|---|---|
| EGG, whole | 80 | 1 |
| white | 15 | 1 |
| yolk | 60 | 1 |
| EGGPLANT, boiled | 39 | 1 cup |
| ENDIVE, Belgian | 10 | 1 stalk |
| curly or chicory, broken | 5 | 1 cup |
| ESCAROLE | 5 | 2 leaves |

**F**

| Food | Calories | Amount |
|---|---|---|
| FARINA, cooked | 100 | 1 cup |
| FIGS, fresh | 90 | 3 small |
| canned, in syrup | 150 | ½ cup |
| calories reduced | 68 | ½ cup |
| dried | 100 | 2 med. |
| FLOUNDER, fillet, fresh, poached | 170 | 8 oz. |
| frozen, poached | 76 | 4 oz. |
| FLOUR, all purpose | 400 | 1 cup |
| cake or pastry, sifted | 365 | 1 cup |
| self rising, enriched | 385 | 1 cup |
| whole wheat | 400 | 1 cup |
| FRANKFURTER (10 to lb.) | 120 | 1 |
| FRENCH DRESSING, low calorie | 16 | 1 tbsp. |
| regular | 65 | 1 tbsp. |
| FRUITCAKE, dark | 215 | 1 sliver |
| FRUIT COCKTAIL, canned, in syrup | 195 | 1 cup |
| calories reduced | 60 | ½ cup |

**G**

| Food | Calories | Amount |
|---|---|---|
| GELATIN, unflavored | 35 | 1 tbsp. |
| flavored | 81 | ½ cup |
| GIN | 160 | 2 oz. |
| GINGER ALE | 80 | 8 oz. |
| GINGERBREAD | 175 | 1 piece |
| GRAPEFRUIT, fresh | 45 | ½ med. |
| fresh, sections | 75 | 1 cup |
| canned, sections | 175 | 1 cup |
| calories reduced | 70 | 1 cup |
| Grapefruit juice, fresh | 95 | 1 cup |
| canned, sweetened | 130 | 1 cup |
| canned, unsweetened | 100 | 1 cup |
| frozen concentrate, sweetened reconstituted | 115 | 1 cup |
| unsweetened reconstituted | 100 | 1 cup |
| GRAPES, fresh, Niagara, Concord, Delaware, Catawaba, Scuppernong Malaga, Muscat, Thompson seedless | 65 | 1 cup |
| Emperor, Flame, Tokay | 95 | 1 cup |
| Grape juice, bottled or canned | 165 | 1 cup |

**H**

| Food | Calories | Amount |
|---|---|---|
| HADDOCK, fresh, broiled | 100 | 6 oz. |
| frozen, broiled | 88 | 4 oz. |
| frozen, fish sticks, breaded | 280 | 5 |
| HALIBUT, fresh, broiled | 217 | 8 oz. |
| frozen, broiled | 144 | 4 oz. |
| HAM, baked | 253 | 1 slice |
| boiled, sliced | 135 | 2 oz. |
| HERRING, pickled | 127 | 2 oz. |
| HOMINY GRITS, cooked | 120 | 1 cup |
| HONEY, strained | 65 | 1 tbsp. |
| HONEYDEW melon, | 73 | ⅛ med. |
| cubes | 58 | 1 cup |

**I**

| Food | Calories | Amount |
|---|---|---|
| ICE CREAM, chocolate | 200 | ⅔ cup |
| vanilla | 193 | ⅔ cup |
| brick | 145 | 1 slice |
| ICE MILK, chocolate | 144 | ⅔ cup |
| vanilla | 136 | ⅔ cup |

**J and K**

| Food | Calories | Amount |
|---|---|---|
| JAMS, jellies, preserves | 55 | 1 tbsp. |
| KALE, cooked | 30 | 1 cup |
| KIDNEY, cooked, beef | 118 | 3 oz. |
| lamb | 111 | 3 oz. |
| pork | 130 | 3 oz. |

**L**

| Food | Calories | Amount |
|---|---|---|
| LAMB chop, loin, raw | 223 | 6 oz. |
| rib, raw | 240 | 5 oz. |
| shoulder, raw | 252 | 5 oz. |
| Lamb roast, leg | 165 | 1 slice |
| Lamb shank, raw | 275 | 10 oz. |
| LARD | 125 | 1 tbsp. |
| LEEKS, chopped, cooked | 25 | ½ cup |
| LETTUCE, head | 47 | 1 lb. |
| LEMON | 20 | 1 med. |
| Lemonade concentrate, reconstituted | 110 | 1 cup |
| Lemon juice, fresh | 5 | 1 tbsp. |
| LIMEADE concentrate, reconstituted | 105 | 1 cup |
| Lime juice, fresh | 4 | 1 tbsp. |
| | 65 | 1 cup |
| LIQUEURS | 165 | 1 oz. |
| LIVER, cooked beef | 117 | 3 oz. |
| calf's | 136 | 3 oz. |
| lamb | 171 | 3 oz. |
| pork | 115 | 3 oz. |
| LIVERWURST | 100 | 1 slice |
| LOBSTER, fresh, boiled | 108 | ¾ lb. |
| canned, meat | 80 | ½ cup |
| frozen tails, boiled | 81 | 3 small |

**M**

| Food | Calories | Amount |
|---|---|---|
| MACARONI, cooked | 155 | 1 cup |
| Macaroni and cheese, baked | 470 | 1 cup |
| MANDARIN oranges, canned, in syrup | 55 | ⅓ cup |
| calories reduced | 29 | ⅓ cup |
| MANGO | 133 | 1 med. |
| MANHATTAN | 165 | 2½ oz. |
| MARGARINE | 100 | 1 tbsp. |
| MARTINI | 145 | 2½ oz. |
| MAYONNAISE | 100 | 1 tbsp. |
| imitation | 55 | 1 tbsp. |
| MELBA TOAST | 17 | 1 slice |
| MILK | | |
| buttermilk | 90 | 1 cup |
| condensed, sweetened | 980 | 1 cup |
| dry, instant nonfat | 250 | 1 cup |
| evaporated | 345 | 1 cup |
| evaporated skim | 80 | ½ cup |
| skim | 90 | 1 cup |
| whole | 160 | 1 cup |
| MIXED VEGETABLES, frozen, cooked | 55 | ½ cup |
| MOLASSES | 50 | 1 tbsp. |
| MUFFINS, plain | 140 | 1 |
| MUSHROOMS, fresh | 14 | 6 |
| canned, with liquid | 40 | 1 cup |
| MUSTARD, prepared | 4 | 1 tsp. |

**N**

| Food | Calories | Amount |
|---|---|---|
| NECTARINES | 50 | 1 med. |
| NOODLES, egg, cooked | 200 | 1 cup |

**O**

| Food | Calories | Amount |
|---|---|---|
| OAT CEREAL, ready to eat | 100 | 1 cup |
| Oatmeal | 130 | 1 cup |
| OKRA, fresh, cooked | 25 | 8 pods |
| frozen, sliced, cooked | 26 | ½ cup |
| OLIVES, green unpitted | 15 | 4 med. |
| ripe, unpitted | 15 | 2 large |
| OLIVE OIL | 125 | 1 tbsp. |
| ONION, green | 20 | 6 small |
| raw, whole | 40 | 1 med. |
| raw, chopped | 60 | 1 cup |
| Onion soup mix, dry | 150 | 1 env. |
| ORANGE, fresh | 70 | 1 med. |
| sections | 50 | ½ cup |
| Orange juice, fresh | 110 | 1 cup |
| canned, unsweetened | 120 | 1 cup |
| frozen concentrate, reconstituted | 110 | 1 cup |
| OYSTERS, raw | 160 | 15 med. |
| Oyster stew | 200 | 1 cup |

**P**

| Food | Calories | Amount |
|---|---|---|
| PANCAKES, buckwheat | 55 | 1 cake |
| plain, home recipe | 60 | 1 cake |
| PAPAYA, fresh, cubed | 70 | 1 cup |
| PARSLEY, fresh, chopped | 1 | 1 tbsp. |
| PARSNIPS, cooked, diced | 100 | 1 cup |
| PEACHES, fresh, whole | 35 | 1 med. |
| fresh, sliced | 65 | 1 cup |
| canned, in syrup | 90 | 2 halves |
| calories reduced | 54 | 2 halves |

| Food | Calories | Measure |
|---|---|---|
| dried, uncooked | 420 | 1 cup |
| cooked, unsweetened | 220 | 1 cup |
| frozen, sweetened | 99 | 1/3 cup |
| Peach nectar, canned | 120 | 1 cup |
| PEANUTS, roasted, | 100 | 20 med. |
| chopped | 55 | 1 tbsp. |
| dry roasted | 170 | 1/4 cup |
| Peanut butter | 95 | 1 tbsp. |
| PEARS, fresh, whole | 100 | 1 med. |
| canned, in syrup | 98 | 2 halves |
| calories reduced | 62 | 2 halves |
| Pear nectar, canned | 130 | 1 cup |
| PEAS, blackeye, frozen, | | |
| cooked | 95 | 1/2 cup |
| Peas, green, cooked | 115 | 1 cup |
| canned | 146 | 1 cup |
| frozen, cooked | 60 | 1/2 cup |
| PECANS, halves | 100 | 12 |
| chopped | 376 | 1/2 cup |
| PEPPERS, sweet, green, | | |
| raw | 15 | 1 med. |
| green, raw, diced | 16 | 1/2 cup |
| red, raw | 20 | 1 med. |
| PERSIMMONS | 75 | 1 med. |
| PICKLES, dill | 15 | 1 (5") |
| sweet | 30 | 1 (3") |
| PIES | | |
| apple | 306 | 1/8 |
| blueberry | 255 | 1/8 |
| cherry | 299 | 1/8 |
| custard | 233 | 1/8 |
| lemon meringue | 269 | 1/8 |
| mince | 298 | 1/8 |
| pecan | 479 | 1/8 |
| pumpkin | 230 | 1/8 |
| PIMIENTO, canned | 10 | 1 med. |
| PINE NUTS (pignolias) | 671 | 1/2 cup |
| PINEAPPLE, fresh | 75 | 1 cup |
| canned, sliced, in syrup | 90 | 2 slices |
| crushed, in syrup | 195 | 1 cup |
| cubes, juice-pack | 57 | 1/2 cup |
| Pineapple juice, canned | 135 | 1 cup |
| frozen, reconstituted | 125 | 1 cup |
| PLUMS, fresh, whole | 25 | 1 med. |
| canned, in syrup | 100 | 3 plums |
| calories reduced | 75 | 3 plums |
| PORK, chop, rib, raw | 250 | 6 oz. |
| roast, loin | 330 | 1 chop |
| luncheon meat | 165 | 2 oz. |
| POPCORN, with | | |
| oil and salt | 40 | 1 cup |
| plain | 24 | 1 cup |
| sugar-coated | 135 | 1 cup |
| POTATOES, baked, | | |
| without skin | 90 | 1 med. |
| boiled, without skin | 90 | 1 med. |
| French fried, frozen | 125 | 10 pcs. |
| mashed, with milk only | 70 | 1/2 cup |
| Potato chips | 115 | 10 |
| PRUNES, | 70 | 4 med. |
| cooked, unsweetened | 295 | 18 med. |
| Prune juice | 200 | 1 cup |
| PUMPKIN, canned | 75 | 1 cup |

### R

| Food | Calories | Measure |
|---|---|---|
| RADISHES | 5 | 4 |
| RAISINS | 460 | 1 cup |
| RASPBERRIES, fresh | 70 | 1 cup |
| canned, in syrup | 100 | 1/2 cup |
| frozen, sweetened | 115 | 1/2 cup |
| RHUBARB, cooked with sugar | 385 | 1 cup |
| RICE, cooked, brown | 100 | 2/3 cup |
| precooked, cooked | 140 | 2/3 cup |
| long-grain, white | 212 | 1 cup |
| wild | 73 | 1/2 cup |
| Rice cereal, ready to eat | 115 | 1 cup |
| puffed | 55 | 1 cup |
| ROLLS, | | |
| frankfurter | 120 | 1 |
| French | 118 | 1 |
| hamburger | 123 | 1 |
| Parker house | 114 | 1 |
| RUM | 160 | 2 oz. |

| Food | Calories | Measure |
|---|---|---|
| RUTABAGAS, cooked | 25 | 1/2 cup |
| RYE WAFERS | 63 | 3 |

### S

| Food | Calories | Measure |
|---|---|---|
| SALAD DRESSINGS | | |
| blue cheese, low calorie | 16 | 1 tbsp. |
| regular | 65 | 1 tbsp. |
| Italian, low calorie | 16 | 1 tbsp. |
| regular | 65 | 1 tbsp. |
| mayonnaise, imitation | 55 | 1 tbsp. |
| regular | 100 | 1 tbsp. |
| Thousand Island, | | |
| low calorie | 16 | 1 tbsp. |
| regular | 75 | 1 tbsp. |
| SALAMI | 130 | 3 slices |
| SALMON, fresh, steak, | | |
| broiled | 430 | 6 oz. |
| canned | 120 | 1/2 cup |
| SARDINES, canned, in oil | 100 | 4 |
| SAUERKRAUT, canned | 32 | 1 cup |
| SCALLOPS, sea, fresh, | | |
| steamed | 105 | 6 med. |
| frozen, steamed | 210 | 1 cup |
| SESAME SEEDS | 10 | 1 tbsp. |
| SHERBET, orange, milk | 260 | 1 cup |
| SHORTENING, vegetable | 125 | 1 tbsp. |
| SHRIMP, fresh, poached | 100 | 7 med. |
| canned | 167 | 5 oz. |
| frozen, poached | 100 | 9 med. |
| cocktail, tiny, canned | 33 | 15 |
| SOLE, fillet, fresh, | | |
| poached | 177 | 1 piece |
| fillet, frozen, | | |
| poached | 88 | 4 oz. |
| SOUPS, canned condensed, | | |
| prepared with water, | | |
| following label directions, | | |
| asparagus, cream of | 51 | 1 cup |
| bean with bacon | 130 | 1 cup |
| beef broth | 22 | 1 cup |
| beef noodle | 55 | 1 cup |
| black bean | 80 | 1 cup |
| celery, cream of | 75 | 1 cup |
| cheese | 142 | 1 cup |
| chicken broth | 85 | 1 cup |
| chicken, cream of | 85 | 1 cup |
| chicken gumbo | 48 | 1 cup |
| chicken noodle | 54 | 1 cup |
| chicken vegetable | 60 | 1 cup |
| chicken with rice | 44 | 1 cup |
| chili beef | 133 | 1 cup |
| clam chowder | 60 | 1 cup |
| consommé | 25 | 1 cup |
| grean pea, cream of | 110 | 1 cup |
| madrilène | 27 | 1 cup |
| minestrone | 85 | 1 cup |
| mushroom, cream of | 113 | 1 cup |
| onion | 52 | 1 cup |
| pepper pot | 83 | 1 cup |
| potato, cream of | 59 | 1 cup |
| Scotch broth | 74 | 1 cup |
| split pea | 130 | 1 cup |
| tomato | 74 | 1 cup |
| tomato rice | 82 | 1 cup |
| turkey noodle | 65 | 1 cup |
| turkey vegetable | 58 | 1 cup |
| vegetable | 63 | 1 cup |
| vegetable beef | 61 | 1 cup |
| Soups, packaged mix | | |
| prepared with water, | | |
| following label directions, | | |
| beef | 87 | 1 cup |
| chicken noodle | 60 | 1 cup |
| chicken rice | 55 | 1 cup |
| green pea | 128 | 1 cup |
| mushroom, cream of | 46 | 1 cup |
| onion | 40 | 1 cup |
| potato, cream of | 90 | 1 cup |
| tomato vegetable | 69 | 1 cup |
| vegetable | 69 | 1 cup |
| SOY SAUCE | 10 | 1 tbsp. |
| SOYBEAN OIL | 125 | 1 tbsp. |
| SPAGHETTI, cooked | 155 | 1 cup |

| Food | Calories | Measure |
|---|---|---|
| SPINACH, fresh, cooked | 40 | 1 cup |
| canned | 45 | 1 cup |
| frozen | 24 | 1/2 cup |
| SQUASH, yellow, zucchini, | | |
| crookneck, patty pan, | | |
| sliced, cooked | 30 | 1 cup |
| frozen, cooked | 20 | 1/2 cup |
| Squash, acorn, banana, | | |
| hubbard, baked, mashed | 130 | 1 cup |
| frozen, cooked | 50 | 1/2 cup |
| STRAWBERRIES, fresh | 55 | 1 cup |
| Strawberries, frozen, | | |
| whole, unsweetened | 55 | 1 cup |
| sliced, sweetened | 140 | 1/2 cup |
| SUCCOTASH, frozen, cooked | 87 | 1/2 cup |
| SUGAR, brown, firmly | | |
| packed | 820 | 1 cup |
| | 51 | 1 tbsp. |
| granulated | 770 | 1 cup |
| | 45 | 1 tbsp. |
| lump | 25 | 1 |
| 10X (confectioners | | |
| powdered) | 495 | 1 cup |
| | 30 | 1 tbsp. |
| SWEET POTATOES, baked | | |
| or boiled | 155 | 1 med. |
| canned, without syrup | 235 | 1 cup |
| SYRUP, | | |
| corn, light, or dark | 60 | 1 tbsp. |
| maple | 61 | 1 tbsp. |
| maple blended, | | |
| regular | 54 | 1 tbsp. |
| pancake | 55 | 1 tbsp. |
| sorghum | 55 | 1 tbsp. |

### T

| Food | Calories | Measure |
|---|---|---|
| TANGERINE | 40 | 1 large |
| Tangerine juice, canned | | |
| unsweetened | 105 | 1 cup |
| TAPIOCA, quick cooking, | | |
| uncooked | 35 | 1 tbsp. |
| TOMATOES, fresh | 35 | 1 med. |
| canned | 50 | 1 cup |
| Tomato juice, canned | 45 | 1 cup |
| TUNA, canned, in oil, | | |
| drained | 170 | 1/2 cup |
| canned, in water | 109 | 1/2 cup |
| TURNIPS, yellow, cooked, | | |
| diced | 50 | 1 cup |
| white, cooked, diced | 35 | 1 cup |
| TURKEY, roast | 134 | 1 slice |
| Turkey potpie, frozen | 429 | 8 oz. |
| Turkey TV dinner | 325 | 1 pkg. |

### V

| Food | Calories | Measure |
|---|---|---|
| VEAL, chop loin, raw | 251 | 8 oz. |
| chop, rib, raw | 240 | 6 oz. |
| roast, leg | 159 | 1 slice |
| scallopini, sautéed | 172 | 3 pieces |
| VINEGAR | 2 | 1 tbsp. |

### W

| Food | Calories | Measure |
|---|---|---|
| WALNUTS, chopped | 50 | 1 tbsp. |
| halves | 794 | 1 cup |
| WATERMELON, | 115 | 1 wedge |
| cubed | 40 | 1 cup |
| WHEAT CEREAL, cooked | 175 | 1 cup |
| flakes, ready to eat | 100 | 1 cup |
| puffed | 83 | 1 cup |
| puffed, presweetened | 105 | 3/4 cup |
| shredded | 90 | 1 biscuit |
| WHEAT GERM | 27 | 1 tbsp. |
| WHISKEY | 160 | 2 oz. |
| WINE, dry | 85 | 3 oz. |
| sweet | 160 | 3 oz. |

### Y and Z

| Food | Calories | Measure |
|---|---|---|
| YAMS, pared, cubed, | | |
| cooked | 90 | 1/2 cup |
| YOGURT, skim milk | 120 | 1 cup |
| whole milk | 176 | 1 cup |
| ZWIEBACK | 31 | 1 slice |

# MARY ANN CRENSHAW'S EATING FOR BEAUTY

Eating your way to beauty is a lot easier for us all these days, thanks to the health awareness of the '70's generation. For, the good whole grains, the healthful unprocessed foods, the fresh, organically grown vegetables that once were almost impossible to find are now available in most supermarkets. And it's all the better for that famous American Beauty and for America's health as well.

Health awareness is the forerunner to beauty, all right—for without health, there simply can be no beauty.

### American Eating Habits

Before we get into the specifics of what can, and will, improve all of you —your health as well as your looks —let's first take a hard look at our eating habits. They leave much to be desired.

There is malnutrition in this land of plenty, and it is on the move as much among the affluent as among the poor. In some cases, even more so. The reason for this sort of malnutrition is usually lack of information.

The mother who lets her children munch and crunch on nutritionally empty snacks is certainly not trying to starve her family. But that is, in fact, exactly what she is doing. And childhood is where good nutrition habits start. And where beauty begins as well—for, good bones, healthy skin and hair are basic to good looks.

### We're All Protein

Beauty is what I want to talk about. So let's get right down to the facts.

Fact No. 1—the most important one for you to remember—is that *you*, your hair, your skin, your nails, all have one essential ingredient. And that's *protein*. That means protein must be No. 1 on your list of foods to get plenty of.

Experts have not yet determined the exact amount of protein you should have every day. A pretty safe recommendation is anywhere from 56 to 75 grams each day, depending on your size. Naturally, a strapping man is going to need more protein than a small child. But no one from teen-age on should have less than 45 grams.

Protein is meat, of course. But protein is also fish, fowl, cheese, milk, eggs and—don't forget them—seeds, nuts and beans. And because some of these vegetable proteins contain other beauty-building minerals in extraordinary amounts, they should be considered excellent sources (cheaper, too) of some of the protein you must have each and every day of your life. And put emphasis on *every* day, for protein *cannot be stored* in your body.

### Protein-Hungry Hair?

Your hair is one place where any protein deprivation is going to show up. Because if your body needs that protein to maintain its general health, it really isn't going to care whether your hair is looking its best. But *you* certainly care!

One of the best protein sources for the health of your hair is contained in the simple, so-available egg. Not only that; the egg also contains two of the most important B vitamins to your hair. They are *choline* and *inositol*, part of the B complex, but not always present with other B vitamins.

Now, I realize that there has been a lot of scare literature about eggs— "cholesterol can kill you" and all that. If you're really frightened of eggs, I suggest you have your physician keep a close check on that cholesterol level of yours. Because eggs are such an important food for beauty, you should never be without them.

### You Need Some Fats

Many women shy away from the very thought of "fats." You'd better not if you expect high-gloss, healthy hair. For there is no way to get it unless you include some fats in your diet. And the same goes double when we come to dewy skin!

I have been told by nutritionists that most of the complaints and questions about dry skin or dry hair come from women who are convinced that "fats" put fat on them. Not true! Fats are essential for beauty.

The fats we are talking about are the unsaturated sort—the best kind for you, your cholesterol level, your health, your hair and your skin. These are the fats that come from vegetable oils, such as corn oil, safflower oil, soybean oil. (The exception is coconut oil, which, for some reason, is saturated.)

These fats should give you no cholesterol worries. They move through the body, taking that cholesterol with them so that it has little chance to clog up your arteries. Not only that! The unsaturated fats are full of vitamin E, which, you will soon see, is an essential vitamin for the health of your hair.

### Get Your B Vitamins

The *B-complex vitamins* are perhaps the most important vitamins for good hair. Without them, that hair will look like a thatched-roof mess.

B vitamins are found in unprocessed whole grains, in liver, in leafy dark-green vegetables, in yeast (which is why so many nutritionists recommend yeast as an important source of all the B vitamins) and in eggs. And B vitamins also turn up in those seeds and nuts.

There are now on your grocer's shelves new breads made from B-rich whole-grain flours, in some cases with sprouted grains included, and without preservatives of any kind. This means you have to keep them refrigerated, but the B-vitamin and other beauty benefits you'll reap will make it well worth the small effort.

If you're unsure of your B's, you may want to take a B-complex capsule. The B vitamins *are* complex, and separating them into their various components requires real expertise. As nature put them together for our convenience, and the B's all work together in harmony to do the beauty job you want, you can take them all together in one easy-to-swallow capsule.

There is now available a *stress* formula of B vitamins. Good thing, too. For stress is one of the worst beauty killers of all. It can even make you lose your hair, and that's not what we're heading for.

### Nature's Calmative

And while you're remaining calm, for your beauty's sake, consider one of nature's own tranquilizers—*calcium*.

Remember all those tales about warm milk before bedtime for a sound sleep? Surprise! They were all true. For calcium has marvelous tranquilizing abilities. And here again, don't be misinformed into believing that calcium might produce arthritis. In some cases, it has been known to have the opposite effect.

Calcium is found, of course, in milk, cheese, yogurt and some dark-green vegetables. If you don't like any of those things, you'd best ask your doctor about calcium tablets, for the tension you might be living under is sure to destroy the good looks your good diet is going to build up. If you stay calm, it will show up in your shining hair, your radiant skin, your relaxed and coolly confident manner.

### Vitamin E for Hair

There's another vitamin that's essential for healthy hair. That is *vitamin E*. Remember those unsaturated fats that you're already eating to high-gloss your hair? Well, they're chock-full of vitamin E as well, doing double duty for beauty.

Wheat germ is one of the best natural sources of vitamin E, and it's full of protein besides. If you want plenty of healthy, beautiful hair, then learn to love wheat germ. Toasted wheat germ is great; raw wheat germ is even better, and your supermarket will, no doubt, have the wheat germ of your choice. If you don't want wheat germ as your dish, then start nibbling on seeds—sunflower seeds or pumpkin seeds. Both contain vitamin E and minerals that are great for keeping hair healthy.

### Feeding Your Skin

When it comes to skin, we come back to protein. Skin may look different from hair, but it's still protein. And as for vitamins, the B vitamins are just as basic for beautiful skin as they are for hair. Remember that if you're headed for a beach weekend, because the sun, it seems, tends to eat up your body's supply of vitamin B.

While you're in the sun, your own body is going to manufacture another skin vitamin for you. That's *vitamin D*. And about the only way you'll get it is from sunshine, unless you find it added in synthetic form in milk.

Still, there's no better way to get that skin-vitamin D than to get lots of healthy sunshine. But not too much, you understand. Because we said "healthy sunshine," and the kind that roasts your skin till it looks like leather is most certainly not healthful and decidedly not beautiful.

*Vitamin C* is the skin strengthener. Surely you're aware citrus fruits are full of vitamin C. But so are tomatoes and berries and even potatoes. An important thing to remember with C is that it often hides out close to the peel of, say, a potato. You'll also find extra C and other nutrients in that white part of an orange—a part you probably used to throw away.

Vitamin C is the vitamin that strengthens your capillaries and thereby just possibly helps avoid broken veins. The stronger those capillaries are, the less likely they are to break.

And remember, too, that your vitamin C goes up in smoke. Which means that, if you are a smoker, you'd better make allowances. Cigarettes eat it up, according to some reports, at the rate of 25 milligrams per smoke.

### The Skin Vitamin

I've saved the obvious skin vitamin for last. And that is *vitamin A*. I hope everyone knows that A is the skin vitamin—the one that can help all sorts of problems from breakouts to rashes. It is the skin-soother of the

vitamin world, and without it, or enough of it, you're not likely to come even close to beautiful skin. Leafy dark-green vegetables contain vitamin A—as do all the dark-yellow vegetables, such as squash or carrots. Butter has it, and so do eggs, cheese, liver and kidney.

And speaking of liver, it's one of the best skin-beauty foods around. If you don't like it, then buy the dried sort—the kind known as "desiccated" liver, found in most health-food shops. It makes for luminous skin.

### High-Vitamin Cookery

All vitamins, with the exception of vitamins A and D which are fat-soluble therefore remain in your body for a period of time, need to be replenished each day and every day, just like protein.

Vitamins are quite delicate, too. If you tend to overcook your vegetables, you're delivering those vitamins up to steam. So cook them just to the tender point and then stop. And never, never pour the juice down the drain—unless you want the vitamin there as well.

That's why it's a good idea to cook vegetables with as little water as possible. Try it the French way—waterless, with your vegetables covered by a few lettuce (full of "E") leaves. These give off precisely the right amount of moisture for cooking to

save those valuable vitamins.

### Salt-Shaker Beauty Aid

Don't, meanwhile, overlook the advantages of using iodized salt. For iodine is the great thyroid normalizer, and the thyroid gland works for beautiful skin *and* hair. Unless you have a real thyroid problem and your doctor has forbidden iodine, you can make real beauty use of this item.

As for nails—there are plenty of myths surrounding those. Did you, for example, believe—as I once did—that your nails are made of calcium? The simple truth is that nails are protein, just like the rest of you, and protein is quite simply the only thing that makes them strong.

Gelatin, as you've probably heard, *is* a protein—but only a "partial" protein. With it you need some "complete" protein—the kind you get from meat, cheese, eggs, fish, fowl—to help your nails grow out strong. Some jellied desserts are made with algins —which are carbohydrates, not proteins—instead of gelatin. So don't count on these to help your nails.

All this only shows further how much *balance* is everything in eating for beauty and health. ∎

By Mary Ann Crenshaw
Ms. Crenshaw is the author of "The Natural Way to Beauty."

## SUGGESTED WEIGHTS FOR HEIGHTS

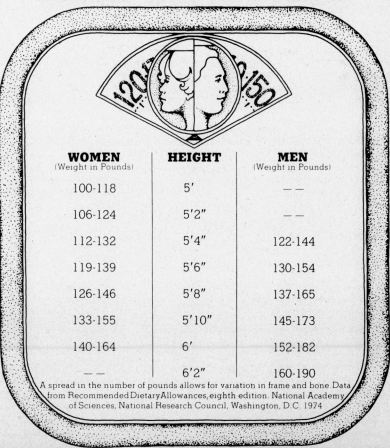

| WOMEN (Weight in Pounds) | HEIGHT | MEN (Weight in Pounds) |
|---|---|---|
| 100-118 | 5' | — — |
| 106-124 | 5'2" | — — |
| 112-132 | 5'4" | 122-144 |
| 119-139 | 5'6" | 130-154 |
| 126-146 | 5'8" | 137-165 |
| 133-155 | 5'10" | 145-173 |
| 140-164 | 6' | 152-182 |
| — — | 6'2" | 160-190 |

A spread in the number of pounds allows for variation in frame and bone. Data from Recommended Dietary Allowances, eighth edition. National Academy of Sciences, National Research Council, Washington, D.C. 1974

# EXPLODING SOME OF THE VITAMIN MYTHS

Many health-conscious Americans have misconceptions about the proper role of vitamins. While vitamins are assuredly essential for good health, more *isn't* better. Actually, excessive amounts are not only unnecessary; they can also be harmful.

According to some of the latest "pop" literature, a hefty helping of vitamins will cure everything from the common cold to a lagging sex life. But medical research indicates otherwise. Exhaustive studies evaluated by the National Academy of Sciences have shown that amounts greater than the Recommended Dietary Allowance (RDA) provide nothing of value for normal individuals. Only people with definite, medically diagnosed vitamin deficiencies can benefit from amounts greater than the RDA, and in the U.S., vitamin deficiencies are rare.

In fact, taking too many vitamins can produce such adverse reactions as rashes, diarrhea or headaches, and, in extreme cases, can even kill you.

The myth that since vitamins are good for you, the more the better, is just one of many accepted by a lot of health-conscious Americans. Another popular myth is that vitamins are an "insurance" policy guaranteeing good health. People who follow this line of reasoning usually believe that even a balanced diet cannot provide adequate nutrients, that modern farming methods have depleted the soil, and that we need vitamin supplements to make up for what's lacking in our food.

Actually, through modern farm practices, more is done today to protect and enrich the soil than ever took place back in "the good old days." In addition, the protein, carbohydrates, fat, fiber and vitamins in food are primarily controlled by the plant's genetic structure, not by the soil in which it grows.

## Much Ado about Vitamin E

Vitamin E seems to be the "miracle" vitamin these days. Among the claims made for it are that it promotes physical endurance and sexual potency, prevents heart attacks and slows down the aging process.

But, a careful examination of research studies shows there are no bases for these claims. In laboratory experiments, male rats deprived of vitamin E *did* become sterile—but the use of large doses has never proved to have any effect on human sterility or impotence (except perhaps a psychological one). Similarly, E is known to be essential to *maintaining* pregnancy, but it has not been found to be a factor in fertility. Vitamin E supplements have been found useful in only two conditions—for premature babies who, because of poor placental transfer, may have received too little of the vitamin before birth, and for persons with intestinal disorders in which fats (the major source of the vitamin) are poorly absorbed.

One reason that so little is known about this vitamin is that E-deficiency is almost impossible to produce in humans. To withdraw all sources of E for purposes of experimentation is virtually to withdraw food itself, since the vitamin is present to some extent in almost everything we eat.

## C for Colds?

Vitamin C has many proven benefits. It helps hold body cells together and strengthens blood vessels; it helps heal wounds; it helps tooth and bone formation, and it helps build resistance to infection.

But, there is no evidence that vitamin C will cure or even prevent colds. In several clinical studies, people who believed they were being given C but who were actually receiving inert tablets reported fewer colds than they expected to have, while some of those who were actually taking C reported no change. The most favorable studies suggest a 25 percent benefit—one less cold out of four, and one less sick day out of four. You certainly wouldn't rely on an antibiotic with this kind of record—and yet, many continue to swear by C as a good cold tablet.

Furthermore, some research has indicated that there may be hazards involved in taking large doses of C, including destruction of vitamin $B_{12}$ in the body, severe diarrhea, kidney stones and possible danger to those who have diabetes. None of these studies is conclusive—but to play it safe, your wisest course is to absorb the RDA of 45 milligrams a day. (Doctors do prescribe increased doses of vitamin C for alcoholism, hemolytic anemia, anti-convulsant therapy, or chronic infection—but these are disease conditions.)

## B Vitamins

A common myth about B vitamins is that if you feel rundown, swallowing $B_{12}$ supplements will act as a pick-me-up. But, again, unless there's an actual deficiency, amounts beyond the RDA won't help. In fact, they're useless, since where there is a deficiency, the vitamin is usually administered through injection, because it isn't very effective when taken orally.

Another far-fetched claim says that an insufficiency of pantothenic acid (one of the B vitamins) makes your hair turn gray. It is true that in the laboratory a severe pantothenic acid deficiency has caused male rats' hair to turn gray, and when they were given pantothenic acid, the original color was restored. However, that doesn't mean that human beings' hair turns gray because of inadequate supplies of pantothenic acid. Although gray hair may occur when there is a severe deficiency, this is very rare. There are many other reasons for gray hair (most of them genetic). But there is still nothing we know of that you can take to prevent your hair from going gray.

## Vitamins A and D

An excess of certain vitamins can be toxic. In 1974, London scientist Basil Brown died after consuming 70 million units of vitamin A in 10 days—along with a gallon of carrot juice a day during that period. His entire skin turned bright yellow, and pathologist Dr. David Haler, who performed the autopsy, listed the cause of death as "an enormous intake of vitamin A," which is indistinguishable from alcoholic poisoning. "It produces the same result," he said, "as cirrhosis of the liver."

In less severe cases, large doses of vitamin A taken over extended periods have been known to retard growth in children and cause dry, cracked skin, headaches and bone pain, among other symptoms. In fact, an overdose often produces virtually the *same symptoms as a severe deficiency*.

As far as vitamin D goes, excessive doses have been known to retard mental and physical growth in children. They can also cause nausea, weakness, stiffness, constipation, hypertension, and even death.

Because of this, the government decided to limit the potency of A and D tablets you can buy without a prescription to daily intakes of not more than 10,000 International Units (IU) and 400 IU, respectively. You can still buy and consume as much at one time as you want—but these vitamins are being sold in smaller dosages in an attempt to minimize the overconsumption and serve as a warning to buyers.

# DR. JEAN MAYER'S GUIDE TO BETTER NUTRITION

### Are Natural Vitamins Superior?

Still another myth is that natural vitamins are superior to those synthesized by man. "Getting back to nature" can be an expensive trip. People have paid close to $6 for tablets of vitamin C from "pure rose hips," or "Acerola cherries," or for a host of combinations with natural but irrelevant ingredients when the same amount of pure ascorbic acid can be bought for less than $1. Apart from that, most of these products still use synthetic vitamin C (watch for that little word "with"—rosehips *with* vitamin C). A tablet containing 100 mg. of vitamin C derived only from natural sources would weigh at least 5 grams (about the size of a rounded teaspoon of sugar).

In reality, each vitamin has a particular molecular structure that remains the same whether it's synthesized in a laboratory or extracted from an animal or plant, or consumed as part of an animal or plant. And it is the structure, not the source from which it has been derived, that determines whether a substance is a vitamin and which vitamin it is.

### Getting Vital Nutrients

Since much of the preoccupation with taking supplements stems from the fear of not getting enough nutrients, how do you make sure you are being properly nourished? The answer is, of course, by eating a balanced diet.

When it comes down to it, most people can easily have a balanced diet that generally meets the RDA vitamin requirements of A, B₁, B₂, C and D. When these five are obtained in sufficient amounts from ordinary foods, they almost always provide the needed amounts of other vitamins, and supplements are not needed.

It's perfectly possible to get a good, balanced diet from many different types of foods—because there is such a wide variety containing similar nutrients. Just choose wisely, and be sure to include enough of each of the "Basic Seven" food groups in your daily meals. Read labels carefully and pay particular attention to products using the new nutrition labels. To find out which vitamins are present in specific foods, and the amounts required for good nutrition, see the Recommended Dietary Allowances Chart on page 116. ∎

By Jane Heenan
Ms. Heenan, a free-lance writer living in Alexandria, Virginia, has been a health writer for the Federal Drug Administration and was editor of the United States Labor Department's special publication, *Job Safety and Health*.

## How You Should Eat to Feel Your Best

We belong to the most diet-conscious nation in the world. Americans have an enormously wide range of foods to choose from, and every week a new theory is advanced about which foods we should eat. It's so hard to sort out fact from fad concerning good nutrition—how can you know if you are getting the best possible diet?

In the following article I shall try to show you that practicing good nutrition need not be dreary or difficult. It is simply the habit of buying, preparing and consuming a wide range of good foods to ensure yourself of getting the necessary nutrients for your health needs.

### Which Nutrients Are Necessary?

Nutrients are all the components of food—including proteins, fats, carbohydrates, vitamins, minerals and water—that your body needs for health and well-being. (In addition to nutrients, the body needs roughage for good intestinal function.)

Nutrients are needed for three vital functions:
1. For energy to keep you warm, to help your organs function, to help you move, think and work.
2. For the utilization of all foods.
3. For growth and for replacement of worn-out cells.

In general, if you eat a variety of basic foods—fruits, vegetables, animal products, whole-grain cereals, vegetable oils—you are unlikely to be deficient in any major nutrients.

### A Primer on Proteins

Proteins are the main raw materials used for building body tissues. The 20 building blocks of protein (amino acids) in animal products are closer than those in vegetable products to the proportions the human body needs to form its own proteins for cell growth and function. By consuming animal and vegetable proteins in the right combinations, you can get all the amino acids your body requires.

In selecting foods for protein, you should consider:
1. protein content
2. calorie, fat and cholesterol content
3. cost

*Sources of animal proteins:* Meat, poultry, fish, milk, cheese and eggs.
*Sources of vegetable proteins:* Legumes (peas, beans and lentils), nuts, seeds, cereals (whole-grain in particular), and cereal-based foods.
*"Cholesterol factor":* Many sources of animal protein are also high in saturated fats and cholesterol, which may increase the risk of heart disease by raising blood cholesterol. For reasons that are not fully understood, most women who have not undergone menopause do not build up cholesterol in the walls of their arteries, even though they may eat high-cholesterol foods and their blood cholesterol level may be as high as men's. After menopause, cholesterol accumulates in the arteries of women just as it does with men—a good reason why women should get into healthy eating habits early on.

Eggs are a particularly good food for young children and young women (especially during pregnancy and nursing). But males from 15 on should go easy unless their blood cholesterol is low and tested frequently. Emerging evidence suggests that damage to arteries—from a build-up of cholesterol in the bloodstream—occurs at a much earlier age than previously supposed.

Red meat is higher in saturated fat, cholesterol and calories than poultry and fish. Whatever fat there is in fish is generally high in polyunsaturated acids, which actually help to lower cholesterol levels in the blood.
*Good cheap protein combinations:* Bread and cheese; rice and beans (serve with milk or a little meat, fish or poultry); whole-grain cereals (add milk and fresh fruit); rice and soybeans (Chinese style, complemented by a little poultry, meat or fish).

### Facts about Fats

Fats are the richest source of energy. Many sources of fats provide important nutrients, such as fat-soluble vitamins and polyunsaturated fatty acids, which are essential to life itself. High-fat foods such as butter and fortified margarine, for example, give you vitamin A; vegetable oils supply vitamin E.

Why then are you constantly told

to cut down on fats? In the first place, fats are packed with calories—they contain approximately twice as many calories per gram or per ounce as you find in proteins and carbohydrates. Secondly, saturated fats can raise your blood cholesterol level. In terms of blood cholesterol, however, it's not just the amount but the kind of fat you eat that matters. Here is a rundown of the four different kinds of dietary fats:

• *Saturated fats:* Generally obtained in meat and dairy products, including butter, eggs, milk and cheese. These fats tend to raise blood cholesterol levels. Such fats (except for coconut oil) do not melt at room temperature.
• *Unsaturated fats:* Found in fish, nuts, olive and peanut oils. Unsaturated fats contain less hydrogen than saturated fats and have little effect on blood cholesterol levels. Such fats are liquid when kept at room temperature.
• *Polyunsaturated fats:* Found in soybean, corn and safflower oils. These fats contain less hydrogen than unsaturated fats and tend to lower blood cholesterol levels. Such fats are liquid at room temperature.
• *Hydrogenated fats:* Unsaturated fats that have been hardened by the addition of hydrogen. They are often found in shortening and in some margarines and tend to raise blood-cholesterol levels.

### It's the Cholesterol in Your Blood That Counts

Cholesterol is a wax-like substance which tends to deposit in the arteries, particularly in teen-age boys, men and postmenopausal women. It is also found in animal products.

*Cholesterol and fat:* Accumulation of cholesterol can lead to hardening of the arteries, high blood pressure and obstruction of the vessels of the heart (coronary) or of the brain (stroke). Your blood cholesterol level may become elevated through eating foods high in cholesterol and saturated fat, and also by being overweight and not getting enough exercise. Polyunsaturated fats tend to lower blood cholesterol. People differ in their ability to handle saturated fats and cholesterol—but the advice here applies to the great majority of the population.

If your cholesterol and/or blood pressure levels are high, pay careful attention to the fats in your diet. Studies have shown that people whose cholesterol is 250 or more have a three- to four-time greater risk of having a coronary than those with a cholesterol level of only 150. And since excessive salt in the diet can raise blood pressure, don't oversalt food— learn to season with spices and herbs

instead. Or, try lemon juice for a refreshing change.

*"No" foods:* For cholesterol watchers, foods to be eaten sparingly include: eggs, beef (choose lean cuts, and eat no more than three or four times a week), sausage, cold cuts, organ meats, goose, lamb, pork, frankfurters, whole milk, ice cream, sour cream, butter, high-fat cheeses, solid shortening, coconut oil, most commercially baked goods, any homemade desserts not made with polyunsaturated fat or oil. Also go easy on commercially fried foods, sauces and gravies, fish roe, candies made with chocolate, butter or cream.

*"Yes" foods:* By contrast, poultry, fish, fruits and vegetables, wholegrain products and low-fat cheeses are excellent foods that you can eat to your heart's content, provided you don't exceed your calorie limits.

Obviously it makes no sense nutritionally to reject whole categories of foods. Without being unduly harsh on yourself with foods you love, try to lower the fat content of your diet in general, and your intake of saturated fat and cholesterol in particular. Remember that diet is only one of many factors—including heredity, life-style and stress—that play a part. Why not have all the odds you can control in your favor?

### Taking the Confusion Out of Carbohydrates

Carbohydrates (starches and sugars) are the main source of energy for most people worldwide. Starches are found in cereals (wheat, rice, corn, oats), sorghum and tuber roots (potatoes, beets, yams and turnips). Beans, peas and other legumes are high in carbohydrates as well as in proteins. Sugars include table sugar (sucrose), fruit sugar (fructose) and milk sugar (lactose).

Carbohydrates are almost entirely the products of plants—the only significant carbohydrate of animal origin is lactose. Except for liver, meats are almost devoid of carbohydrates.

*Starchy foods:* Cereal grains, rice, potatoes, pasta, breads, flour, beets and turnips.

*Sugars:* Honey, syrup and table sugar are chief dietary sources. The average American eats 105 pounds of cane and beet sugar and 15 pounds of corn syrup annually.

Glucose, another sugar, is required for the brain to function, but the body makes all it needs from starch and proteins. Table sugar, whether it comes from beets or cane, is almost pure sucrose and contains nothing except empty calories; the same goes for brown sugar and raw sugar. Honey and maple syrup are also essentially sugars with no special health value,

contrary to what some people think. Sugar is hidden in many prepared foods that you buy, as you can discover by checking the labels.

It won't hurt you to have an occasional sweet dessert, but too much or too often can have deletrious effects on the teeth.

### Bread: A Misunderstood Food

The nutritional value of breads depends on the type. Eaten in moderation, bread is by no means as fattening as is commonly supposed. An ordinary slice of bread has about 70 calories; it's what you put on it that drives up the calorie count. To help you buy better bread, here is a quick guide:

*Whole-grain breads:* Contain bran fiber, B vitamins and trace minerals; are extremely nutritious, but are not liked by everyone.

*Enriched white breads:* Contain vitamin $B_1$, $B_2$, and niacin and iron which have been added up to the levels found in whole grain. White bread is usually fortified with skim milk as well. Though less nutritious than wholegrain breads, enriched white bread is not just "empty calories."

*Brown breads:* Vary widely in nutritional content; some are rich in vitamins, but others are essentially white breads with caramel flavoring and coloring matter added.

*French and Italian breads:* Sometimes made of very white flour, not enriched with vitamins or minerals or supplemented with skim milk. Many people prefer them to packaged enriched white bread, but be sure to read the label and buy breads made with enriched flour.

### Start the Day with Cereal

Hot or cold, whole-grain cereals such as oats, wheat, rice or whole-grain blends, especially when combined with milk and fruit, are an excellent source of protein. Bran cereals, in addition, contain fiber that is needed for bowel regularity. Regular consumption of fiber (also found in raw carrots and lettuce) may help reduce your chances of getting diverticulitis and cancer of the large intestine.

You can make a delicious and nutritious breakfast cereal by combining a variety of cereal grains with dried fruits and unsalted nuts. (For a recipe, see page 99.) It's much cheaper than the health-food store variety, and healthier too, since it doesn't contain sugar.

Most cereals are excellent breakfast foods. But even though they may contain 100 percent of the daily requirements of some (or even all) vitamins and iron, this doesn't mean that you can ignore the quality of your diet for the rest of the day. There are a great many other nutrients you require, including up to 20 minerals.

## Facts about Vitamins and Minerals

Vitamins are needed in tiny amounts for cell function. Minerals are required in minute quantities for building bone, teeth, red pigment of red blood cells and other tissue structures.

Unfortunately, many Americans are not getting all the vitamins and minerals they need because they are consuming too many non-nutritious processed foods. By processed foods I don't mean canned or frozen fruits and vegetables or frozen fish—these provide essentially the same nutrients as fresh ones. I do mean snack foods, soft drinks, highly sugared foods and the like.

In recent years, new deficiencies in the American diet have been emerging that are different from the classical ones. There's a high incidence of folic acid deficiency, especially among pregnant women. And there are some children who are deficient in zinc. One study found that several middle-class children suffered retarded growth and development and lost their sense of taste—symptons which were reversed by zinc supplements.

For a quick look at the major sources of important vitamins and minerals, consult the following list. It's not intended as a rigid guide to meal planning but rather as a reminder of the importance of variety:

*Vitamin C:* Found in orange juice (freshly squeezed, commercially bottled or in cartons, or frozen concentrate), lemons, limes, green peppers, grapefruit, fresh strawberries, raw cabbage, crisp salad greens and tomato juice. Baked and boiled potatoes are also good sources of vitamin C.

*B Vitamins:* Though there are nine of them, some are better known than others. The "big-three" B vitamins are thiamin ($B_1$), riboflavin ($B_2$), and niacin. A diet high in proteins as well as fruits and vegetables generally insures against a deficiency of these vitamins. Back-up insurance comes from the enrichment of flours. Enriched breakfast cereals and enriched bread contribute significantly to daily requirements of thiamin, riboflavin and niacin. Whole-grain bread has not only these vitamins but other vitamins and minerals as well.

Vitamin $B_{12}$, found amply in the average American diet, is plentiful in meat, poultry, fish, eggs, milk and cheese. Vegetarians who do not eat any of these products have no source of vitamin $B_{12}$ and may develop a deficiency.

Folic acid, also a B vitamin, is found primarily in green vegetables, dried legumes, nuts, whole wheat and liver. Deficiencies sometimes occur in pregnant women.

*Vitamin A:* Probably the only vitamin that can be seen in many of its food sources! Three of the chemical sources from which the body manufactures vitamin A, called carotenes, are yellow or orange-yellow. Carotene gives a characteristic color to carrots, pumpkins, apricots, nectarines and corn, plus butter, Cheddar cheese and egg yolk. Carotene is used to color as well as to enrich margarines. Vitamin A itself (also found in milk, butter, some enriched margarines, eggs and liver) is colorless.

*Vitamin D:* The one vitamin that's hard to get enough of in ordinary foods unless they are fortified. Yet just moderate exposure to sun seems to provide the vitamin D needs of most adults. Best food source is fortified milk or margarine.

Other food sources include liver, egg yolks, fish and butter.

*Vitamin E:* Found in a great variety of foods—vegetable oils, green leafy vegetables, legumes, nuts, meats, eggs and wheat germ.

*Vitamin K:* Plentiful in all green leafy vegetables, liver, egg yolks, cauliflower and cabbage.

*Calcium:* Found in milk and milk products.

*Phosphorus:* In general, almost every good source of calcium provides phosphorus. Other foods, including meat and cereal, are phosphorus-rich.

*Sodium, potassium and magnesium:* These minerals are omnipresent in the average American diet.

*Iron:* Among the best sources are red meats (especially organ meats), eggs, dark whole grains, prunes, raisins, molasses and green leafy vegetables. Deficiency often occurs in females who have heavy periods and may need an iron supplement.

*Copper:* Only minute amounts are needed. Deficiency is unlikely with a varied diet.

*Zinc:* This mineral is found in fruits, vegetables, whole-grain cereals and animal products.

*Iodine:* Deficiency can cause goiter. This can be avoided by the use of iodized salt in the diet.

## How to Turn Nutrients into Good Nutrition for All the Family

How do you take the information about nutrients and translate it into healthy, delicious meals for your family? First of all, don't exclude whole classes of foods—potatoes and breads, for example—which many people avoid when they're dieting. These foods in themselves do not add many calories to your diet if eaten in moderation. A plain potato, for example, has only about 100 calories; serve it hashed-browned and it can have as many as 400 calories.

If you've held on to the notion of the Basic Four food groups all these years, it's time to discard it. The Basic Four, in case you've forgotten, consists of the energy group (cereals and potatoes); the protein group (meat and fish); the milk group (milk and milk products); and the fruit and vegetable group. The problem with the Basic Four is that it excludes fats and lumps together foods that are nutritionally different and cannot be substituted for each other. For example, spinach and oranges are both part of the vegetable group—but each provides something different and essential. Even if you followed the Basic Four devotedly, you might still be deficient in certain key vitamins. If your dinner consisted of meat, cooked carrots, bread and skimmed milk, you've fulfilled the Basic Four, but you've had no vitamin C or polyunsaturated fats.

## Back to the Basic Seven Food Groups

Your family will be eating well to stay healthy if they get at least one food from each of the seven major food groups every day:

1) Green, yellow and leafy green vegetables.
2) Citrus fruits, tomatoes, raw cabbage and salad greens.
3) Noncitrus fruits, potatoes and all vegetables not included in Group 1.
4) Milk and milk products.
5) Meats, poultry, fish, eggs, nuts and dried beans and peas.
6) Bread and flour (whole-grain or enriched) and cereals.
7) Butter and margarine or oil.

People always ask me whether they have to eat all seven kinds of foods every day. I tell them that different members of the family have different needs, depending upon their age and sex. For example growing children certainly need a rich source of protein every day. Adults, except for pregnant women and nursing mothers, don't need such large amounts.

In general, you may run into nutritional difficulty if you eliminate a whole category of food. Post a list of the Basic Seven in your kitchen as a reminder of what foods to serve.

## How to Shop with Nutrition in Mind

• Spend more of your food budget on a variety of less expensive high-nutrition foods. For example, buy a variety of whole-grain or enriched breads and cereals, a variety of dried beans, and a smaller amount of meat.

• Plan to serve fish and poultry at least twice a week.

- Buy fresh fruits and vegetables when in season, but avoid stale, wilted or overripe items which have lost some of their nutrients.
- Buy canned or frozen vegetables to provide variety or save money.
- Don't pass over fruits and vegetables at the supermarket because they are not the variety to which you are accustomed. For example, yellow tomatoes have the same nutritional content as red.
- Buy real fruit juices; they do not cost more than imitation fruit juice, which contain very little juice and a lot of sugar and calories.

### Cooking for Best Nutrition

Fortunately, the same methods of preparation and cooking that preserve nutrients preserve taste. In fact, flavor disappears from food as rapidly as nutrients, with the possible exception of vitamin C.

The three basic factors in preparing and cooking food for best nutrition are:

1) Short storage of fresh fruits and vegetables before preparing and serving them.
2) Shortest possible cooking time.
3) The least amount of water.

Become familiar with these simple guidelines and you're on your way to eating right:

*Vegetables and fruits:*
- Wash fruits and vegetables quickly and avoid soaking them.
- Don't overdo chopping and peeling; many nutrients are lost, including vitamin C.
- Don't thaw frozen vegetables and fruits before cooking or they'll lose nutrients.
- Cook vegetables whenever possible. Contrary to what most people believe, cooked vegetables are sometimes more nutritious than raw ones. Uncooked vegetable cells have a cellulose layer around them that is not easily digested. The vitamins and minerals are more available to you in spinach, chard, carrots and cabbage in their cooked state than when eaten raw.
- Add fruits and vegetables to water that is already boiling, and preheat the oven before broiling or baking them. Save cooking liquids for sauces and soups—they are high in vitamins and minerals.
- Bake or boil potatoes in their skins.
- Trim leafy vegetables like lettuce and cabbage as little as possible. The greatest concentration of nutrients is in the outer, not inner, leaves.
- Don't use baking soda for cooking yellow or green vegetables. It preserves color but, at the same time, destroys vitamin $B_1$.
- Try steaming vegetables with either a steamer or an improvised model (put a colander inside a large pot). The water should not touch the vegetables. Or, use a pressure cooker that requires little water.

*Meats:* The higher the temperature at which meat is cooked, the greater the shrinkage and drying, and the greater the loss of nutrients. As a rule, cook at slow to moderate temperatures from 300° to 350°. Try not to overcook. One common mistake is to overcook pork; many homemakers, aware of the danger of trichinosis from undercooked pork, go to the other extreme and overcook it, thus losing valuable nutrients. Trichinae are destroyed at 140°, so pork cooked at 325° for 30 minutes per pound, or to 170° on a meat thermometer, is flavorful, nutritious and safe.

Roasting and broiling are the most nutritional ways of cooking meat. In broiling, much of the fat drips off and can be discarded. Frying may double the calorie count and add cholesterol, depending on what fat or cooking oil is used.

Don't stew meat until it becomes stringy—you'll end up with meat that is not only tasteless but low in nutrition. If the meat is tough when purchased, marinate it for 24 to 48 hours in wine, lemon juice or a marinade of vinegar and polyunsaturated oil.

*Fish and shellfish:* When baking or broiling fish, cook at high temperatures (400° or more) for rapid doneness. Leave on the skin to seal in nutrients and flavor and brush fish lightly with margarine or butter. When fish flakes with a fork, it is done.

Lobsters or crabs steamed in their shells are more nutritious. Shrimp can be shelled because cooking time is so short—only 3 to 5 minutes.

*Cereals and pasta:* Simmer rice, barley and other cereals in a minimum of water—usually twice as much water as cereal.

Cook pasta in already boiling water, drain quickly and serve.

### How to Read a Food Label

As of January 1975, an increasing number of packaged foods in the supermarket are carrying new labels describing the nutritional value of their contents. For the first time you can get precise information on the amount of calories and nutrients (proteins, carbohydrates, vitamins and minerals) in each serving. You will also find information on polyunsaturated and saturated fats in margarine and on sodium in dietetic products.

At present, nutritional labeling for most packaged and canned products is voluntary. But if any nutrients have been added to a food product, or if any nutritional claims are made about it (for example, "low in saturated fats, high in vitamin C") the package must contain not only numerical data on this information, but the entire nutritional label. No manufacturer can make a claim if it is not substantiated.

Here is a listing of common terms used on the new labels and what they mean:

*Enriched:* Certain nutrients—thiamin, riboflavin and niacin removed by the milling of grain in cereal products (flour, pasta, etc.)—have been replaced, according to levels set by the government. If the product is labeled "enriched," it simply means that some of the nutrients which were lost in the preparation process have been replaced, not that other nutrients have been added.

*Fortified:* Nutrients not found in the original product have been added or are found in greater amounts than in the original product. For example, vitamin D is added to milk, iodine to salt.

*Gram:* Basic unit of weight in the metric system, equal to about 1/30th of an ounce. Amounts of nutrients are listed in parts or multiples of grams.

*Grade:* The Department of Agriculture employs grading systems which generally have to do with size and appearance of food and not nutrition. For example, beef is graded for taste and fat content, vegetables such as peas for size, and eggs for size and appearance.

*U.S. Recommended Daily Allowance (U.S. RDA):* Replaces outmoded Minimum Daily Requirement. The U.S. RDA is the amount of protein and some of the vitamins and minerals that a person needs each day, with a comfortable margin of safety. (See chart; page 116.) The RDA for some nutrients has not yet been established.

*Percentages of vitamins and minerals:* Percentages of at least seven (vitamins A and C, thiamin, riboflavin, niacin, calcium and iron) nutrients must be given. Mention of others is optional. If a single serving contains less than 2 percent of RDA requirement, it will either be listed as "0" or marked with an asterisk.

*Ingredients:* Listed by weight in decreasing order.

*Cholesterol content:* Information on content of cholesterol, fats and fatty acids is optional and may be given for individuals who have been advised by their physicians to lower their dietary intake of cholesterol.

### Food Additives

Suddenly everyone is talking about food additives. On the one hand, some people stress that additives are a necessary ingredient in certain foods to keep them from spoiling. On the other, some people point out that some additives are not necessary.

Most experts agree that the usefulness and safety of additives must be studied on the basis of each individual substance. Many food additives had been widely used for years without much study, until the White House Conference on Food, Nutrition and Health in 1969, which called for a review of the safety of all food additives. So about all the nutrition-wise consumer can do is become familiar with the different additives and their purposes, keep informed about any of their reported side effects, and read food labels carefully.

To my way of thinking, additives can be used if there is a good reason for their use, particularly as related to safety or nutrition. This is certainly the case with preservatives and antioxidants. There is far less justification for the use of dyes and flavorings if any evidence suggests they may be harmful.

One reassurance: If a food additive is definitely proved to be harmful in amounts close to those used in food products, or if it produces cancer at *any* dose in animals, it must be removed from the market under government regulations.

Here is a rundown of common food additives:

*Preservatives:* These make foods safe by inhibiting the growth of bacteria or fungi. A group of preservatives, known as antioxidants, prevent the spoilage of fat and protect against the formation of dangerous peroxides.

*Flavoring agents:* Used in some foods and beverages, from ice cream to pickles.

*Improving agents:* This group includes chemicals such as lecithin for improving taste and consistency of many foods, including bakery goods.

*Taste enhancers:* Monosodium glutamate is the main additive in this category and is responsible for the so-called "Chinese Restaurant Syndrome." Following a Chinese meal, some people develop hot flushes, headaches and rapid breathing. Major manufacturers of baby food removed MSG from their products after it was shown that very large doses caused changes in the brains of baby animals.

*Jelling agents and stabilizers:* These keep ice cream creamy and jellies in a gel state and so on.

*Coloring matter:* Dyes are used in many foods that lose their natural color when processed and look less appetizing. Ice creams, orange peel and many soft drinks contain such dyes. Nitrite, used mostly as a preservative (it prevents the growth of the botulism organism), has also been used simply as a dye (to make canned meat pink instead of brown). Some scientists feel that the latter is not justified.

## Nutrition and Dieting

Excess weight is caused by eating in excess of need. To lose weight, you have to take in fewer calories than you burn up—and exercise regularly. One pound of body fat equals 3,500 calories. By reducing your caloric intake 500 calories each day, you'll lose a pound in one week.

Proteins and carbohydrates have 4 calories per gram, or 120 calories per ounce. Fat has 9 calories per gram, or 270 per ounce. People have different caloric needs depending upon their sex, age and life-style. Adult males need around 2,500 calories a day; a teen-age male who participates in active sports may need 3,000 or more. One of the best guides to the calorie content of foods is the government nutrition guide, Agricultural Handbook 8, entitled *Composition of Food.* It is available for $3.60 from the Superintendent of Documents, Government Printing Office, Capitol and G Streets, N.W., Washington, D.C. 20402.

When dieting, eat a variety of food-stuffs—you need the same assortment of nutrients as the non-dieter, and you must get similar amounts in fewer calories. Keep limits on portion size. Eat plenty of fruits and vegetables and stay away from fatty meats, fried foods and rich desserts. Polyunsaturated margarine is preferable to butter because of its effect on cholesterol, but it contributes as many calories and should not be eaten in excessive amounts.

Fad reducing diets are generally useless, may even be harmful. Anyone who excludes whole categories of foods in the basic seven for a long time may be headed for disaster.

And remember that nutrition and exercise go hand in hand as related components of good health. ■

By Dr. Jean Mayer, with Judith Ramsey

---

# COOK'S GUIDE

*Page 64:* Vegetable Spray on—Mazola® No Stick, Pam®.
*Page 78:* Frozen San Francisco-style vegetable combination—Birds Eye® Americana Recipe San Francisco Style Vegetables.
*Page 83:* Frozen Japanese-style vegetable combination—Birds Eye®

Japanese Stir-Fry Vegetables with Seasoning.
*Page 94:* High Protein rice and wheat cereal—Kellogg's Special K®
*Page 99:* Four-grain multivitamin and iron supplement cereal—Kellogg's Product 19®; shreds of wheat bran cereal—Kellogg's All-Bran®.

# BUYER'S GUIDE

*Page 34:* Levy Shea "Stretch into Your Day" morning and evening exercise tape, 30 minutes per side, plus instruction guide. (To order by mail, send check or money order for $6.95 to Levy Shea Inc., 100 E. 16th Street, New York, NY 10003.)
*Page 60:* "Basket" porcelain platters and soup tureen by Villeroy and Boch, 225 5th Avenue, New York, NY 10010; Casserole spoon from "Royal Lace" Hostess Set by Oneida, Ltd., Silversmiths, Oneida, NY 13421.

*Page 62:* "Alice" casual china platter from the "Looking Glass Collection" by Denby Ltd., Inc., 10880 Wilshire Boulevard, Los Angeles, CA 90024. Inset photo: Middle—"Belmont" crystal wine glass by Lenox, Inc., Prince and Meade Streets, Trenton, NJ 08605. Left and right—"Torrino" wine glasses by Villeroy and Boch.
*Page 76:* "Garland Crown" Limoges porcelain platter by Denby Ltd., Inc.
*Page 85:* Glass plates by Imperial Glass Corporation.
*Pages 86-87:* Clockwise from bottom

—"Wild Bouquet" Limoges porcelain plate by Denby Ltd., Inc.; "Ming Jade" Calyx tableware plate by Adams, 211 County Avenue, Secaucus, NJ 07094; "Fruit Sprays" china plates by Wedgewood, 211 County Avenue, Secaucus, NJ 07094; "Strawberry Basket" dish by Spode, 11 East 26th Street, New York, NY 10010.
*Page 88:* "Moonrise" crystal wine glass by Denby Ltd., Inc.
*Page 95:* "Wild Bouquet" Limoges porcelain plates, cup and saucer, teapot, creamer and sugar bowl, and "Arabesque" crystal sherbet glass, all by Denby Ltd., Inc., "Mandarin" sterling silver flatware by Towle Silver-smiths, Newburyport, MA 01950; breakfast tray available at B. Altman and Company, 5th Avenue and 34th Street, New York, NY 10016.
*Page 96:* Platter by Spode.

# CREDITS

**Jacqueline Heriteau,** pages 46-47; **Claudia Jessup,** pages 32-33; **Toni Kosover,** bottom, page 44, cols. 1 and 2, page 45; **Ruth K. Mumbauer,** pages 114-115; **Sally Obre,** pages 8-9.

ACKNOWLEDGEMENTS

The editors gratefully acknowledge the help of: American Lamb Council; Angostura Bitters; California Frozen Vegetable Council; Frozen Southern Vegetable Council; Kellogg's Company; Naional Kraut Packers Association; North Atlantic Seafood Association; RJR Foods; South African Rock Lobster; The Flanagan Brothers Kraut Company; Western Iceberg Lettuce, Incorporated.

# RECIPE INDEX

## A & B

Aloha Lamburgers, 107
Apple and Kraut Bake, 83
Apple French Toast, 100
Apricot Mold, 91
Asparagus Roulade, 79
Baked Corn on the Cob, 81
Baked Maine Lobster, 65
Barbecued Eggplant Slices, 81
Barbecued Franks, 111
Beef Stroganoff, 89
Beef Stuffed Peppers, 106
Belgian Pot Roast, 69
Berry Floating Island, 93
Bitters Baked Vegetables, 80
Blue Cheese Dressing, 80
Blue Cheese Stuffed Celery, 98
Bouillabaisse Salad, 66
Braised Lamb Chops, 66
Braised Pork Steak, 67
Broiled Cornish Hens, 110
Burgundy Burgers, 105

## C & D

Cannelloni Florentine, 64
Cantonese Chicken, 108
Cape Cod Scallop Salad, 104
Cheesecake Mold, 92
Chicken with Watercress, 106
Chilled Cucumber Soup, 101
Chilled Vichyssoise, 100
Chinatown Special, 78
Citrus Salad Dressing, 80
Cheese Omelet, 98
Chocolate Eclairs, 91
Clam Soufflé, 108
Coleslaw Relish Mold, 80
Cold Zucchini Soup, 101
Consommé Madrilène, 101
Continental Chicken Bake, 68
Continental Veal Bake, 68
Corned Beef and Slaw Mold, 78
Country Farm Chicken, 107
Crab Filled Artichokes, 83
Creamed Curry Sauce, 82
Creamed Spinach, 83
"Cream" of Mushroom Soup, 101
Creamy Cheese Sauce, 64
Creamy Egg Sauce, 110
Crunchy Chef's Salad, 110
Crunch Topped Egg Cups, 98
Cucumber Crisps, 83
Curried Fish Bake, 106
Curry Tomato Dressing, 112
Daffodil Cake Ring, 90
Deviled Egg Slices, 97
Devonshire Cream Topping, 100

Diet Crèpes, 64
Dill-Caraway Dip, 97
Dilly Beans and Carrots, 98
Dollar Pancake Stacks, 99
Double Boiler Soufflé, 108
Double Cheese Parfait, 78
Double Cheese Topping, 78
Double Fruit Coupe, 93

## E & F

Easy Veal Parmigiana, 66
Egg Drop Soup, 100
Egg Salad Cups, 109
Eggs en Gelée, 111
Eggplant au Gratin, 113
Eggplant Provençale, 67
Fish in Spinach Nests, 82
Florida Baked Fillets, 105
Fluffy Coconut Pancakes, 99
Franks and Kraut Salad, 102
French Topping, 79
French Veal Ragoût, 67
Frittata di Vegetali, 107
Fruited Ham Steak, 103
Fruit Tarts, 90

## GHI & J

Gazpacho, 101
German Steak Platter, 103
German Sauerkraut, 112
Golden Tomato Cups, 82
Gourmet Beef Patties, 104
Grapefruit Deluxe, 100
Greek Chicken Livers, 104
Grilled Lemon Chicken, 107
Halibut in Yogurt, 107
Ham in Cherry Tomatoes, 97
Ham Omelet, 98
Ham and Potato Boats, 82
Ham "Bacon," 100
Harlequin Parfaits, 91
Honey Baked Pears, 93
Honey Lemon Syrup, 99
Italian Meatballs, 102
Jellied Chicken, 67
Jeweled Melon Wedges, 91

## K & L

Kabob Chicken Livers, 102
Kathy's Ratatouille Mold, 113
Kraut Vegetable Salad, 83
Lamb Chops en Brochette, 104
Lamb Italiano, 105

Leek Sauce, 108
Lemon Chicken, 103
Lemon Dressing, 111
Lemony Lamb Kabobs, 103
Lobster and Eggs, 104
Low Calorie Pastry, 90
Low Calorie Sangria, 97

## M & N

Make Your Own Yogurt, 99
Marinated Artichokes, 112
Marinated Bean Bowl, 80
Marinated Beef Rolls, 66
Meatballs in Yogurt Sauce, 106
Meat Loaf Italiano, 111
Michigan Cherry Roll, 113
Minestrone, 100
Mocha Bavarian, 93
Molded Turkey Crown, 112
Mushroom Bouillon, 101
Mushrooms and Squash, 81
Mushrooms en Aspic, 76, 78

## O & P

Omelet with Chives, 98
Oranges Caribe, 98
Oriental Pork Platter, 109
Oriental Vegetable Bowl, 83
Our French Dressing, 79
Oven Fried Chicken, 106
Oven Fried Fish, 111
Oven Roast Potatoes, 65
Paella Granada, 68
Parfait Française, 79
Parfait Verdi, 79
Parsley Cucumbers, 112
Pâté Indienne, 97
Persian Fruit Dessert, 113
Petite Marmite, 64
Piquant Tomato Dressing, 66
Plums Devonshire, 99
Pork Chops Seville, 105
Pork in Wine, 68
Potatoes and Oysters, 102
Puffy Italian Omelet, 110

## Q & R

Quick Moussaka, 106
Raspberry Parfait, 92
Ratatouille Niçoise, 79
Ready-to-Eat Cereal Mix, 99
Red Cabbage Slaw, 112
Rock Lobster Hong Kong, 105
Rosy Pineapple Chicken, 108

## S & T

Salmon Omelet, 98
San Francisco Chioppino, 69
San Francisco Crab Salad, 81
Sautéed Chicken Breasts, 65
Scandinavian Lamb Kabobs, 104
Shanghai Dressing, 81
Sherry Spanish Cream, 90
Shrimp Stuffed Mushrooms, 82

Skillet Gingered Lamb, 108
Skillet Okra and Tomatoes, 112
Skillet Turkey Scramble, 103
Southern Cream Soup, 101
South Seas Cup Custards, 93
Spaghetti with Seafood, 103
Spanish Snapper, 107
Spiced Fruits, 90
Spicy Apple Syrup, 100
Spicy Orange Syrup, 100
Spicy Yogurt Topping, 79
Spring Cheese Salad, 67
Spring Lamb Roll-Ups, 102
Spring Veal Ragoût, 109
Spring Vegetable Bouquet, 65
Squash Bake, 111
Steak with Mushrooms, 66
Steamed Celery Cabbage, 80
Strawberry Filling, 92
Strawberry Salad Bowl, 81
Strawberry Wonder Torte, 92
Sukiyaki Tray, 68
Sun Gold Egg Mold, 109
Supper Ham Salad, 67
Tangy Cooked Dressing, 78
Tart Shells, 90
Thousand Island Dressing, 111
Triple Vegetable Bowl, 81
Tropical Breakfast Blend, 98
Tomato Consommé, 102
Tuna Stuffed Squash, 82
Turkey Hawaiian, 68

## UVWXY

Veal à la Français, 65
West Coast Salad Bowl, 80
White Wine Sauce, 102
Wine Jelly with Fruits, 92
Wine Poached Fish, 110
Wine Salad Dressing, 80
Yankee Clam Broth, 100
Yellow Squash Boats, 69
Yogurt Coleslaw, 81

## & Z

Zucchini Antipasto Rounds, 98
Zucchini Pizzas, 97
Zucchini Provençal, 113